Monitoring and Evaluation of Biomaterials and their Performance In Vivo

Related titles

Biocompatibility and Performance of Medical Devices
(ISBN 978-0-85709-070-6)

Biomedical Imaging
(ISBN 978-0-85709-127-7)

Bio-Tribocorrosion in Biomaterials and Medical Implants
(ISBN 978-0-85709-540-4)

Woodhead Publishing Series in Biomaterials

Monitoring and Evaluation of Biomaterials and their Performance In Vivo

Edited by

Roger J. Narayan

AMSTERDAM • BOSTON • CAMBRIDGE • HEIDELBERG
LONDON • NEW YORK • OXFORD • PARIS • SAN DIEGO
SAN FRANCISCO • SINGAPORE • SYDNEY • TOKYO
Woodhead Publishing is an imprint of Elsevier

Woodhead Publishing is an imprint of Elsevier
The Officers' Mess Business Centre, Royston Road, Duxford, CB22 4QH, United Kingdom
50 Hampshire Street, 5th Floor, Cambridge, MA 02139, United States
The Boulevard, Langford Lane, Kidlington, OX5 1GB, United Kingdom

Notices

Knowledge and best practice in this field are constantly changing. As new research and experience broaden our understanding, changes in research methods, professional practices, or medical treatment may become necessary.

Practitioners and researchers must always rely on their own experience and knowledge in evaluating and using any information, methods, compounds, or experiments described herein. In using such information or methods they should be mindful of their own safety and the safety of others, including parties for whom they have a professional responsibility.

To the fullest extent of the law, neither the Publisher nor the authors, contributors, or editors, assume any liability for any injury and/or damage to persons or property as a matter of products liability, negligence or otherwise, or from any use or operation of any methods, products, instructions, or ideas contained in the material herein.

ISBN: 978-0-08-100603-0 (print)
ISBN: 978-0-08-100604-7 (online)

Library of Congress Cataloging-in-Publication Data
A catalog record for this book is available from the Library of Congress

British Library Cataloguing-in-Publication Data
A catalogue record for this book is available from the British Library

For information on all Woodhead Publishing publications visit our website at https://www.elsevier.com/

Publisher: Matthew Deans
Acquisition Editor: Laura Overend
Editorial Project Manager: Natasha Welford
Production Project Manager: Poulouse Joseph
Designer: Maria Inês Cruz

Contents

List of contributors

J. Bowen The Open University, Walton Hall, Milton Keynes, United Kingdom

J.S. Choi University of Illinois at Urbana-Champaign, Urbana, IL, United States

K. Creber The University of Western Ontario, London, ON, Canada

B.T. Cunningham University of Illinois at Urbana-Champaign, Urbana, IL, United States

D.W. Hamilton The University of Western Ontario, London, ON, Canada

B.A.C. Harley University of Illinois at Urbana-Champaign, Urbana, IL, United States

L. Hermansson Doxa AB and Applied Research Sweden AB, Uppsala, Sweden

H. Hermawan Laval University, Quebec City, Quebec, Canada

I.V. Larina Baylor College of Medicine, Houston, TX, United States

S. Maity National Institute of Technology, Yupia, Papum Pare, Arunachal Pradesh, India

N. Mehrban University College London, London, United Kingdom

P. Morissette Martin The University of Western Ontario, London, ON, Canada

Mrignayani Kotecha University of Illinois at Chicago, Chicago, IL, United States

D. Noviana Bogor Agricultural University, Bogor, West Java, Indonesia

D. Paramitha Laval University, Quebec City, Quebec, Canada

D. Pissuwan Mahidol University, Bangkok, Thailand

A. Purnama Laval University, Quebec City, Quebec, Canada

A. Sarkar National Institute of Technology, Yupia, Papum Pare, Arunachal Pradesh, India

S. Selvam Sree Chitra Tirunal Institute for Medical Sciences and Technology, Thiruvananthapuram, Kerala, India

M.F. Ulum Bogor Agricultural University, Bogor, West Java, Indonesia

S. Wang Baylor College of Medicine, Houston, TX, United States

D.H.B. Wicaksono University of Technology of Malaysia, Johor Bahru, Johor, Malaysia; Swiss-German University, Tangerang, Banten, Indonesia

Y. Zhuo University of Illinois at Urbana-Champaign, Urbana, IL, United States

Part One

Monitoring and evaluation of the mechanical performance of biomaterials in vivo

Nanostructured ceramics

1

L. Hermansson
Doxa AB and Applied Research Sweden AB, Uppsala, Sweden

1.1 Introduction

Ceramics are defined as inorganic nonmetallic materials and are often classified according to Table 1.1. Biomaterials based on ceramics are found within all the classical ceramic families: traditional ceramics, special ceramics, glasses, glass ceramics, coatings, and chemically bonded ceramics (CBC) [1,2]. Examples of bioceramics are given in Table 1.1.

This chapter deals specifically with bioceramics with nanostructures. The nanosize is defined as less than 100 nm. Nanostructured ceramics are found most frequently among the CBC [1] shown in Table 1.2.

The nanostructured chemically bonded ceramics have structures with the same general structure as hard tissue, i.e., small crystals, all surrounded by a softer interlayer, in the case of hard-tissue collagen layers, and in the case of the chemically bonded silicate, aluminate, and phosphate ceramics, nanothin water layers. The structures of all the apatite-based body ceramics (enamel, dentine, and hard tissue) include individual plates just above the nanosized level, approximately 0.2 μm, but composed of nanocrystals of approximately 20 nm in diameter [1,3].

Nanostructured bioceramics are also, to some extent, found within the special ceramics field based on zirconia, titania, silica, or other oxides produced by low-temperature sintering using laser techniques, hot pressing, or hot isostatic pressing [4,31].

This chapter will treat nanostructured ceramics with emphasis on nanostructured materials, not nanostructured particles, needles, wires et cetera.

1.2 Test methods for nanostructured ceramics

As early as 1946, Professor Powers [5] proposed that chemically bonded ceramics, specifically Ca silicate hydrates, ought to have an average crystal size of approximately 14 nm, based on BET measurements, i.e., based on the surface area measurement of dried cements. However, at that time the microscopes did not have efficient resolution to detect this. Approximately 50 years later the first actual micro/nanopictures of chemically bonded ceramics were presented [6], all of which demonstrated that the proposal of Professor Powers was right.

Monitoring and Evaluation of Biomaterials and their Performance in vivo. http://dx.doi.org/10.1016/B978-0-08-100603-0.00001-8

Table 1.1 Classification of ceramics and examples of bioceramics

Ceramics – classification	Examples of bioceramics
Traditional ceramics	Dental porcelain, (K_2O-Al_2O_3-SiO_2)
Special ceramics	Al-, Zr, and Ti-oxides
Glass	Bioactive glasses (Na_2O-CaO-P_2O_5-SiO_2)
Glass ceramics	Apatite (CaO-P_2O_5-H_2O), Wollastonite (CaO-SiO_2), Li-silicate based (Li_2O-SiO_2) and Leucite-based (K_2O-Al_2O_3-SiO_2)
Chemically bonded ceramics	Phosphates, aluminates, silicates, and sulfates

Table 1.2 Chemically bonded bioceramic systems

Group/name	Basic system
Calcium silicates	CaO-SiO_2-H_2O
Calcium aluminates	CaO-Al_2O_3-H_2O
Calcium phosphates	CaO-P_2O_5-H_2O
Calcium sulfates	CaO-SO_3-H_2O
Calcium carbonates	CaO-CO_2

1.2.1 *Micro/nanostructural evaluation*

Methods used in the evaluation of the microstructures, including nanostructures, and phase and elemental analyses are traditional SEM, TEM, HRTEM, XRD, XPS, and STEM with EDX.

To analyze interfaces and calcified tissue at the highest level, transmission electron microscopy (TEM), in combination with focused ion beam microscopy (FIB), for intact site-specific preparation of the TEM samples at very high site-specific accuracy is recommended. This procedure is treated in detail in Ref. [7]. Cross-sectional TEM samples from the interface between, e.g., enamel and a dental filling material are produced by FIB. The system scans over a beam of positively charged gallium ions over the samples, similar to an electron beam in SEM. The ions generate sputtered neutral atoms, secondary electrons, and secondary ions. Here it is possible to increase the beam current of the primary ion beam and use the FIB as a fine-scale micromachining tool to cut TEM samples with high accuracy (see Fig. 1.1). To produce the TEM samples the so-called "lift-out" technique can be used [7]. The thickness of the samples used is approximately 150 nm. The samples in Fig. 1.1 are from the interface between bone and an injectable Ca aluminate-based material.

1.3 Nanostructured bioceramics

There are only a few ways of producing nanostructured ceramics. These methods relate to either low-temperature sintering or chemical low-temperature bonding.

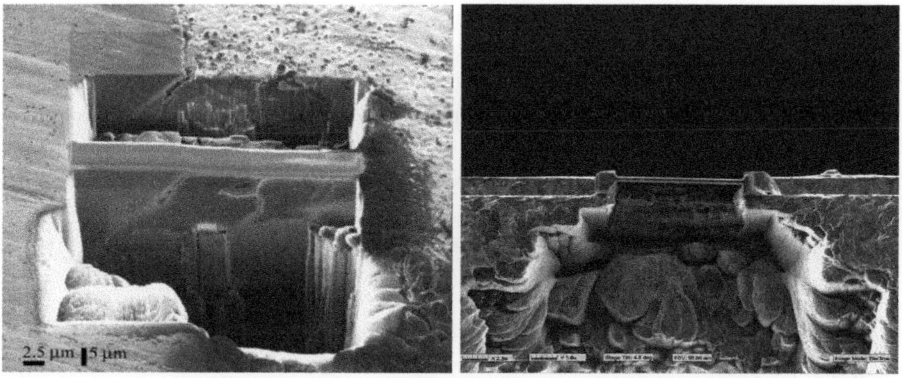

Figure 1.1 Preparation of test samples with the FIB technique; TEM samples ready for lift-out (left), followed by mounting on the TEM grid, and final polishing to electron transparency (FIB electron mode) (right).

In the preparation of all these nanostructured materials, the size of the precursor (the raw material) is crucial. In the case of sintering, the original ceramic particles of course have to be less than 100 nm, and this reduces the applications of sintered nanostructures. For the chemically bonded ceramics the situation is different in that the precursor particles dissolve. However, the size should be less than approximately 10 μm, since the penetration of water into hydrated bioceramics is reduced to almost zero after 5–10 μm. This is treated in more detail in Ref. [8].

1.3.1 Low-temperature chemical bonding

Most ceramics are formed at high temperatures through a sintering process. By using chemical reactions, ceramic biomaterials can be produced at low temperatures (body temperature), which is attractive from several perspectives: cost, avoidance of temperature gradients (thermal stress), dimensional stability, and minimal negative effect on the system with which the material interacts. Notably the hard tissue of bone and teeth (apatite, a Ca phosphate-based material) also is formed via a biological chemical reaction, and is close in composition to some of the chemically bonded bioceramics. The chemistry of the chemically bonded bioceramic systems is similar to that of the hard tissue found in living organisms. One of the first ceramics to be proposed as a biomaterial was gypsum, $Ca(SO_4) \times \frac{1}{2}H_2O$. The first cement to be proposed and used was a Zn phosphate, which is still used as a dental cement. Examples of typical phases formed in the chemically bonded ceramic systems are presented in Table 1.3.

Chemically bonded ceramics constitute ceramics that are being formed due to chemical reactions, in many cases an acid–base reaction, where the powder is the base and the water the weak acid. The precursor material is a ceramic powder (e.g., Ca silicate or Ca aluminate), which is "activated" in the water-based liquid. A chemical reaction takes place in which the initial powder is partly or completely dissolved and new phases precipitate. The precipitated phases are composed of species from both the liquid and the precursor powder. The degree of reaction of the powder depends on the size of the precursor particles and/or the amount of water/liquid presence, as well as the powder (p) to water (w) ratio (the p/w ratio). This is treated in more detail in Ref [9]. The precipitates can be formed in situ in vivo, often in the nanosized scale due to low solubility of the phases formed (details presented later). The nanostructural chemically bonded bioceramics are especially found within the Ca phosphate, Ca aluminate, and Ca silicate systems. The large pores between the original dissolving precursor powders are increasingly filled with nanocrystals, and the material hardens. The dissolution speed and the solubility products of the formed hydrate phases determine the nanosize, the setting time, and the final curing (hardening) of the material. The setting time can be controlled by selection of the precursor grain size and/or by addition of accelerating or retarding substances. Table 1.4 shows a typical time sequence of the different stages in the formation of chemically bonded bioceramics.

Since the material can be formed from a precursor powder mixed with a liquid, the material can be made moldable simply by controlling the amount of liquid (in relation to the powder) and by the possible addition of small amounts of polymers in the liquid. This makes the chemically bonded ceramics useful as injectable biomaterials, where the final biomaterial is formed in situ in vivo.

Also worth mentioning is a relatively new group of ceramics, called geopolymers [10,11]. These are also produced by chemical reactions but do not involve a hydration,

Table 1.3 Chemically bonded ceramic systems

Group/name	Basic system	Typical phases formed
OPC[a]	$CaO-SiO_2-H_2O$ (CSH)	Amorhous CSH, Tobermorite
CA[b]	$CaO-Al_2O_3-H_2O$ (CAH)	Katoite, and Gibbsite
Gypsum plaster	Ca sulfates	$CaSO_42H_2O$
Sorel	$MgO-H_2O$ (Cl)	MgOCl
Bioglasses	$CaO-Na_2O-SiO_2-P_2O_5$	Carbohydroxyapatite
Phosphates	$CaO-P_2O_5-H_2O$ (CPH)	Apaties, Brushite, Monetite
Carbonates	$CaO-CO_2-H_2O$	Calcite, Aragonite
Geopolymers[c]	Aluminosilicates, Metakaolin	Amorphous phases

[a]OPC = Ordinary Portland cements.
[b]CA = High alumina cements, C_3A, $C_{12}A_7$, CA, etc.
[c]Geopolymers = Metakaolin or synthetic aluminosilicates.

Table 1.4 Time sequence of the formation of nanostructured chemically bonded bioceramics

Dissolution and repeated crystallization	Working and setting time	Initial hardening	Ready to use
Starts immediately	5–15 min	5–20 min	5–60 min

i.e., new uptake of water. The geopolymerization is thus not a hydration process in which the water is consumed. Instead the water resides in the pores but plays an active role as a dissolution medium during the reaction, an inorganic polymerization. The most well-known geopolymer is zeolite [11].

The chemically bonded nanostructured ceramics can further be divided into two main groups: resorbable, including partly resorbable (Ca phosphates, bioglasses, Ca sulfates and Ca carbonates), and stable biomaterials (Ca aluminates and Ca silicates).

1.3.2 Why nanostructures in chemically bonded ceramics?

This question can be returned by a bold statement; it is even difficult to avoid nanostructures in chemically bonded bioceramics (CBBCs). The nanostructures developed in some of the CBBCs, especially the $CaO\text{-}Al_2O_3\text{-}H_2O$ (CAH), $CaO\text{-}SiO_2\text{-}H_2O$ (CSH), and the $CaO\text{-}P_2O_5\text{-}H_2O$ (CPH) systems, are a consequence of the low solubility product of the phases formed in these systems [12] (see Table 1.5).

These values correspond to ion concentrations of approximately 10 mM or less. It is interesting that the solubility of apatites is the lowest of all these possible phases. This means that in presence of phosphate ions in contact with the basic system Ca aluminate or Ca silicate systems, possible apatite formation is even likely, and in fact difficult to avoid. This explains the bioactivity seen in these systems, i.e., the formation of apatite in the contact zone to living tissue [8].

A survey presentation, including calculations based on pK values, of how and why nanostructured phases appear is given here. The example is from the Ca aluminate system, and apatite phases appear in the contact zone between the biological surroundings and the biomaterial.

The phase Katoite, $Ca_3[Al(OH)_4]_2(OH)_4$, and Gibbsite, $Al(OH)_3$, are formed in the Ca aluminate system. For Katoite with even the highest solubility of these low-solubility phases, a rough calculation shows the easiness of forming nanosized crystals.

pKs = 22.3 for Katoite, $Ca_3[Al(OH)_4]_2(OH)_4$

- Ion concentration for precipitation is approximately 10 mM
- Approximately 6×10^{21} molecules/liter for precipitation to occur

Table 1.5 The solubility products of some of the phases in the CAH, CSH, and the CPH systems

Phase	Formula	pKs
Octacalcium phosphate	$Ca_8H_2(PO_4)_6.5H_2O$	48.5
Hydroxyapatite	$Ca_2(PO_4)_3(OH)$	58.5
Fluoroapatite	$Ca_2(PO_4)_3F$	59.7
Katoite	$Ca_3[Al(OH)_4]_2(OH)_4$	22.3
Gibbsite	$Al(OH)_3$	32.2
Tobermorite	$Ca_5Si_6O_{16}(OH)_2{\cdot}4H_2O$	–

Actual volume of interest is approximately $10^3\,nm^3$
Number of molecules at saturation $6 \times 10^{21}/10^{24} \times 10^3 = 6$

- Approximately 50–200 ions per $10^3\,nm^3$ = approximately 5 ions per 10 nm

The ions "jump" into the water liquid surroundings, and immediately the condition for saturation is fulfilled, and precipitation of crystals occurs. The surface energy of these approximately 1.5 nm molecules is extremely high, and in the hydrate systems approximately 1000 molecules in a crystal are necessary to reduce the total surface energy to stability at the environmental conditions at body temperature. Nanocrystals of an approximate size of 15 nm appear.

The nanostructures observed in Ca aluminate and Ca silicate systems confirm a typical size in the interval of 10–40 nm. Even the tooth structure in detail reveals the individual crystals of the size of approximately 20 nm.

In addition to phases based on the original biomaterial systems, in contact zones to organic tissue, apatite phases may be found. The following section presents a summary of possible reactions and how the stable (low solubility) phases appear in the bulk material and in the contact zone to hard tissue. The nanoporosity between the precipitated nanocrystals is also discussed. The nanochannels between the nanocrystals are in the range 1–3 nm.

1.3.3 Nanostructures in the Ca aluminate–Ca phosphate system

Six different mechanisms have been found to be involved during the hydration and curing of chemically bonded bioceramics in the Ca aluminate–Ca phosphate (CAPH) system [12]. The biomaterials will be in contact with different tissue—enamel, dentine, hard bone tissue, and soft tissue—as well as other biomaterial contact surfaces. These six mechanisms affect the integration differently depending on (1) what type of tissue the biomaterial is in contact with, (2) in what state (unhydrated or hydrated) the biomaterial is introduced, and (3) what type of application is aimed for (cementation, dental fillings, endodontic fillings, sealants, coatings, or augmentation products). The actual contact zone developed depends on a combination of the discussed mechanisms and the surrounding tissue. The latter varies from a cellular-free high content apatite tissue in the case of a dental enamel, via dentine to a bone structure with cellular and body liquid contact. Both a pure nanostructural, mechanically controlled integration, and a chemically induced integration seem plausible.

Table 1.6 presents a summary of the six mechanisms involved in the integration of CAPH materials toward tissues and implant surfaces.

Figs. 1.2–1.6 show the nanostructure of phases and porosity formed. Fig. 1.2 illustrates the typical nanosized microstructure of the hydrated material with nanosized porosity between precipitated nanosized hydrates [12].

Fig. 1.3 illustrates the integration between the biomaterial and the tissue, in this case dentine. Even in high magnification a complete integration without gaps seems possible [12].

Table 1.6 Chemical reactions of the CaO-Al_2O_3-P_2O_5-H_2O (CAPH) system in contact with different environments [11]

Reaction mechanism	Description	Comments
Mechanism 1. Main reaction	$3\,(CaO\,Al_2O_3) + 12H_2O \rightarrow 3Ca^{2+} + 6Al^{3+} + 4(OH)^- \rightarrow 3Ca^{2+} + 6Al(OH)_4^- \rightarrow Ca_3\left[Al(OH)_4\right]_2(OH)_4$ (katoite) $+ 4Al(OH)_3$ (gibbsite)	Katoite and Gibbsite are formed as the main nanosized hydrates
Mechanism 2. Complementary reaction with phosphate-containing solution	$5Ca^{2+} + 3PO_4^{3-} + OH^- \rightarrow Ca_5(PO_4)_3OH$	Additional phase formed: nanosized apatite
Mechanism 3. Contact zone reaction with body liquid in presence of the basic Ca phase	$HPO_4^{2-} + OH^- \rightarrow PO_4^{3-} + H_2O$ Thereafter the apatite formation reaction occurs as mechanism 2, $5Ca^{2+} + 3PO_4^{3-} + OH^- \rightarrow Ca_5(PO_4)_3OH$	Nanosized apatite formation in the contact zone in presence of body liquid
Mechanism 4. Transformation reaction of the originally formed phase Katoite.	$Ca_3 \cdot \left(Al(OH)_4\right)_2 \cdot (OH)_4 \rightarrow 2Ca^{2+} + HPO_4^{2-} + 2H_2PO_4^- \rightarrow Ca_5 \cdot (PO_4)_3 \cdot (OH) + 2Al(OH)_3 + 5H_2O$	Nanocrystals of apatite and Gibbsite formed in the biomaterial contact zone toward tissue
Mechanism 5. Biologically induced integration and ingrowth	Bone ingrowth toward the biomaterial contact area allows the new bone structure to come into integrated contact with the biomaterial.	New bone formation at the contact zone
Mechanism 6. Mass increase reaction due to presence of unhydrated Ca	$3CaO\,Al_2O_3 + 12H_2O \rightarrow 3CaO\,Al_2O_3\,6H_2O + 2Al_2O_3\,3H_2O$	Mass increase and point welding

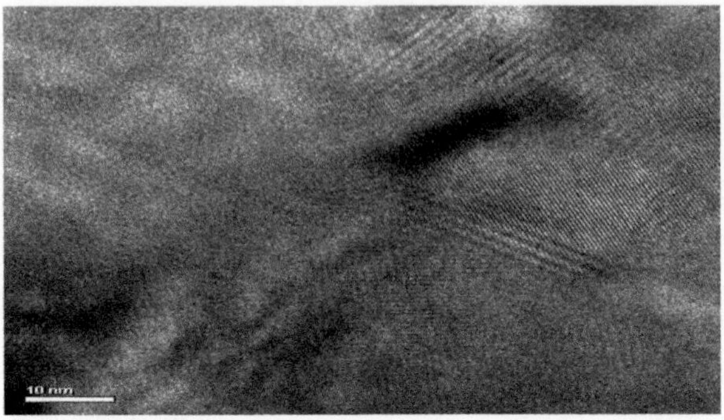

Figure 1.2 Nanostructure of Ca aluminate hydrates. The pore channels are estimated to be 1–2 nanometers and the hydrates in the interval 10–40 nm. (white bar 10 nm).

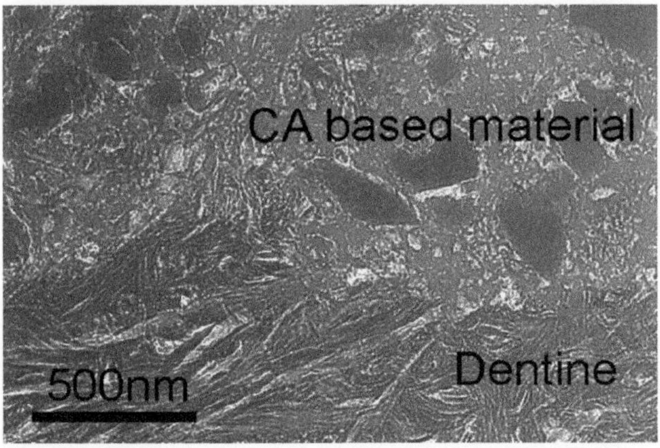

Figure 1.3 Nanostructural integration of CAPH material with dentine (gray particles in the biomaterial are glass particles).

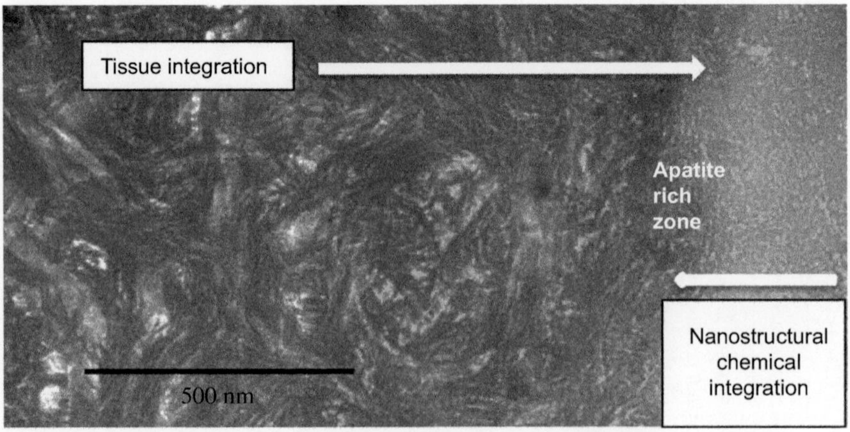

Figure 1.4 Tissue integration toward the nanostructured biomaterial, a hydrated Ca aluminate-based material with nanocrystals in the range 10–40 nm (black bar = 500 nm).

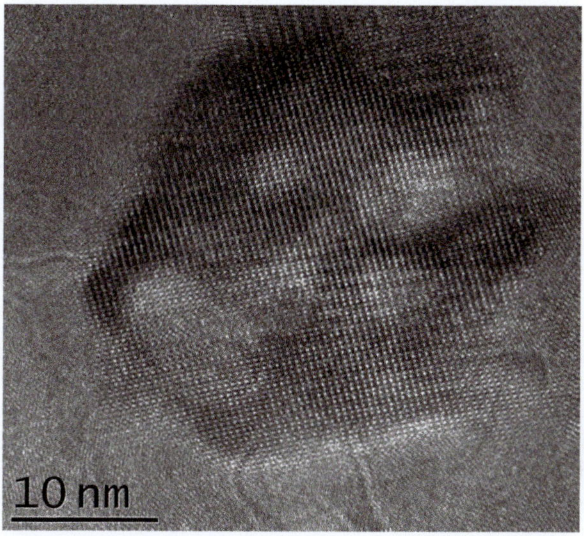

Figure 1.5 HRTEM of a precipitated hydroxyapatite crystal approximately 30 nm in size in the Ca aluminate-phosphate system.

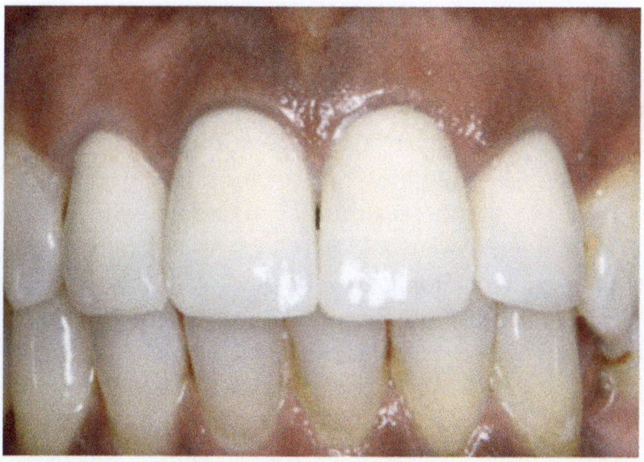

Figure 1.6 Four dental crowns cemented by Ceramir C&B, a Ca aluminate-based chemically bonded bioceramic.

When apatite is formed at the interface according to any of the reaction mechanisms 2–4 above, at the periphery of the bulk biomaterial, the biological integration may start. Bone ingrowth toward the apatite allows the new bone structure to come in integrated contact with the biomaterial. The transition from tissue to the biomaterial is smooth and intricate [12]. For an experimental Ca aluminate-based system the ingrowth is shown in Fig. 1.4.

Fig. 1.5 shows how a nanocrystal of apatite is formed in the contact to tissue [12].

1.4 Application field of nanostructured bioceramics

A short summary of the application possibilities with nanostructured bioceramics is presented in this section. The potential for these ceramics are great, and bioceramics have been addressed as candidate materials for many dental, orthopedic, and drug delivery carrier systems. The chemically bonded ceramic possibilities to produce in situ in vivo products are especially interesting. Another field deals with bioceramic coating materials. One promising feature in the coating technology is related to mechanism 6 (point welding), presented in Table 1.6. A further area with high potential refers to additive manufacturing. Here is the possibility, among others, to use the same kind of materials as implants (blanks) and as cements, as well as a base when the tooth structure has a waist.

Ca aluminate-based biomaterials and, to some extent, Ca silicates are stable and high-strength biomaterials after hydration and can favorably be used for load-bearing applications. The Ca phosphates, Ca sulfates, and Ca carbonates are known to be resorbable or slowly resorbable when inserted in the body, and their main applications are within bone void filling with low mechanical stress upon the biomaterial.

1.4.1 Dental applications including coating products

The nature of the mechanisms utilized by Ca aluminate and silicate materials (especially mechanism 1, see Table 1.6), when integrating and adhering to tooth tissue and other materials, makes these materials compatible with a range of other dental materials, including resin composite, metal, porcelain, zirconia, glass ionomers, and gutta-percha. This expands the range of indications for nanostructured chemically bonded bioceramic products from not only those involving tooth tissue, e.g., cavity restorations, but also to a range of other indications that involve both tooth tissue and other dental materials. Examples here include dental cement, liner/base, base, and core buildup and endodontic sealer/filler materials, which involve contact with materials such as porcelain, oxides, and polymers and metals, and coatings on dental implants such as titanium or zirconia-based materials.

Long-term success of fixed restorations depends on a range of factors, including the quality of the luting agent used, biocompatibility, insolubility, and resistance against degradation; all of which help maintain the seal at the restoration, margins, thus preventing ingress of bacteria leading to leakage, sensitivity, and secondary decay.

The progression of luting agents has evolved with a succession of chemistries over the past century or more, including zinc phosphate, polycarboxylate, glass ionomer, resin, resin-modified glass ionomer, and self-adhesive resin cements [13–15]. These cement compositions are now challenged by a new hybrid calcium aluminate/glass ionomer cement: Ceramir C&B, originally named XeraCem (Doxa Dental AB, Uppsala, Sweden), a luting agent intended for permanent cementation of crowns and fixed partial dentures, gold inlays and onlays, prefabricated metal and cast dowel and cores, and all-zirconia or all-alumina crowns, as well as Li silicate-based crown materials [1]. The cement is a water-based composition comprising calcium aluminate and glass ionomer components and has been demonstrated to be bioactive. The term "bioactivity" refers to a property of this new cement to form hydroxyapatite when immersed in vitro in a physiological phosphate-buffered saline solution.

Figs. 1.7 and 1.8 show examples of the X-ray examination of orthograde and retrograde treatments using an experimental Ca aluminate-based nanostructured material [16].

For successful implantation of implants in bone tissue, early stabilization is of great importance [17–21]. Even small gaps may lead to relative micromotions between the implant and the tissue, which increases the risk of the implant loosening over time due to the formation of zones of fibrous tissues at the implant–tissue interface. Early loading of implants is of particular interest for dental implants. The use of surface coating technology is today an established method to reduce the problem with poor interfacial stability for implants. With coating technology, structural characteristics of the implant (e.g., strength, ductility, low weight, or machinability) may be combined with surface properties promoting tissue integration. There are several established coating deposition techniques, e.g., physical vapor deposition (sputtering) and thermal spraying techniques. Coatings based on calcium phosphates are the most used ones.

The implant coating technique is used in similar ways for dental and orthopedic applications. One specific feature related to nanostructured chemically bonded bioceramics is early retention due to point welding. This is defined as the possibility of early adaption to the implant surface and the hard tissue by the increase of the coating

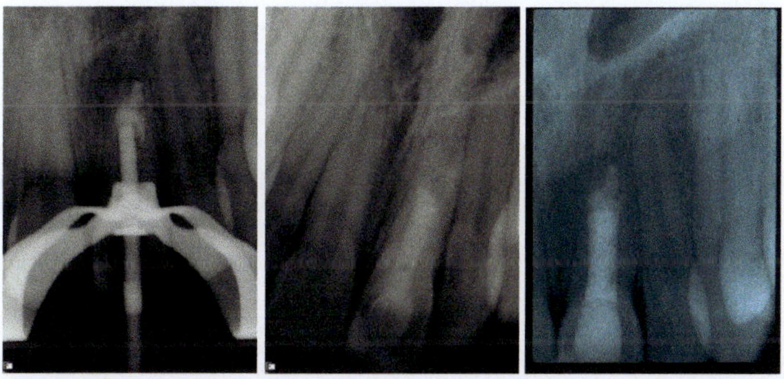

Figure 1.7 Orthograde filling, tooth 21; condensing with a gutta-percha pointer (left), just after treatment (middle) and at two-year control (right).

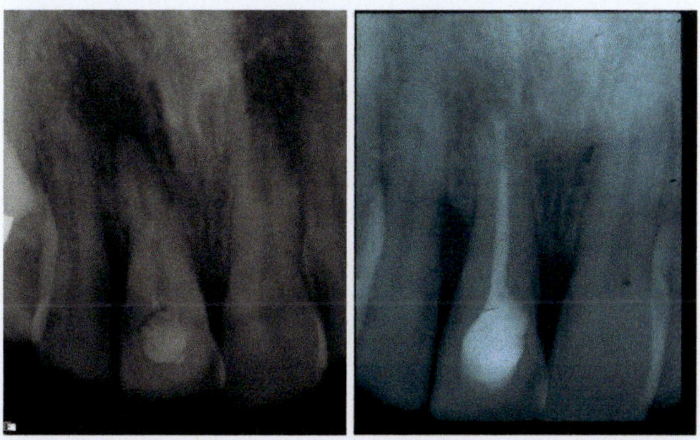

Figure 1.8 Retrograde filling, tooth 21 at treatment (left) and at two-year control (right).

material volume by interaction with the contact liquid. The coating material has a certain amount of unreacted chemically bonded bioceramic, and this part includes body liquid into the formed contact zone material. This contributes to an early fill-up of the void between the original coating material and the tissue wall. Further aspects of coating implants and testing are presented in Ref [22].

1.4.2 Orthopedic applications

The apatite-based biomaterials are excellent for bone void filling but still lack the strength for load-bearing applications. Other aspects of the use of apatite or Ca phosphate biomaterials are related to handling, hardening time, and shelf life. This is studied in a PhD thesis by Åberg [23]. Biomaterials based on Ca sulfate and Ca phosphate are described in a PhD thesis by Nilsson [24]. However, many of these biomaterials are not typical nanostructured materials; in some cases, they are just one of the phases in the multiphase materials.

For load-bearing applications within orthopedics, nanostructured chemically bonded bioceramics such as Ca aluminate and Ca silicate with higher strengths than other CBBCs may be options [25]. Results from the relatively new CBBC material, the Ca aluminate-based biocement are presented in this section.

Within orthopedics the following areas for Ca aluminate biomaterials have been identified: percutaneous vertebroplasty (PVP), kyphoplasty (KVP), and general augmentation.

The rate of the hydration is controlled by (1) the cement phase, (2) the particle size of the cement, (3) the hydration temperature, and (4) processing agents, including temperature rise. This is especially important when larger amounts of injectable materials are necessary, as for some orthopedic applications. The PVP and KVP techniques are shortly described here.

Percutaneous vertebroplasty (PVP): PVP is predominantly performed under local anesthesia by interventional radiologists. The material is injected directly into the fractured vertebra to stabilize it and relieve pain.

Kyphoplasty (KVP): KVP is predominantly performed under anesthesia by orthopedic surgeons and neurosurgeons but increasingly also by interventional radiologists. The fracture of the collapsed vertebra is reduced by inflating a balloon inside it. After deflation and removal of the balloon the stabilizing material is injected.

The calcium aluminate-based material is highly moldable and is applicable to orthopedic cavities with standard syringes and needles. The paste may cure within about 5 min at 37°C and develops strength values comparable to PMMA bone cement. The cured material is stable in the long-term and shows promisingly good biocompatibility. The benefits of the injectable ceramic biomaterials based on Ca aluminate related to orthopedic applications are as follows:

During the surgical procedure [7,26]:

- High radiopacity allows for superior visibility of the cement and increases the probability to detect potential leakages during injection (see Fig. 1.9).
- High and linearly increasing viscosity reduces the risk of leakage and gives a predictable handling.

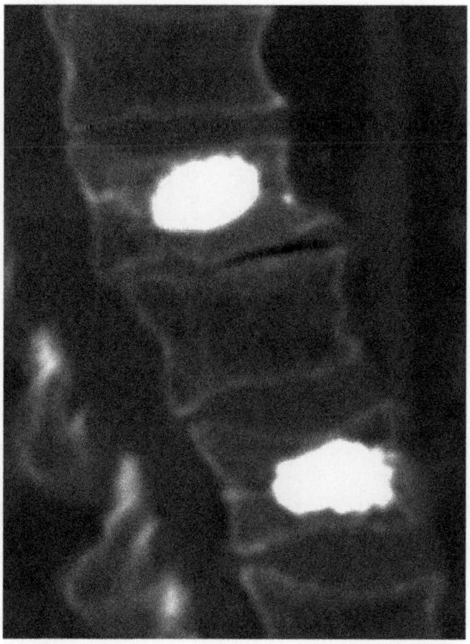

Figure 1.9 Vertebral compression factures restored by a Ca aluminate-based material.

- High cohesiveness optimizes the cement's filling pattern in the vertebrae.
- No toxic or smelling fumes.

After the procedure [9,26,27]:

- High mechanical strength
- Biocompatibility including biological integration
- Long-term stability, i.e., nonresorbable systems

The injectability of the chemically bonded ceramics is mainly controlled by the added water as the reacting phase with the powdered cements. This reaction is an acid–base reaction where water acts as a weak acid, and the cement powder acts as a base. The technological importance of this is that all the water needed for injectability can be consumed in the formation of solid phases, yielding products with low porosity, one of the requirements for high strength.

1.4.3 Drug delivery carrier applications

The ceramic carrier chemistry allows for the loading of almost any medicament. The drugs can favorably be loaded in the water liquid, in the pore system of inert filler particles, and in processing agents. Thus drugs can be loaded both during the formation of hydrates or after hydration by infiltration. For hydrophobic medical agents, the agent can be easily mixed into the precursor powder or together with a second ceramic filler. The nanoporous materials are sometimes divided into micro- (<2 nm), meso- (2–10 nm), and macroporosity (<10 nm). General aspects of materials as drug carriers are treated in the papers [1,10,28–32], among others.

Table 1.7 **Pore size interval for different types of ceramics.**

Pore size intervals	Fully hydrated	Partly hydrated	Sintered ceramics (submicron)	Sintered ceramics	Others
A	1–10 nm				
B		10–100 nm			
C			0.1–1 µm		
D				1–10 µm	
E					10–100 µm

A = fully hydrated, B = partially hydrated or low hydration degree, C = sintered ceramics (submicron), D = sintered ceramics (partially or coarse grain), and E = others.

The carrier material system described exhibits well-controlled microstructures on the nanosized level, which lends the carrier material opportunities for selected and controlled release of the medicament. The release time is controlled mainly by the contents of the hydrated chemically bonded cement phases: the higher the content of the cement, the longer the release time. The longest release time is achieved for fully hydrated phases with water contents close to the water to cement ratio (w/c) required for complete hydration.

By introducing optional additives, or by changing the w/c ratio, the release time can be controlled from a few hours to more than one day. The release time is also dependent upon where the drug is placed in the body. In cortical bone a release time of months seems possible.

The carrier may be used as a vehicle for transport and delivery of the medicament as an injectable implant. The combination of the material as a carrier and implant material makes site-specific placement of drugs and implants possible. Table 1.7 summarizes the pore size intervals obtainable with different ceramics used for drug delivery.

The amount of drug released in a specific case is controlled by the amount of the drug in the carrier and how the carrier material is designed. Using the mixed powder cement and an inert phase opens up the use of combined drugs, e.g., for rapid release based on the inert phase, medium release rate based on partially hydrated phases, and slow release based on fully hydrated cement phases. Test materials have been used with the loading of the drugs in the interval 1–10 mg/100 mg carrier material. Fig. 1.10 shows schematic release rates using corresponding selected pore structures of the carrier material. The material types C, B, and A from Table 1.7 were used.

1.5 Conclusion and summary

The chemically bonded bioceramics, especially the materials based on phosphates, aluminates, and silicates, exhibit a general nanostructure related to both the crystals and pores between the crystals. Due to a low solubility product of the phases formed,

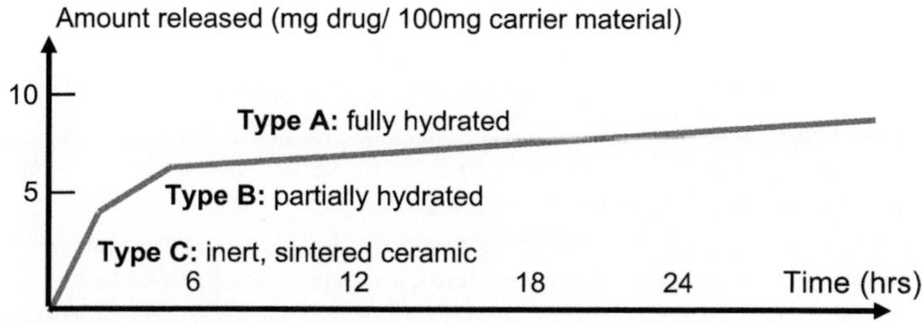

Figure 1.10 Schematic release of drugs using different pore structures.

nanocrystals are easily formed, and it is even difficult to avoid the nanostructured features. The nanocrystal size is often in the range of 10–40 nm with an open porosity with pores in the range of 1–3 nm. A broad range of applications are foreseen within odontology, orthopedics, and drug delivery carrier systems.

Acknowledgments

The author expresses his great gratitude to all the personnel at Doxa AB and Applied Research Sweden AB for input under a ten-year period.

References

[1] Hermansson L. Nanostructural chemically bonded Ca-aluminate based biomaterials. In: Pignatello R, editor. BIOMATERIALS – physics and chemistry. INTECH Publ.; 2011.
[2] Park JB, Lakes. R.S.BIOMATERIALS, an introduction. Springer; 2007.
[3] Martin RB. Bone as a ceramic composite material. In: Shackelford JF, editor. Bioceramics. Switzerland: Trans Tech Publ.Ltd; 1999.
[4] Li J. Development of high-strength bioactive ceramic composites [Ph.D. thesis]. Sweden: The Department of Prosthodontics, Karolinska Institute; 1992.
[5] Powers TC, Brownyard TL. Studies of the physical properties of hardened cement paste. Chicago, USA: Publ. of Res. Lab. of the Portland Cement association; 1946.
[6] Engqvist H, Schultz-Walz JE, Lööf J, Botton GA, Mayer D, Phaneuf MW, et al. Chemical and biological integration of a mouldable bioactive ceramic material capable of forming apatite in vivo in teeth. Biomaterials 2004;25:2781–7.
[7] Engqvist H, Botton GA, Couillard M, Mohammadi S, Malmström J, Emanuelsson L, et al. A new tool for high-resolution transmission electron microscopy of intact interfaces between bone and metallic implants. J Biomed Mater Res 2006;78A:20–4.
[8] Hermansson L. NANOSTRUCTURAL BIOCERAMICS – advances in chemically bonded ceramics. Pan Stanford Publ.; 2015.
[9] Engqvist H, Hermansson L. Chemically bonded bioceramics based on Ca-aluminates and silicates. Ceram Trans 2006;172:221–8.
[10] Davidovits J. GEOPLYMER, Chemistry & Applications. Institut Géopolmère; 2008.
[11] Duxson P, et al. Geopolymer technology: the current state of the art. J Mater Sci 2007;42(9):2917–33.

[12] Hermansson L, Lööf J, Jarmar T. Integration mechanisms towards hard tissue of Ca-aluminate based materials. Key Eng Mater 2009;396–398:183–6.
[13] Pameijer CH, Jefferies S, Loof J, et al. Microleakage evaluation of XeraCem in cemented crowns. J Dent Res 2008;87(B):3098.
[14] Pameijer CH, Zmener O, Alvarez Serrano S, et al. Sealing properties of a calcium aluminate luting agent. Am J Dent 2010;23:121–4.
[15] Loof J, Svahn F, Jarmar T, Engqvist H, Pameijer CH. A comparative study of the bioactivity of three materials for dental applications. Dent Mater 2008;24:653–9.
[16] Kraft L, Saks i M, Hermansson L, Pameijer CH. A five year retrospective clinical study of a calcium-aluminate in retrograde endodontics. J Dent Res 2009;88(A):1383.
[17] Ellingsen JE, Lyngstadaas SP. Bioimplant interface, improving biomaterials and tissue reactions. New York: CRC Press, Taylor&Francis; 2003.
[18] Vercaigne S, Wolke JG, Naert I, Jansen JA. Bone healing capacity of titanium plasma-sprayed and hydroxylapatite coated oral implants. Clin Oral Implants Res 1998;9:261.
[19] Liu X, Ding C, Wang Z. Apatite formed on the surface of plasma sprayed Wollastonite coating immersed in simulated body fluid. Biomaterials 2001;22:2007–12.
[20] Rickerby DS, Matthews A. Advanced surface coatings. New York: Chapman & Hall; 1991.
[21] Schneider JM, Rohde S, Sproul WD, Matthews A. Recent developments in plasma assisted physical vapour deposition. J Phys D Appl Phys 2000;33:173–86.
[22] Axén N, Engqvist H, Lööf J, Thomsen P, Hermansson L. In vivo hydrating calcium aluminate coatings for anchoring of metal implants in bone. Key Eng Mater 2005;284–286:831–4.
[23] Åberg J. Premixed acidic calcium phosphate cements [Ph.D. thesis]. Uppsala University; 2011.
[24] Nilsson M. Injectable calcium sulphates and calcium phosphates as bone substitutes [Ph.D. thesis]. Lund University; 2003.
[25] Lööf J. Calcium aluminate as biomaterial [Ph.D. thesis]. Sweden: Uppsala University; 2010.
[26] Jarmar T, Uhlin T, Höglund U, Thomsen P, Hermansson L, Engqvist H. Injectable bone cements for Vertebroplasty studied in sheep vertebrae with electron microscopy. Key Eng Mater 2008;361–363:373–6.
[27] Hermansson L, Engqvist H, Gomez-Ortega G, Abrahamsson E, Björklund K. Nanosize biomaterials based on Ca-aluminate. Key Eng Mater 2006;49:21–6.
[28] Ravaglioli A, Krajewski A. J Mater Sci Mater Med 2000;11(12):763–7.
[29] Lasserre A, Bajpaj PK. Critical reviews. Ther Drug Carr Sys 1998;15:121–6.
[30] Yang L, Sheldon B, Webster TJ. Nanophase ceramics for improved drug delivery. Am Ceram Soc Bull 2010;80(2):24–31.
[31] Forsgren J. Functional ceramics in biomedical applications [Ph.D. thesis]. Uppsala University (Acta Universitatis Upsaliensis); 2010.
[32] Nilsson E. Development of new nanomaterials syntheses for mesostructured TiO_2 and SiO_2 [Ph.D. thesis]. Chalmers University of Technology; 2011.

Monitoring degradation products and metal ions in vivo

2

D. Paramitha[1], M.F. Ulum[2], A. Purnama[1], D.H.B. Wicaksono[3,4], D. Noviana[2], H. Hermawan[1]
[1]Laval University, Quebec City, Quebec, Canada; [2]Bogor Agricultural University, Bogor, West Java, Indonesia; [3]University of Technology of Malaysia, Johor Bahru, Johor, Malaysia; [4]Swiss-German University, Tangerang, Banten, Indonesia

2.1 Introduction

Along with the advances in biomedical science and technology, biomaterials and medical implants are evolving toward a direction where they are no longer required to be inert but actively interact with the living implantation sites [1,2]. The development of bioactive biomaterials is evident in all classes of traditional materials (metals, polymers, ceramics, and composites) for use as implants to tissue engineering supports [3,4]. One of the recent advances in metallic biomaterials is the development of biodegradable metals. These metals bear a concept where instead of keeping them inert, they are purposely designed to degrade within the in vivo setting [5,6]. Implants made of these metals are expected to corrode gradually in vivo, with an appropriate host response elicited by released corrosion products, then dissolve completely upon assisting tissue healing of temporary clinical problems [7].

Proposing biodegradable metal implants certainly opposes the established paradigm of inert metallic biomaterials. The released corrosion products and metal ions may disturb the local and systemic physiological equilibrium of the implanted host. Therefore the biosafety of each kind of degradation product has to be carefully evaluated and an insight into the in vivo monitoring of degradation products and released metal ions is essentially needed. This chapter introduces the state of the art of biodegradable metals, discusses the current in vivo implantation and monitoring techniques of biodegradable metal implants, and proposes new techniques for monitoring degradation products and metal ions in vivo.

2.2 Biodegradable metals: state of the art

Biodegradable metals have the potential to revolutionize current and future healthcare products, and they have been attracting researchers from both academics and medical industries. Among the three known types of biodegradable metals (iron, magnesium, zinc), magnesium alloys are the most elaborated ones, where advanced clinical tests and product

Monitoring and Evaluation of Biomaterials and their Performance in vivo. http://dx.doi.org/10.1016/B978-0-08-100603-0.00002-X

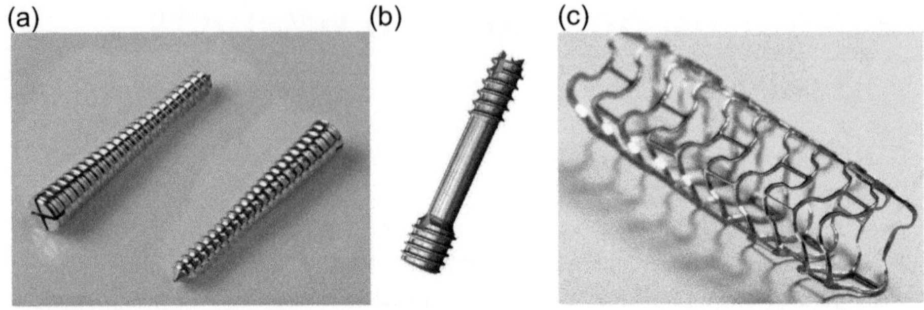

Figure 2.1 Examples of biodegradable metal products made of magnesium alloys: (a) Korean K-Met headless screw, (b) German Syntellix compression screw, and (c) German Biotronik absorbable stent.

development have already been done. Iron and its alloys as the first introduced type are still facing the challenge of slow in vivo degradation rate, while new interests are arising for zinc and its alloys [7]. New standards on materials, processes, and testing procedures are under development by the ASTM subcommittee F04.15 [8]. The term "bioabsorbable" is being preferentially used by the ASTM; however, in this chapter we continue to use the term biodegradable. Recently, there are at least three companies that have launched their commercial biodegradable metal products or prototypes, as shown in Fig. 2.1.

When discussing biodegradable metal implants, one will derive at least three key features. They are: (1) the metal from which an implant is made, (2) the implant used for treating a temporary clinical problem, and (3) the degradation, which refers to the corrosion of the metal in in vivo environment. The following sections briefly describe these three features.

2.2.1 The metals and their alloys

Since their first introduction in the early 2000s, there have been three groups of metallic materials studied as biodegradable metals: pure metals, metal alloys, and metal matrix composites. Iron, magnesium, and zinc are the three types of metal and their alloys that have been studied so far. Nonetheless, every element in a biodegradable metal implant must not cause adverse effect to the healing process and the body system. The most recent development of these three metals is described in the following paragraphs. More detailed discussion can be found in a recent review by Zheng et al. [7].

Iron is one of the essential elements in the human body that is involved in oxygen transport and is a component of metalloprotein with a daily allowance level up to 20 mg [9,10]. Iron has attractive mechanical properties approaching those of stainless steels, which makes it suitable for implants that require high strength such as coronary stents [6,11]. However, iron degrades very slowly in in vivo setting due to the formation of a complex iron phosphate layer [12,13]. Attempts to accelerate its degradation rate have been done by alloying with elements such as manganese and palladium [14], by implanting silver using a vapor vacuum arc technique [15], and by making composites with its oxides or bioceramics [16,17], resulting in a little improvement. A different direction has been taken by utilizing iron in its porous structure for potential scaffold applications [18,19] and is recently enhanced by creating a nanoporous surface via a dealloying zinc-diffused process on Fe Mn alloys [20].

Magnesium is an essential element with a high daily allowance level up to 700 mg, and it acts as protein coregulator and cofactor in more than 300 enzymatic reactions [21,22]. Magnesium is a lightweight metal with a density of 1.74 g/cm^3 and has a low elastic modulus of 45 GPa, near to that of bone (~30 GPa), which makes it very attractive for bone applications [23]. The main challenges with magnesium are its relatively low strength and ductility, and rapid corrosion rate producing hydrogen gas in physiological conditions [24,25]. Improvements have been made by purifying the metal from detrimental trace elements like iron, copper, and nickel [26]; by alloying with calcium, zinc, zirconium, and rare earth elements [27–29]; or by changing the microstructure to nanocrystalline and amorphous state [30]. Other methods for delaying its corrosion include surface coating with bioceramics and biopolymers [31,32].

Zinc has been proposed as a biodegradable metal, considering its essential role in many enzymes and in cell metabolic activity, proliferation, and differentiation [33]. It has a medium level of daily allowance at 15 mg, and possible neurotoxicity occurs if it is present in excess [34]. The cytocompatibility of zinc and its alloy was studied in view of its applications for bone and vascular implants [35,36]. Pure zinc has a less attractive mechanical property, but it degrades at a rate between magnesium and iron [37]. Alloying zinc with a low amount of magnesium (up to 3 wt%) improved mechanical properties to the level of some magnesium alloys and were further enhanced with severe plastic deformation processing techniques [38,39].

2.2.2 The temporary functional implants

The basic concept of biodegradable metal implants is providing a mechanical support to the healing process of an injured or diseased tissue and degrading away thereafter. Some clinical problems in cardiovascular, orthopedic, and pediatric care require only temporary support for eventual healing. A stented arterial blockage undergoes vessel remodeling, thus its permanent presence becomes unnecessary if not causing long-term disadvantages [40]. A set of mini plate and screws for bone fracture fixation that degrades after a complete bone reconstruction will avoid local biomechanic disturbance and patient discomfort and nullify the need for a second surgery [41]. Ideally, a biodegradable metal implant will have an optimum compromise between maintaining its mechanical integrity for a required period and progressing its degradation over time, as illustrated in Fig. 2.2.

Referring to Fig. 2.2, the inflammatory process starts rapidly within 1–7 days after fracture followed by soft callus formation in 2–3 weeks. Once the soft callus links fracture tips, the hard callus stage starts and lasts until the fragments are firmly united by new woven bone (3–4 months). Until this stage, the biodegradable metal plate must retain its mechanical integrity. The woven bone is then slowly replaced by lamellar bone through the osteonal remodeling process, which may take a few months to several years until the bone has completely returned to its original morphology [42,43].

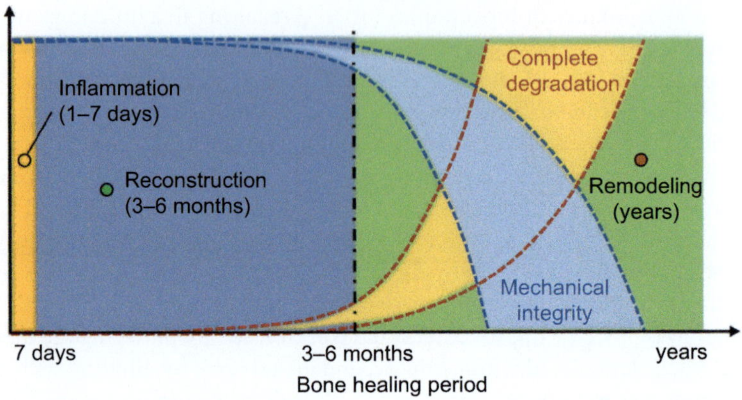

Figure 2.2 Illustration of ideal compromise between mechanical integrity and degradation rate of a biodegradable metal bone implant.

In the case of stent applications, the mechanical integrity and degradation must suit the period of the vessel's healing process. Inflammation occurs following the implantation of a stent for several days and is followed by a granulation period where endothelial cells migrate to cover the injured surface and the proliferation of smooth muscle cells (1–2 weeks). Furthermore, the remodeling period takes place with the deposition of extracellular matrix. The total time required for a stent to mechanically support the whole process has not been clearly defined, but a period of 6–12 months has been suggested [44,45].

2.2.3 The in vivo degradation

A biodegradable metal implant is continuously exposed to the extracellular tissue fluid once implanted into the human body. This exposure causes an electrochemical dissolution of metal at which the body responds via a cascade process of protein absorption, coagulation, acute inflammation, chronic inflammation, and foreign body response, as illustrated in Fig. 2.3. Acute interaction occurs shortly after implantation related to the corrosion process that induces the formation of an interspace (dead space) between the implant and the tissue filled with a large volume of body fluid. Cellular inflammation follows during the first-week postimplantation, which then decreases over a prolonged time, where the dead space is filled with proliferation of the surrounding tissue [46,47].

Corrosion is the typical process of degradation for biodegradable metals. It is initiated at any site on the surface that has a potential difference created from metallurgical inhomogeneity such as phase variation, grain boundaries, impurities, or from geometrical and environmental variation such as crevice, notch, scratch, coating defect, oxygen level gradient, etc. In the physiological environment, corrosion of metal (M) generally involves the following reactions:

Anodic reaction: $$M \rightarrow M^{n+} + ne^- \quad (2.1)$$

Cathodic reaction: $$2H_2O + 2e^- \rightarrow H_2 + 2OH^- \quad (2.2)$$ or

$$2H_2O + O_2 + 4e^- \rightarrow 4OH^- \quad (2.3)$$

Product formation: $$M^{n+} + nOH^- \rightarrow M(OH)n \quad (2.4)$$

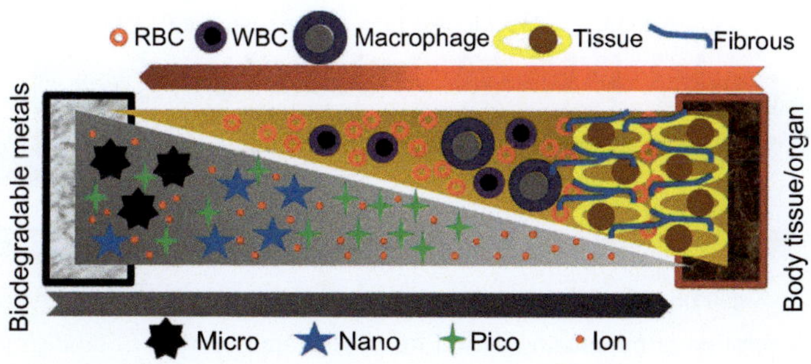

Figure 2.3 Illustration of possible interaction between a degrading metal implant with the local tissue and systemic body response.

The physiological solution contains various anions and cations, dissolved oxygen, organic compounds, amino acids, proteins, and so on. The released metal ions interact with water and other species, creating a layer of degradation products from as simple as metal hydroxides (M(OH)*n*) to metal complexes. Meanwhile, the produced electrons flow in the metal and are consumed by the reduction of water and/or oxygen to form hydrogen gas or hydroxide ions. A decrease in pH to 5.3–5.6 around the implantation site, due to inflammatory response, may accelerate the corrosion process of the metal and reduce local oxygen concentration [48]. The inorganic ions in physiological solutions such as Cl^-, one of the most abundant solutions, aggressively breaks down the M(OH)*n* layer, leading to continuous corrosion and mostly localized attack [49]. Similar effect as that of Cl^- is also observed for $SO_4{}^{2-}$, meanwhile other ions such as $HPO_4{}^{2-}/PO_4{}^{3-}$, $HCO_3{}^{-}/CO_3{}^{2-}$, and Ca^{2+} help to passivate magnesium and iron due to the precipitation of phosphate and carbonate salts on the metal surface [50,51]. Adsorption of organic molecules such as albumin on the metal surface delays the corrosion process of magnesium in the initial stage only [52]; meanwhile, amino acid reduces the barrier effect of the insoluble salt layer against the dissolution of magnesium [50].

The nature of the corrosion process that produces a flow of electrons (Eq. (3.1)) has been long exploited as a tool for measuring kinetics of corrosion by means of electroanalytical tools such as potentiostat/galvanostat. However, this measurement, which requires electrical connection wires and the insertion of reference and counter electrodes, is not applicable for in vivo corrosion monitoring. On the other side, the nature of metal ion release to the extracellular fluid around the implant can be used to approximate the degradation rate by measuring their concentration over time. By combining a kind of fluid sampling tool and electroanalytical apparatus, this approach can become an effective system for monitoring in vivo degradation of biodegradable metal implants. Details of this approach are discussed in the next section.

2.3 In vivo implantation study of biodegradable metals

When material testing and in vitro degradation studies produce promising results, an in vivo study is required to comprehensively examine the body's response to

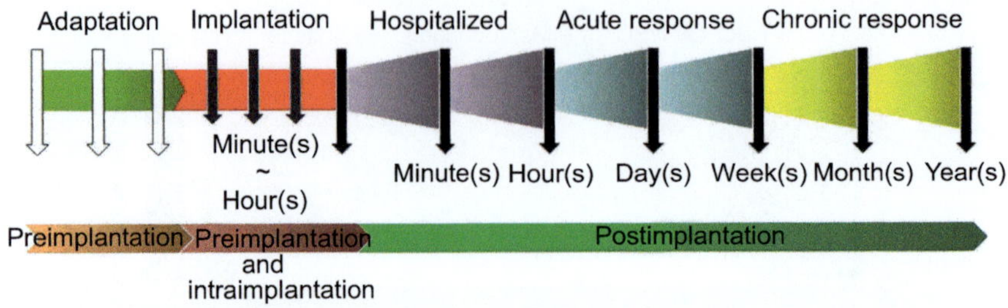

Figure 2.4 Illustration of monitoring period for in vivo animal study of biodegradable metals.

biodegradable metal implantation, before going further to clinical trials. An ethical clearance must be obtained prior to conducting an animal experiment. The experiment must be carefully designed starting from selecting the animal model (small to large mammals) and its number based on the type of implant specimen and the collection of expected data until the determination of pre- and postimplantation procedures. The preimplantation protocols include animal acclimatization and health state synchronization, implant and surgical device sterilization, presurgical medication, preanesthesia, analgesia, and anesthesia. After surgical implantation, the animal is subjected to peri-/intrasurgical monitoring, postsurgical hospitalization, and monitoring until a full recovery [53,54]. As illustrated in Fig. 2.4, monitoring of implant degradation is matched with the corresponding short- and long-term body responses.

Considering the implant tissue interaction, the postsurgical monitoring can be done by collecting information from the implant itself and its corrosion products, local cellular, and organ or systemic responses. Radiographic techniques such as X-ray radiography, ultrasonography, microcomputed tomography (μCT), and magnetic resonance imaging (MRI) scans can be used to indirectly detect the degree of corrosion and corrosion product formation and the changes in the tissue structure around the implant [55]. The results are then confirmed by direct analysis after sacrificing the animal. This can be done on the retrieved implant by measuring weight loss, observing surface morphology, and checking chemical composition of the corrosion product and on the surrounding tissue by performing histology. The systemic response can be determined by analyzing the blood and extracellular fluid for possible ion content released during implant degradation or for changes on the blood profile related to acute response [56]. At the same time, the tissue healing progress can be monitored through related biomarkers contained in the blood. Biomarkers such as estrogen, testosterone, and progesterone may be detected and quantified for monitoring bone healing progress after implantation [57–59].

In general, monitoring of degradation and tissue healing can be done using offline and online systems for both local and systemic monitoring, as illustrated in Fig. 2.5. Offline monitoring assesses the affected tissue in segmental form (not real time), for example, by using radiographic imaging (a noninvasive method) or by taking a fluid sample (an invasive method) from tissue around the implant (local) or from circulating blood (systemic). Online monitoring is done in real time, for example, by using radiography in combination with rapid image processing software and by sampling blood in combination with online mass spectroscopy.

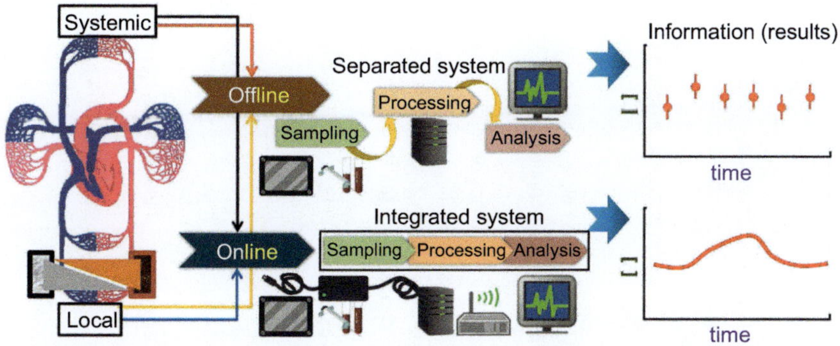

Figure 2.5 Illustration of offline and online in vivo monitoring system for biodegradable metals.

2.4 Current in vivo techniques for monitoring degradation

Numerous methods have been used to evaluate in vivo corrosion behavior of biodegradable metals, involving both qualitative and quantitative measurement. So far, these methods are the adoption from common protocols for in vivo corrosion evaluation of inert metallic biomaterials using various analytical tools ranging from radiography, blood analysis to histology. Table 4.1 summarizes the principal in vivo studies on biodegradable metal implants and their assessment methods capable of monitoring the degradation process, degradation product, and metal ions.

The following paragraphs provide a highlight on selected in vivo studies of magnesium and iron-based implants and the methods they used and its analysis. Fischerauer et al. demonstrated the use of online μCT to monitor the degradation of magnesium alloy ZX50 pins combined with histological analysis [58]. The pins were implanted into the femoral bone of SD rats and an online μCT scan was performed every week after implantation up to 24 weeks. The μCT images showed that the degradation rate is dependent on the surface topography. The increasing degradation rate correlated with increasing surface area per volume of implants. Any form of pits, pores, cracks, or calderas increased the surface area of the implant, thus facilitating the penetration of physiological fluid and thus corrosion attack. The μCT also showed the images of gas formation around the implants leading to callus formation, while the released magnesium ions induced new bone formation. This concluded that the absence of gas formation facilitates the contact of bone implant, leading to the formation of new bone.

Zhao et al. harnessed H_2 evolution from different magnesium (Mg8H, ZK40 and AZ31) using a H_2 microsensor as a tool for measuring degradation in vivo [61]. Disks of the alloys were implanted subcutaneously into the back part of specific pathogen free female athymic nude mice. The level of H_2 gas was observed every week after implantation using H_2 microsensor up to 8 weeks. Measurement was done by placing the sensor tip above the skin at several different points (near, immediately adjacent, and far) from the H_2 gas cavity. The microsensor showed a sensitive reproducible measurement in a quite short time (30 s) detecting very low H_2 concentration (30–400 μM).

Table 4.1 Summary of the principal in vivo implantation studies of biodegradable metal implants

Study	Method and analytical tools	Principal finding
ZX50 magnesium alloy pins in femoral legs of Sprague–Dawley (SD) rats [60]	Degradation monitoring by using μCT and histological analysis over 24 weeks	Increasing degradation rate correlates with increasing surface area-to-volume ratio of implants
Subcutaneous implantation of pure magnesium (Mg8H) and its alloys (ZK40, AZ31) in nude mice [61]	Degradation monitoring via H_2 gas evolution transdermally using electrochemical H_2 microsensor up to 8 weeks	H_2 level correlates with the degradation rate and weight loss of implants
Magnesium alloy plates (WE43) with and without coating in calvarial bone of miniature pigs [62]	Radiography, CT, μCT, and histological analysis up to 24 weeks	Slower degradation of coated plate is associated with broader bone implant contact area
BioDe MSM in femoral shaft and muscle of New Zealand White (NZW) rabbits [63]	Radiography, hemolysis test, and histological analysis over 10 weeks	Corrosion rate of the alloy varies depending on implantation position and site
ZX50 and WZ21 magnesium alloy in femoral bone of SD rats [64]	μCT and histological analysis over 24 weeks	Increasing H_2 gas produced by fast implant degradation correlates with the increasing callus formation
ZEK100 magnesium alloy in femoral bone of NZW rabbits [65]	Radiography, μCT, magnesium serum ion evaluation, and fluorochrome histological analysis over 12 months	Admiring in vivo degradation is not necessarily associated with good biocompatibility
CMZSY HE-BMG magnesium alloy rods in femoral shaft of C57BL/6 mice [66]	Radiography, μCT, and histological analysis up to 4 weeks	Osteogenesis and new bone formation is not necessarily associated with an obvious degradation
W4 short fiber magnesium alloy scaffolds in femoral bone of NZW rabbits [67]	μCT, ICP-OES blood evaluation, and histological analysis over 12 weeks	The initial corrosion rate of the alloys has been too fast for its high initial surface area
Mg-Ca-Si alloy for bone graft in tibial bone and subcutaneous area of Wistar rats [68]	Radiography, μCT, colorimetric method for metal ion blood evaluation and histological analysis over 4 weeks	Different reactivity and degradation shown by implants in the different implantation site

Mg-Sr alloy bone graft implantation in tibial bone of NZW rabbits [69]	Radiography up until 8 weeks	The degradation rate and bone formation correlates with different status preparation of implants
MgYREZr alloy screws for ligament reconstruction in tibial bone of NZW rabbits [70]	Radiography μCT, ICP-MS blood evaluation, and histological analysis up until 24 weeks	Degradation and gas formation surrounding the screw did not affect the attachment of fixed tendon
Iron-based pins in femoral bone of SD rats [71]	μCT and histological analysis up to 52 weeks	Degradation rate mainly influenced by in vivo condition rather than implant composition
Nitride iron-based scaffolds in abdominal aorta of NZW rabbits [72]	μCT, OCT, MRI, and histological analysis over 13 months	The corrosion rate of scaffolds examined by OCT and MRI are in accordance with that of μCT and histological analysis
Porous pure magnesium tablets in femoral legs of SD rats [25]	H_2 gas measurement using radiography analysis over 3 weeks	Rapid degradation resulting in excessive H_2 gas and leading to the high mortality of rats
Implantation of Fe-bioceramic composite chips in femoral and tibial legs of Indonesian thin tailed sheep [17,55]	Radiography, B-mode ultrasonography, blood evaluation, and histological analysis over 10 weeks	Degradation rate of the bioceramic composites are lower than pure iron, yet showed higher bioactivity
Rolled iron sheet in tail venous of mice [73]	μCT and histological analysis over 36 weeks	Degradation occurred after 1 month of implantation, progressively, and the corrosion product is metabolically inactive
Iron and magnesium wire in artery wall and lumen of SD rats [74]	Histological analysis over 36 weeks	Degradation of iron and magnesium wires directed by the arterial environment (blood vs matrix contact)
Pure iron wire in muscle of mice [75]	Scanned parafinized block of tissue sample and histological analysis up to 14 days	Distribution particle speed of the degradation product correlates with oxide diameter area
Zinc wire in abdominal aorta of SD rats [76,77]	SEM and histological analysis over 24 weeks	Increasing degradation rate correlates with increasing cross-sectional area reduction

The H_2 concentration was correlated to the weight loss and degradation rate of each sample. Albeit it seems very promising for monitoring in vivo degradation, this technique is specific to magnesium-based implants that produce H_2 gas during degradation. It is still limited to thin skin and tissue and will need an optimization for application to bigger animals or humans and to implant in a deeper tissue.

Kraus et al., determined the in vivo degradation rate of iron-based (pure Fe, Fe-10Mn-1Pd, and Fe-21Mn-0.7C-1Pd) pins by implant volume and mass losses [71]. The pins were implanted into the cortical area of the femoral bone of rats, and observation was done up to 52 weeks using reconstructed μCT, surface analysis of the retrieved implants, and tissue histological analysis. The results showed that until 52 weeks of implantation, there were no significant degradation that occurred on the pins as the formed degradation product layer inhibited further degradation process. Degradation analysis was difficult to perform by μCT since the very little degradation product scattered the images. This finding demonstrated that in vivo degradation of iron-based implants was mainly influenced by composition of degradation products and oxygen availability at the implant site, rather than the composition of the implant.

Lin et al. [72] performed observation of nitrided iron-based stents in the abdominal aorta of NZW rabbits up to 13 months using μCT, MRI, optical coherence tomography (OCT), and histological analysis. The results showed that the corrosion examination by MRI and OCT on the living animals was in accordance with the results from μCT and histological analysis of the explants and tissues. This study showed a way for online in vivo degradation monitoring by using OCT and MRI. The OCT provides qualitative information on degradation, even though it can only work for implants located near to the skin surface due to the use of semicoherent infrared light. The MRI provides good visualization of the dark artifact resulting from iron ferromagnetism that gives the semi-quantitative degradation measurement. Nevertheless, they admitted that μCT was more effective to visualize and quantitatively monitor the degradation on small animals or ex vivo. However, this combination of OCT and MRI seems less suitable for monitoring degradation of nonmagnetic substances or nonferrous metal implants.

According to the mentioned studies (Table 4.1), there are at least six modalities that are generally used to monitor the degradation of biodegradable metal implants. Those modalities are usually used in combination with each other to obtain comprehensive results. The following section describes the six modalities in more detail.

2.4.1 Radiography

Radiography is the most used and cost-effective diagnostic tool that can distinguish different body tissues based on an X-ray photon attenuation. It is a very versatile tool for the examination of hard tissue, such as bone and teeth, and for a routine check after orthopedic implant placement mostly made of metals. Bone healing, inflammation at the implant interface, and implant position can be assessed by comparing the degree of radiodensity in the two-dimensional (2-D) radiogram. The difference in the radiodensity level can indicate the formation of degradation products in relation to the tissue reaction toward degradation of a metal implant. A high radiodensity value is commonly found for iron implants as it highly absorbs the X-ray energy, making a radiopaque image [55], while a low radiodensity is found for magnesium implants related

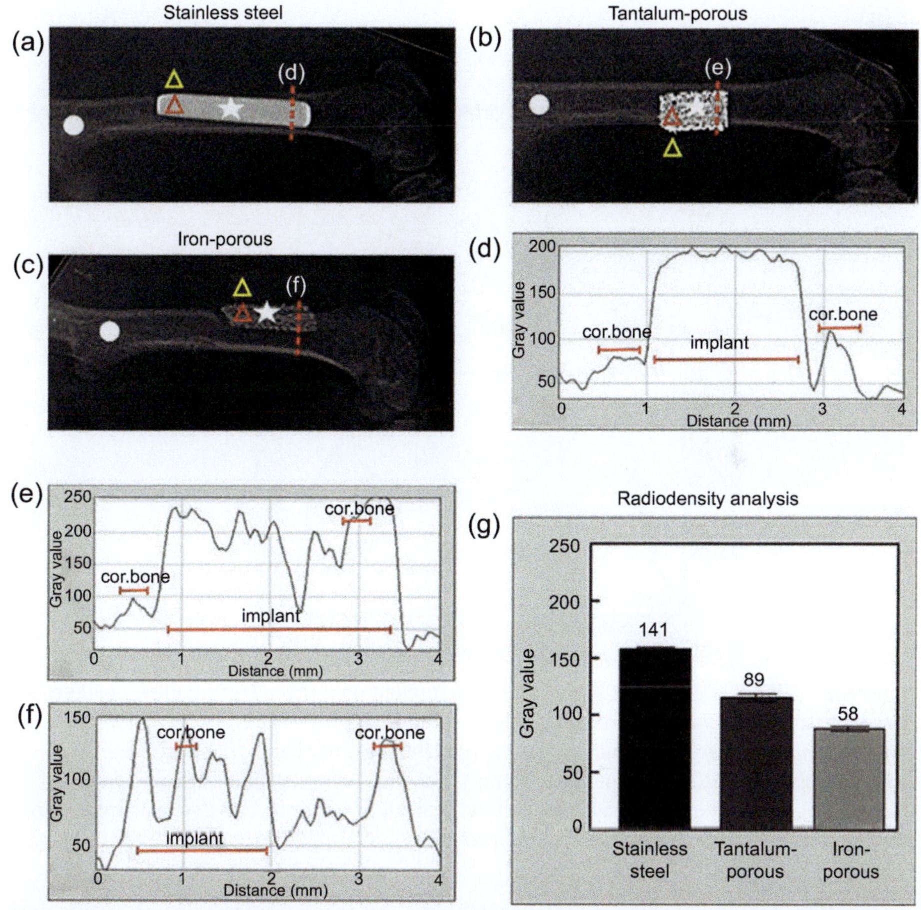

Figure 2.6 Digital radiogram of different metal implants on a mice femur: (a, d) stainless steel, (b, e) porous tantalum, (c, f) porous iron, and (g) their corrected total intensity. *Star*, implant; *circle*, bone; *broken red line*, analysis area "line plot profile" using software of ImageJ; *red triangle*, implant analysis area; and *yellow line triangle*, background analysis area.
Adapted from Noviana D, Estuningsih S, Ulum MF. Animal study and pre-clinical trials of biomaterials. In: Mahyudin F, Hermawan H, editors. Biomaterials and medical devices: a perspective from an emerging country. Cham: Springer International Publishing; 2016. p. 67–101.

to hydrogen gas evolution surrounding the implant [25]. However, radiographic analysis is mostly qualitative and is limited to resolution at the microscopic level. Additional tools such as a densitometer to read the radiograph, especially for implant sizes smaller than 1 mm, and image processing software can enhance the assessment at the peri-implant area, as illustrated in Fig. 2.6.

2.4.2 Ultrasonography

Ultrasonography utilizes high-frequency sound wave energy (ultrasound) to image any particularity in the soft or hard tissues. It is readily available in almost every

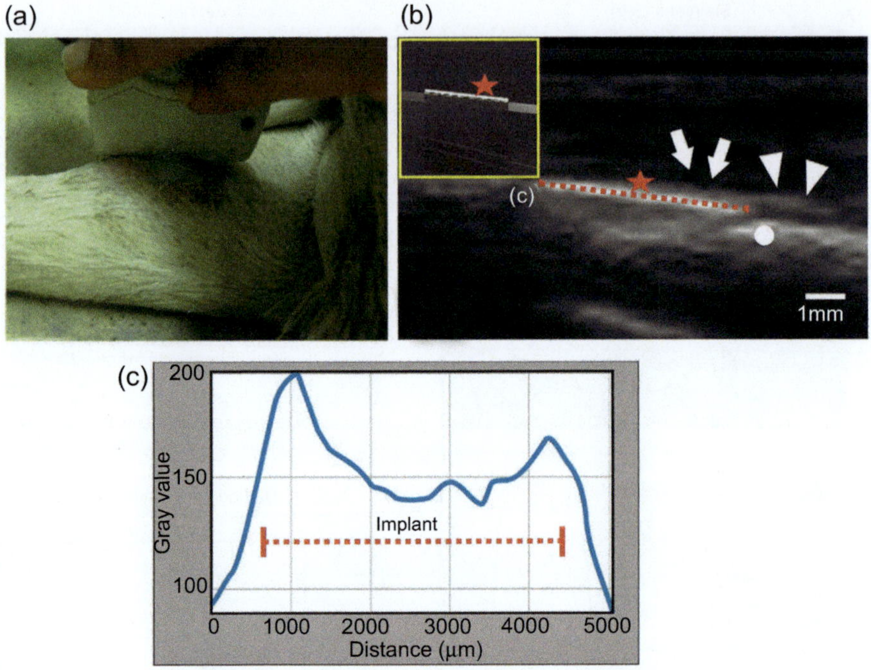

Figure 2.7 Ultrasonography of iron bioceramic implant on a sheep leg: (a) ultrasound probe, (b) sonogram, and (c) analysis of echogenicity using ImageJ software. *Arrow head*, new bone around the implant; *arrow*, liquid around the implant; *star*, implant; *circle*, bone.
Adapted from Noviana D, Estuningsih S, Ulum MF. Animal study and pre-clinical trials of biomaterials. In: Mahyudin F, Hermawan H, editors. Biomaterials and medical devices: a perspective from an emerging country. Cham: Springer International Publishing; 2016. p. 67–101.

medical facility and has been used widely, especially for the imaging of pregnancy and internal disease. Under ultrasonography, degradation products of a metal implant appear as a bright white color image (called hyperechoic) [78,79], while bone and soft tissue appear darker, as illustrated in Fig. 2.7.

The accumulated degradation products induce a local inflammatory reaction, which is imaged by ultrasonography as multitextures (black to white or anechoic to hyperechoic), as illustrated in Fig. 2.8. Sonogram can provide real-time imaging quantification when combined with image analyzer software for radiography [55]. However, it is limited to semiquantitative analysis and low resolution to clearly distinguish degradation products.

2.4.3 Microcomputed tomography

As mentioned in Table 4.1, μCT is the most used diagnostic tool to observe the degradation of biodegradable metal implants. It uses the differences in X-ray attenuation properties of materials to reconstruct 3-D structures. Its high X-ray energy can nondestructively penetrate the microarchitecture of the implant with voxel sizes down to 1 μm or smaller, and thus it can be used to perform both qualitative and quantitative

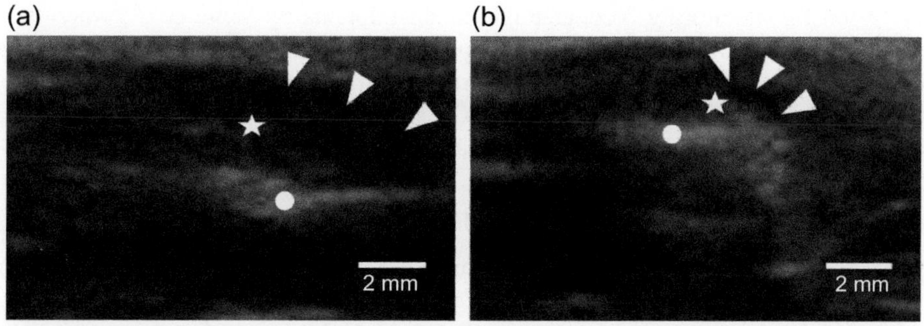

Figure 2.8 Sonogram of porous magnesium implant on rat bone: (a) the long cutting and (b) cross cutting. *Arrow head*, cavity filled with fluid; *star*, implant; *circle*, bone.
Adapted from Noviana D, Estuningsih S, Ulum MF. Animal study and pre-clinical trials of biomaterials. In: Mahyudin F, Hermawan H, editors. Biomaterials and medical devices: a perspective from an emerging country. Cham: Springer International Publishing; 2016. p. 67–101.

measurement [80]. Equipped with finite element analysis software, μCT can measure local density related to intrinsic mechanical properties of certain implants and tissues and generate 2-D and 3-D reconstructed images, as illustrated in Fig. 2.9.

Further enhancement to its image resolution has been done by combining synchrotron radiation (SRμCT), where the higher signal-to-noise ratio enables a simultaneous observation of bone microstructure and the mineralization process [81]. SRμCT was

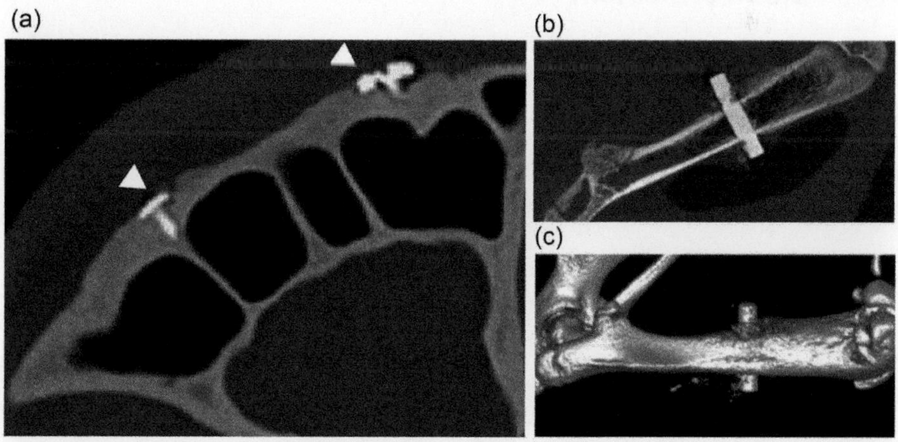

Figure 2.9 μCT images of: (a) WE43 magnesium alloy screws on a minipig's calvarial bone, (b, c) ZX50 magnesium alloy pin in Sprague–Dawley rat's femoral bone.
Adapted from Schaller B, Saulacic N, Imwinkelried T, Beck S, Liu EW, Gralla J, et al. In vivo degradation of magnesium plate/screw osteosynthesis implant systems: soft and hard tissue response in a calvarial model in miniature pigs. Journal of Craniomaxillofacial Surgery 2016;44:309–17 and Kraus T, Fischerauer SF, Hanzi AC, Uggowitzer PJ, Loffler JF, Weinberg AM. Magnesium alloys for temporary implants in osteosynthesis: in vivo studies of their degradation and interaction with bone. Acta Biomaterialia 2012;8:1230–8.

first used for monitoring biodegradable metal implants by Witte et al., where they were able to differentiate degradation products (oxides) from the magnesium metal implants, qualitatively approximate degradation rate, and distinguish degradation mechanism [82]. However, even though μCT is becoming a popular diagnostic tool, it is not widely available in most medical facilities.

2.4.4 Magnetic resonance imaging

MRI utilizes a strong magnetic field to spin and expose the protons of hydrogen atoms naturally present in living tissue to a beam of radio waves, which then produce a faint signal and process it into images. The produced image and resolution is quite detailed and can detect tiny changes of structures within the body, which can be further enhanced by the use of contrast agents. However, the use of MRI to monitor the degradation of biodegradable metal implants is still very limited. The presence of a metal implant can generate heat in the surrounding tissue, leading to thermal damage and signal distortion. It then produces images with artifacts that interfere with the interpretation. Lin et al. were able to turn this limitation into an advantage by utilizing the artifact to monitor the degradation of iron-based stents with a method developed by Koch et al. [72,83]. As shown in Fig. 2.10 the degraded iron and its corrosion products created dark area artifact due to their ferromagnetic property. Applicability of this method for other biodegradable metals such as magnesium and zinc alloys could be challenged by the nonferromagnetism of degradation products of these metals.

2.4.5 Blood evaluation

The degradation of metal produces metal ions that are eventually transported by the blood. The concentration of metal ions in the blood can be used as an indirect measure of degradation over time and an indication of its systemic impact. This invasive procedure is an easy and cost-effective way to monitor the degradation of the metal implant. Following implantation, a blood sample can be taken from veins and then analyzed by means of mass spectrometry such as atomic absorption spectrophotometry (AAS) and inductive couple

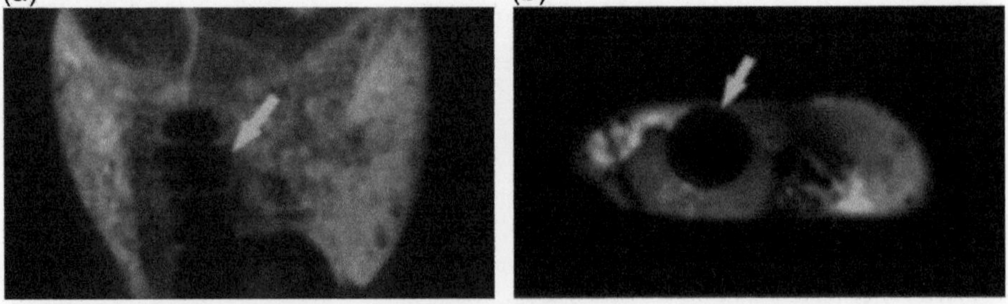

Figure 2.10 MRI images showing the axial (a) and lateral (b) artifacts created by an iron-based stent in a rabbit's abdominal aorta (*white arrow*).
Adapted from Lin WJ, Zhang DY, Zhang G, Sun HT, Qi HP, Chen LP, et al. Design and characterization of a novel biocorrodible iron-based drug-eluting coronary scaffold. Materials & Design 2016;91:72–9.

plasma mass spectrometry (ICP-MS). The ICP-MS has a lower detection limit (higher sensitivity) than AAS and can detect multiple elements at one measurement [84]. Other means that were used for detecting metal ion concentration in blood are a kind of chemistry analyzer using a specific reagent for a magnesium-based implant [65], and colorimetric assay, where the metal ions are determined as inorganic phosphates [68].

2.4.6 Histological analysis

Histological analysis is the gold standard for tissue examination, either for research or diagnostic purposes, for both qualitative and quantitative measure. It is used to assess the inflammation or healing stage and to monitor the presence and distribution of degradation products that dissolved into the surrounding tissue. Different staining is used to identify certain structures, cells, tissues, or even metal components. The most common staining is Hematoxylin-Eosin, in which the cytoplasm of cells are shown in pink and the nucleus in blue. Other staining, which is usually used in the study of biodegradable metals are Masson's Trichrome to distinguish the connective tissue, tartrate resistant acidic phosphatase for osteoclast, Levai-Laczko for bone mineralization detection, periodic acid shift, fluorochrome, and immunofluorescence stain, Quinke reaction, Turnbull blue, and Prussian blue to evaluate iron ions in the tissue [62,68,71,85]. This staining may require long sample preparation until it can finally be observed under the microscope. Fig. 2.11 shows examples of different staining used for iron- and magnesium-based implants.

Overall, the mentioned radiography, μCT, and MRI produce images that are static as the emitted energy takes place in disconnected or segmental time frame [87]. They provide the best imaging but are limited to offline monitoring only. X-ray fluoroscopy and ultrasonography can be developed to become noninvasive online monitoring systems by pairing them with automated image processing software, although long-term imaging procedures may pose a danger from X-ray radiation and from excessive heat generation of high-frequency sound waves [88,89]. Therefore new methods for the online degradation monitoring of biodegradable implants need to be developed.

2.5 Proposed new in vivo monitoring techniques

The previously mentioned radiological imaging techniques have been widely used for the offline monitoring of implant degradation. However, their use for online real-time monitoring is limited due the following factors:

- Continuous or long-term exposure to radiation poses a dangerous effect to living tissue. Imaging thus can only be carried out intermittently and any important changes to implant tissue conditions may be unmonitored.
- The modalities mentioned in previous sections require heavy instrumentation that requires specific handling by specially trained personnel. Their expensive acquisition as well as operational costs make continuous in vivo monitoring of implants not feasible economically. To monitor implant tissue conditions continuously and in vivo, alternative methods, which use low-cost materials and easy to handle operation, are necessary.

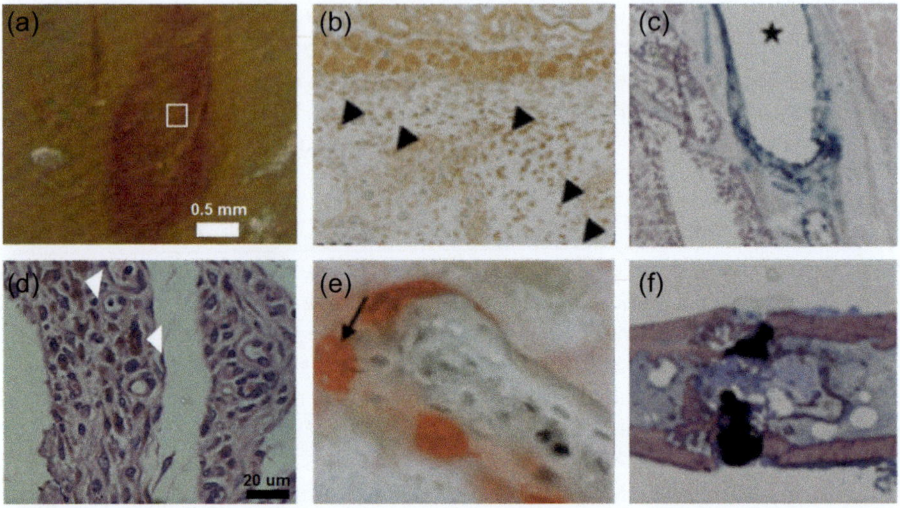

Figure 2.11 Histological images of tissue around a biodegradable metal implant: (a) distribution of degradation products of iron wire in mice skeletal muscle (*rectangle* = implant interface), (b) macrophage-specific F4/80 staining of subcutaneous copper-coated disc implant site in Crl-SKH1-hr mice (*arrow head* = macropages), (c) Quinke reaction staining to detect Fe^{3+}/Fe^{2+} ion at the interface of a Fe-based pin in femoral bone of Sprague–Dawley rats (*star* = implant site), (d) histological analysis at the implant interface of (a) showing degradation products seen as brownish spots (*arrow head*), (e) tartrate resistant acidic phosphatase staining of New Zealand white rabbit's bone implanted with magnesium alloy, (*arrow* = multinucleated osteoclast), (f) Levai-Laczko staining of WZ21 magnesium alloy pin showing the degraded implant in femoral bone of SD rats.
Compiled from Kraus T, Fischerauer SF, Hanzi AC, Uggowitzer PJ, Loffler JF, Weinberg AM. Magnesium alloys for temporary implants in osteosynthesis: in vivo studies of their degradation and interaction with bone. Acta Biomaterialia 2012;8:1230–8; Kraus T, Moszner F, Fischerauer S, Fiedler M, Martinelli E, Eichler J, et al. Biodegradable Fe-based alloys for use in osteosynthesis: outcome of an in vivo study after 52 weeks. Acta Biomaterialia 2014;10:3346–53; Paramitha D, Estuningsih S, Noviana D, Ulum MF, Hermawan H. Distribution of Fe-based degradable materials in mice skeletal muscle. European Cells & Materials 2013;26:1; Ragamouni S, Kumar JM, Mushahary D, Nemani H, Pande G. Histological analysis of cells and matrix mineralization of new bone tissue induced in rabbit femur bones by Mg-Zr based biodegradable implants. Acta Histochemica 2013;115:748–56; and Bartsch I, Willbold E, Yarmolenko S, Witte F. In vivo fluorescence imaging of apoptosis during foreign body response. Biomaterials 2012;33:6926–32.

- The instrumentations used in current in vivo monitoring techniques are not miniaturized, thus the monitoring can only be carried out in a special environment in a clinical platform. Many of the steps that are required to be performed to prepare the monitoring must also be conducted in a specially prepared environment. To do monitoring, the subject who has the implant must be brought to this special environment. The specific place where the implant is located must be prepared, and body fluid must also be sampled using special procedures. Overall, it is not possible to conduct a continuous in vivo monitoring at the original location of the subject who bears the implant, i.e., at the point of care.
- In order to get a clear prognosis on implant tissue interaction, postanalysis is required to understand the raw data obtained in radiology and other imaging modalities techniques.

This postprocessing requires some amount of time. For 3-D μCT the analysis may require a considerable length of time to reconstruct the 3-D model and recognize degradation. Similarly, systemic blood analysis of the implant tissue condition also usually requires a significant amount of time to prepare the samples, e.g., to separate plasma or serum from the whole blood sample. This time factor makes real-time continuous monitoring of implants unfeasible. For continuous in vivo monitoring, new techniques that can be attached to the subject with integrated data processing or sample purification need to be developed.

- Special expertise is usually required to handle and operate the current in vivo monitoring techniques. This is unavoidable since they rely heavily on complex instrumentations or procedures. For continuous point-of-care monitoring however, a new approach with simplified steps and procedures needs to be invented, so that continuous monitoring by the subject who has the implant is made possible.

To be able to conduct real-time online monitoring, different approaches that could overcome the aforementioned limitations should be developed. The proposed new techniques can monitor the degradation process either through monitoring the local changes of the tissue environment surrounding the implantation or through monitoring systemic changes of the body indicated by released ion content or biomarker concentration in blood.

2.5.1 Monitoring local changes surrounding an implantation site

Following the insertion of an implant, local changes manifest around the implantation site caused by the inflammatory reaction as well as by the corrosion process. These changes include chemical content and cell activity, which can be monitored. Examples of chemical changes due to the corrosion of a magnesium implant are the release of Mg^{2+} and OH^- ions, H_2 gas evolution and formation of $Mg(OH)_2$. As mentioned previously, by using an electrochemical sensor, Zhao et al. detected the level of subcutaneous H_2 gas generated from a magnesium implant in rats. The sensor detected H_2 concentration as low as 30 μM and as fast as 30 s, correlated to the degradation rate of the implant [61]. Kapnisis et al. injected fluorescent-labeled donor monocytes as a novel in vivo imaging technique to assess the occurrence of inflammation in a mouse stent implantation model [90]. Differences were found between mice having corroded and noncorroded nitinol stents with respect to the numbers of recruited monocytes and the intensity of the resulting fluorescent signal. Through image analysis, they revealed a subtle increase in matrix metalloproteinase activity in corroded compared with the normal stented aortas. This cell activity observation method seems applicable for monitoring degradation of biodegradable implants.

Another local change that can be monitored is the characteristic of the biodegradable metal implant itself over time. Boutry et al. developed miniaturized wireless operation biodegradable radiofrequency-driven resistor–inductor–capacitor (RLC) resonators made of biodegradable metals (Mg, Mg alloy, Fe, and Fe alloys) and biodegradable conductive polymer composites (polycaprolactone–polypyrrole, polylactide–polypyrrole) [91]. Fig. 2.12 shows the resonator design. The study showed that magnesium alloy is the most promising candidate to fabricate RLC resonators, since it combines high conductivity (high Q), faster degradation rate, and higher mechanical performance [92]. Further analysis seems required to validate the idea and its utilization for monitoring degradation of biodegradable metal implants.

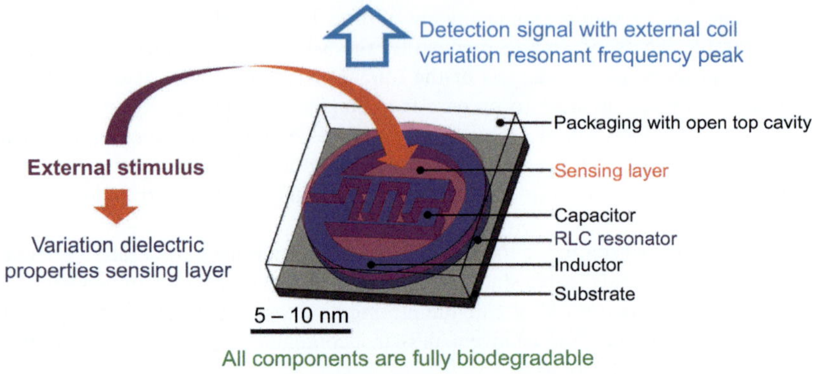

Figure 2.12 Schematic design of a fully biodegradable sensor (wireless telemetry with inductive link).
Adapted from Boutry CM, Chandrahalim H, Streit P, Schinhammer M, Hanzi AC, Hierold C. Towards biodegradable wireless implants. Philosophical Transactions of the Royal Society A: Mathematical Physical and Engineering Sciences 2012;370:2418–32.

Another promising method to monitor degradation via the detection of metal ion release is the utilization of microdialysis. It is a well-established method for continuous monitoring of the targeted substrates both in vitro and in vivo. Schumacher et al. used microdialysis to investigate the reaction interface between pure magnesium and tissue in an isolated perfused bovine udder model and examined its biocompatibility using PGE_2 and TNF-α, which served as indicators of inflammation [93]. Although their work has managed to elucidate the in vivo behavior of the implant, the results were not measured in real time. Another work by Ulrich et al. used microflow capillary, which is online-coupled via a flow injection analyzing system to an ICP-MS setup with an electrochemical control to investigate the corrosion behavior of magnesium alloys [94]. However, the generated hydrogen bubbles were suspected to prevent sufficient mixing in the circulating solution within the capillary and thus may lead to inaccurate results.

As an in situ sampling tool, we used microdialysis to collect local extracellular fluid surrounding an implantation site in vivo. The fluid was collected every 6 h after a subcutaneous implantation of pure iron and magnesium pins on NZW rabbits (Fig. 2.13). The microdialysis probe was inserted subcutaneously parallel to the implant, the NaCl 0.9% solution was injected into the microdialysis inlet, and the effluent from the outlet was collected for ion analysis. The microdialysate samples were then simply analyzed by using an AAS for iron and magnesium ion concentration. A more advanced study was done by coupling the microdialysis with an electrochemical enzymatic biosensor based on the requirement of magnesium ions during kinase enzymatic reactions, which provides the required selectivity to the technique [95]. The system can detect magnesium ions in a range from 5 to 1000 μM with a sensitivity of 0.001 μA/μM and limit of detection at 10.16 μM, which shows a capability of detecting magnesium ion concentration in blood serum. However, further studies are necessary to translate the system for in vivo monitoring of biodegradable metal implants.

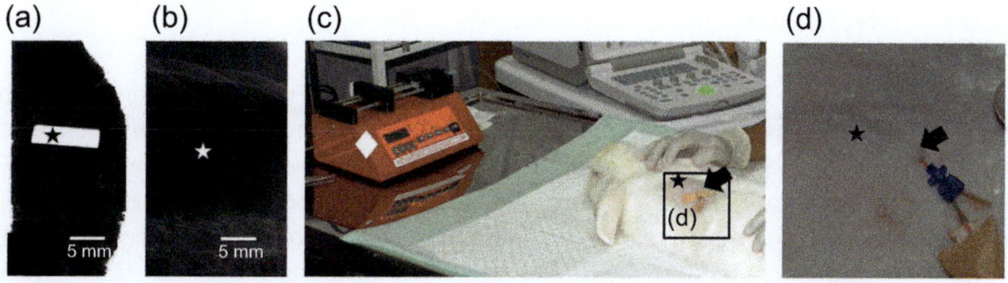

Figure 2.13 Microdialysis system for in situ sampling of metal ions: (a, b) radiogram of iron and magnesium implants, (c) microdialysis probe insertion into a rabbit, (d) highlight on the probe. *Star*, implant; *arrow*, microdialysis probe.

2.5.2 Monitoring systemic changes in body fluid

The interactions between biodegradable metals with the local tissue induce biological responses, e.g., local cell proliferation and systemic cellular migration to a local implantation site, as illustrated in Fig. 2.3. Cellular differentiation and proliferation was considered by specific biochemical substrates that utilized the specific cells for each body event during cellular communication. The form of biochemical substrates that are used for cell communication include growth factors, hormones, and other specific substrates that are released in the extracellular fluid [96,97]. These substrates could be analyzed and also can be used as biomarkers in order to monitor the progression of degradation.

Body fluids are a potential source of many biomarkers that can be collected from living animals in many ways, both noninvasive (i.e., sweat, saliva, milk, and urine) and invasive (i.e., blood, cerebrospinal fluid). Some biomarkers are currently assessed by using immunoassay based analysis such as enzyme immunoassay, enzyme-linked immunosorbent assay, and radio immunoassay. Implantation of different types of biomaterials shows a different trend of growth factors that are released from the microenvironment. For example, osteoblast cells release transforming growth factor-β1 (TGF-β1) in higher concentration after in contact with acrylic bone cement compared to bioinert metallic-based biomaterials such as titanium and cobalt chromium [98,99]. This kind of biomarker has the potential to be utilized as a marker for monitoring the degradation of biodegradable metal implants with specific molecular biological responses after insertion in the body.

2.5.3 Off-clinic point-of-care implant monitoring

Point-of-care diagnostics using the microfluidic system have been introduced in order to speed up the diagnosis process on the site of assessment [100]. A microfluidic technology is considered as a simple, compact (integrated system), rapid, specific, sensitive, and low-cost analytical device with the microvolume of samples provided from invasive or noninvasive procedures. In a point-of-care system, patients can monitor their health status using a simple diagnostic tool, such as a portable blood glucose monitoring device. The patients can directly collect their blood samples using a lancet, and the device will measure the glucose level. The same colorimetric-based principle may also be applicable for monitoring metal ions released from a biodegradable metal implant.

2.6 Conclusion

An ideal implant made of biodegradable metals must fit its degradation kinetics within the window of the tissue-healing period. One of the challenges to fulfill this ideal requirement is to obtain comprehensive data of in vivo degradation behavior as the valid input for optimum material design process. The implant degradation product formation and metal ion release has to be monitored. Current techniques that are used for this purpose include radiography, ultrasonography, μCT, MRI, and blood and histological analysis. Radiography and ultrasonography can provide quantitative degradation measurement and are accessible in most medical facilities. The μCT and MRI provide higher resolution imaging for small implants but at a higher cost and low accessibility compared to radiography and ultrasonography. Analysis of metal ion concentration in the blood over time is considerably easy and an inexpensive way to give indirect indication of degradation. Meanwhile, histological analysis is an invasive way to get direct evidence of degradation, complete history of healing stage, and distribution of the degradation product surrounding the implantation site. Among the proposed new techniques that allow real-time or online monitoring of degradation and metal ions in vivo are biosensors that detect local changes, such as hydrogen evolution and dimensional changes of the implant, and microdialysis that samples fluid around the implant for further detection by mass spectroscopy. Online monitoring can also be applied to systemic changes by utilizing biomarkers sensitive to homeostasis changes caused by the implant degradation event. Another proposed technique is related to off-clinic point of care diagnostics using a microfluidic system to speed up the diagnosis process on the site of assessment. Learning from minimally invasive devices such as blood glucose monitors, this system may be applicable for the indirect monitoring of later routinely used biodegradable metal implants.

Acknowledgments

The authors acknowledge the financial support from the Canadian Natural Sciences and Engineering Research Council (NSERC), the Indonesian Ministry of Research, Technology, and Higher Education (RISTEKDIKTI), and the Malaysian Ministry of Higher Education (MOHE). This work is part of an international research collaboration between Laval University, Canada, Bogor Agricultural University, Indonesia and Universiti Teknologi Malaysia, Malaysia.

References

[1] Hench LL, Thompson I. Twenty-first century challenges for biomaterials. Journal of The Royal Society Interface 2010;7:S379–91.

[2] Brody H. Outlook on biomaterials. Nature 2015;519:S1–19.

[3] O'Brien FJ. Biomaterials & scaffolds for tissue engineering. Materials Today 2011;14: 88–95.

[4] Niinomi M, Nakai M, Hieda J. Development of new metallic alloys for biomedical applications. Acta Biomaterialia 2012;8:3888–903.

[5] Yun Y, Dong Z, Lee N, Liu Y, Xue D, Guo X, et al. Revolutionizing biodegradable metals. Materials Today 2009;12:22–32.

[6] Hermawan H. Biodegradable metals: from concept to applications. Heidelberg: Springer; 2012.

[7] Zheng YF, Gu XN, Witte F. Biodegradable metals. Materials Science and Engineering R: Reports 2014;77:1–34.

[8] ASTM. ASTM WK52640: new guide for in-vitro degradation testing of absorbable metals, West Conshohocken. ASTM International 2016.

[9] Seiler HG, Sigel H, Sigel A. Handbook on toxicity of inorganic compounds. New York: Mercel Dekker; 1988.

[10] Fontcave M, Pierre JL. Iron: metabolism, toxicity and therapy. Biochimie 1993;73:767–73.

[11] Francis A, Yang Y, Virtanen S, Boccaccini A. Iron and iron-based alloys for temporary cardiovascular applications. Journal of Materials Science: Materials in Medicine 2015;26:1–16.

[12] Drynda A, Hassel T, Bach FW, Peuster M. In vitro and in vivo corrosion properties of new iron-manganese alloys designed for cardiovascular applications. Journal of Biomedical Materials Research Part B: Applied Biomaterials 2015;103:649–60.

[13] Yusop AH, Daud NM, Nur H, Kadir MRA, Hermawan H. Controlling the degradation kinetics of porous iron by poly(lactic-co-glycolic acid) infiltration for use as temporary medical implants. Scientific Reports 2015;5:11194.

[14] Schinhammer M, Hänzi AC, Löffler JF, Uggowitzer PJ. Design strategy for biodegradable Fe-based alloys for medical applications. Acta Biomaterialia 2010;6:1705–13.

[15] Huang T, Cheng Y, Zheng Y. In vitro studies on silver implanted pure iron by metal vapor vacuum arc technique. Colloids and Surfaces B: Biointerfaces 2016;142:20–9.

[16] Cheng J, Huang T, Zheng YF. Microstructure, mechanical property, biodegradation behavior, and biocompatibility of biodegradable Fe–Fe_2O_3 composites. Journal of Biomedical Materials Research Part A 2014;102:2277–87.

[17] Ulum MF, Arafat A, Noviana D, Yusop AH, Nasution AK, Abdul Kadir MR, et al. In vitro and in vivo degradation evaluation of novel iron-bioceramic composites for bone implant applications. Materials Science and Engineering: C 2014;36:336–44.

[18] Čapek J, Vojtěch D. Microstructural and mechanical characteristics of porous iron prepared by powder metallurgy. Materials Science and Engineering: C 2014;43:494–501.

[19] Daud NM, Sing NB, Yusop AH, Majid FAA, Hermawan H. Degradation and in vitro cell–material interaction studies on hydroxyapatite-coated biodegradable porous iron for hard tissue scaffolds. Journal of Orthopaedic Translation 2014;2:177–84.

[20] Heiden M, Johnson D, Stanciu L. Surface modifications through dealloying of Fe–Mn and Fe–Mn–Zn alloys developed to create tailorable, nanoporous, bioresorbable surfaces. Acta Materialia 2016;103:115–27.

[21] Saris N-EL, Mervaala E, Karppanen H, Khawaja JA, Lewenstam A. Magnesium: an update on physiological, clinical and analytical aspects. Clinica Chimica Acta 2000;294:1–26.

[22] Vormann J. Magnesium: nutrition and metabolism. Molecular Aspects of Medicine 2003;24:27–37.

[23] Staiger MP, Pietak AM, Huadmai J, Dias G. Magnesium and its alloys as orthopedic biomaterials: a review. Biomaterials 2006;27:1728–34.

[24] Chen Y, Xu Z, Smith C, Sankar J. Recent advances on the development of magnesium alloys for biodegradable implants. Acta Biomaterialia 2014;10:4561–73.

[25] Noviana D, Paramitha D, Ulum MF, Hermawan H. The effect of hydrogen gas evolution of magnesium implant on the postimplantation mortality of rats. Journal of Orthopaedic Translation 2016;5:9–15.
[26] Qiao Z, Shi Z, Hort N, Zainal Abidin NI, Atrens A. Corrosion behaviour of a nominally high purity Mg ingot produced by permanent mould direct chill casting. Corrosion Science 2012;61:185–207.
[27] Wan Y, Xiong G, Luo H, He F, Huang Y, Zhou X. Preparation and characterization of a new biomedical magnesium–calcium alloy. Materials & Design 2008;29:2034–7.
[28] Zhang S, Zhang X, Zhao C, Li J, Song Y, Xie C, et al. Research on an Mg–Zn alloy as a degradable biomaterial. Acta Biomaterialia 2010;6:626–40.
[29] Hort N, Huang Y, Fechner D, Störmer M, Blawert C, Witte F, et al. Magnesium alloys as implant materials – principles of property design for Mg–RE alloys. Acta Biomaterialia 2010;6:1714–25.
[30] Zberg B, Uggowitzer PJ, Loffler JF. MgZnCa glasses without clinically observable hydrogen evolution for biodegradable implants. Nature Materials 2009;8:887–91.
[31] Zhang Y, Zhang G, Wei M. Controlling the biodegradation rate of magnesium using biomimetic apatite coating. Journal of Biomedical Materials Research Part B: Applied Biomaterials 2009;89B:408–14.
[32] Wong HM, Yeung KWK, Lam KO, Tam V, Chu PK, Luk KDK, et al. A biodegradable polymer-based coating to control the performance of magnesium alloy orthopaedic implants. Biomaterials 2010;31:2084–96.
[33] McCall KA, Huang C-c, Fierke CA. Function and mechanism of zinc metalloenzymes. The Journal of nutrition 2000;130:1437S–46S.
[34] Fosmire GJ. Zinc toxicity. The American Journal of Clinical Nutrition 1990;51:225–7.
[35] Murni NS, Dambatta MS, Yeap SK, Froemming GRA, Hermawan H. Cytotoxicity evaluation of biodegradable Zn–3Mg alloy toward normal human osteoblast cells. Materials Science and Engineering: C 2015;49:560–6.
[36] Shearier ER, Bowen PK, He W, Drelich A, Drelich J, Goldman J, et al. In vitro cytotoxicity, adhesion, and proliferation of human vascular cells exposed to zinc. ACS Biomaterials Science & Engineering 2016;2:634–42.
[37] Vojtech D, Kubasek J, Serak J, Novak P. Mechanical and corrosion properties of newly developed biodegradable Zn-based alloys for bone fixation. Acta Biomaterialia 2011;7:3515–22.
[38] Kubásek J, Vojtěch D, Jablonská E, Pospíšilová I, Lipov J, Ruml T. Structure, mechanical characteristics and in vitro degradation, cytotoxicity, genotoxicity and mutagenicity of novel biodegradable Zn–Mg alloys. Materials Science and Engineering: C 2016;58:24–35.
[39] Mostaed E, Sikora-Jasinska M, Mostaed A, Loffredo S, Demir AG, Previtali B, et al. Novel Zn-based alloys for biodegradable stent applications: design, development and in vitro degradation. Journal of the Mechanical Behavior of Biomedical Materials 2016;60:581–602.
[40] Endo A, Hirayama H, Yoshida O, Arakawa T, Akima T, Yamada T, et al. Arterial remodeling influences the development of intimal hyperplasia after stent implantation. Journal of the American College of Cardiology 2001;37:70–5.
[41] Ahmad K, Katballe N, Pilegaard H. Fixation of sternal fracture using absorbable plating system, three years follow-up. Journal of Thoracic Disease 2015;7:E131–4.
[42] Salter RB. Textbook of disorders and injuries of the musculoskeletal system: an introduction to orthopaedics, fractures, and joint injuries, rheumatology, metabolic bone disease, and rehabilitation. Lippincott Williams & Wilkins; 1999.

[43] Ito K, Perren SM. Biology of fracture healing. AO principles of fracture management. AO Foundation; 2016.

[44] Pasterkamp G, de Kleijn DPV, Borst C. Arterial remodeling in atherosclerosis, restenosis and after alteration of blood flow: potential mechanisms and clinical implications. Cardiovascular Research 2000;45:843–52.

[45] Schwartz Md RS. Pathophysiology of restenosis: interaction of thrombosis, hyperplasia, and/or remodeling. The American Journal of Cardiology 1998;81:14E–7E.

[46] Kim YK, Chen EY, Liu WF. Biomolecular strategies to modulate the macrophage response to implanted materials. Journal of Materials Chemistry B 2016;4:1600–9.

[47] Yu T, Tutwiler VJ, Spiller K. The role of macrophages in the foreign body response to implanted biomaterials. Biomaterials in regenerative medicine and the immune system. Springer; 2015. p. 17–34.

[48] Witte F, Eliezer A. Biodegradable metals. In: Eliaz N, editor. Degradation of implant materials. New York, NY: Springer; 2012. p. 93–109.

[49] Xin Y, Huo K, Tao H, Tang G, Chu PK. Influence of aggressive ions on the degradation behavior of biomedical magnesium alloy in physiological environment. Acta Biomaterialia 2008;4:2008–15.

[50] Yamamoto A, Hiromoto S. Effect of inorganic salts, amino acids and proteins on the degradation of pure magnesium in vitro. Materials Science and Engineering: C 2009;29:1559–68.

[51] Xu L, Zhu S, Huang N, Li X, Zhang Y. The corrosion of pure iron in five different mediums. Sheng wu yi xue gong cheng xue za zhi = Journal of Biomedical Engineering = Shengwu yixue gongchengxue zazhi 2009;26:783–6.

[52] Liu C, Xin Y, Tian X, Chu PK. Degradation susceptibility of surgical magnesium alloy in artificial biological fluid containing albumin. Journal of Materials Research 2007;22:1806–14.

[53] Fossum TW. Small animal surgery textbook. Elsevier Health Sciences; 2013.

[54] Noviana D, Estuningsih S, Ulum MF. Animal study and pre-clinical trials of biomaterials. In: Mahyudin F, Hermawan H, editors. Biomaterials and medical devices: a perspective from an emerging country. Cham: Springer International Publishing; 2016. p. 67–101.

[55] Ulum MF, Nasution AK, Yusop AH, Arafat A, Kadir MRA, Juniantito V, et al. Evidences of in vivo bioactivity of Fe-bioceramic composites for temporary bone implants. Journal of Biomedical Materials Research Part B: Applied Biomaterials 2015;103:1354–65.

[56] Schiopu D, Girard J, Soenen M, Krantz N, Migaud H. Metal ions levels measurements for early total hip replacement malfunction diagnosis with "plasma-sprayed ceramic" bearings couple. Orthopaedics & Traumatology, Surgery & Research: OTSR 2010;96:75–9.

[57] Chow J, Tobias J, Colston K, Chambers T. Estrogen maintains trabecular bone volume in rats not only by suppression of bone resorption but also by stimulation of bone formation. Journal of Clinical Investigation 1992;89:74.

[58] Seifert-Klauss V, Prior JC. Progesterone and bone: actions promoting bone health in women. Journal of Osteoporosis 2010:2010.

[59] Vanderschueren D, Sinnesael M, Gielen E, Claessens F, Boonen S. Testosterone and bone. Testosterone: Action, Deficiency, Substitution 2012:177.

[60] Fischerauer S, Kraus T, Wu X, Tangl S, Sorantin E, Hänzi A, et al. In vivo degradation performance of micro-arc-oxidized magnesium implants: a micro-CT study in rats. Acta Biomaterialia 2013;9:5411–20.

[61] Zhao D, Wang T, Guo X, Kuhlmann J, Doepke A, Dong Z, et al. Monitoring biodegradation of magnesium implants with sensors. JOM 2016;68:1204–8.

[62] Schaller B, Saulacic N, Imwinkelried T, Beck S, Liu EW, Gralla J, et al. In vivo degradation of magnesium plate/screw osteosynthesis implant systems: soft and hard tissue response in a calvarial model in miniature pigs. Journal of Craniomaxillofacial Surgery 2016;44:309–17.
[63] Hou L, Li Z, Pan Y, Du L, Li X, Zheng Y, et al. In vitro and in vivo studies on biodegradable magnesium alloy. Progress in Natural Science: Materials International 2014;24:466–71.
[64] Kraus T, Fischerauer SF, Hanzi AC, Uggowitzer PJ, Loffler JF, Weinberg AM. Magnesium alloys for temporary implants in osteosynthesis: in vivo studies of their degradation and interaction with bone. Acta Biomaterialia 2012;8:1230–8.
[65] Dziuba D, Meyer-Lindenberg A, Seitz JM, Waizy H, Angrisani N, Reifenrath J. Long-term in vivo degradation behaviour and biocompatibility of the magnesium alloy ZEK100 for use as a biodegradable bone implant. Acta Biomaterialia 2013;9:8548–60.
[66] Li HF, Xie XH, Zhao K, Wang YB, Zheng YF, Wang WH, et al. In vitro and in vivo studies on biodegradable CaMgZnSrYb high-entropy bulk metallic glass. Acta Biomaterialia 2013;9:8561–73.
[67] Bobe K, Willbold E, Morgenthal I, Andersen O, Studnitzky T, Nellesen J, et al. In vitro and in vivo evaluation of biodegradable, open-porous scaffolds made of sintered magnesium W4 short fibres. Acta Biomaterialia 2013;9:8611–23.
[68] Trincă LC, Fântânariu M, Solcan C, Trofin AE, Burtan L, Acatrinei DM, et al. In vivo degradation behavior and biological activity of some new Mg–Ca alloys with concentration's gradient of Si for bone grafts. Applied Surface Science 2015;352:140–50.
[69] Han J, Wan P, Ge Y, Fan X, Tan L, Li J, et al. Tailoring the degradation and biological response of a magnesium-strontium alloy for potential bone substitute application. Materials Science and Engineering C: Materials for Biological Applications 2016;58:799–811.
[70] Diekmann J, Bauer S, Weizbauer A, Willbold E, Windhagen H, Helmecke P, et al. Examination of a biodegradable magnesium screw for the reconstruction of the anterior cruciate ligament: a pilot in vivo study in rabbits. Materials Science and Engineering C: Materials for Biological Applications 2016;59:1100–9.
[71] Kraus T, Moszner F, Fischerauer S, Fiedler M, Martinelli E, Eichler J, et al. Biodegradable Fe-based alloys for use in osteosynthesis: outcome of an in vivo study after 52 weeks. Acta Biomaterialia 2014;10:3346–53.
[72] Lin WJ, Zhang DY, Zhang G, Sun HT, Qi HP, Chen LP, et al. Design and characterization of a novel biocorrodible iron-based drug-eluting coronary scaffold. Materials & Design 2016;91:72–9.
[73] Mueller PP, Arnold S, Badar M, Bormann D, Bach FW, Drynda A, et al. Histological and molecular evaluation of iron as degradable medical implant material in a murine animal model. Journal of Biomedical Materials Research Part A 2012;100:2881–9.
[74] Pierson D, Edick J, Tauscher A, Pokorney E, Bowen P, Gelbaugh J, et al. A simplified in vivo approach for evaluating the bioabsorbable behavior of candidate stent materials. Journal of Biomedical Materials Research Part B: Applied Biomaterials 2012;100:58–67.
[75] Paramitha D, Estuningsih S, Noviana D, Ulum MF, Hermawan H. Distribution of Fe-based degradable materials in mice skeletal muscle. European Cells & Materials 2013;26:S1.
[76] Bowen PK, Drelich J, Goldman J. Zinc exhibits ideal physiological corrosion behavior for bioabsorbable stents. Advanced Materials 2013;25:2577–82.
[77] Bowen PK, Guillory 2nd RJ, Shearier ER, Seitz JM, Drelich J, Bocks M, et al. Metallic zinc exhibits optimal biocompatibility for bioabsorbable endovascular stents. Materials Science and Engineering C: Materials for Biological Applications 2015;56:467–72.

[78] Noviana D, Nasution AK, Ulum MF, Hermawan H. Monitoring of early biodegradation of Fe-bioceramic composites by B-mode ultrasonography imaging in sheep animal model. European Cells & Materials 2013;26:S57.

[79] Mattoon JS, Nyland TG. Small animal diagnostic ultrasound. Elsevier Health Sciences; 2014.

[80] Boerckel JD, Mason DE, McDermott AM, Alsberg E. Microcomputed tomography: approaches and applications in bioengineering. Stem Cell Research & Therapy 2014;5:144.

[81] Larrue A, Rattner A, Peter ZA, Olivier C, Laroche N, Vico L, et al. Synchrotron radiation micro-CT at the micrometer scale for the analysis of the three-dimensional morphology of microcracks in human trabecular bone. PLoS One 2011;6:e21297.

[82] Witte F, Fischer J, Nellesen J, Crostack HA, Kaese V, Pisch A, et al. In vitro and in vivo corrosion measurements of magnesium alloys. Biomaterials 2006;27:1013–8.

[83] Koch KM, Hargreaves BA, Pauly KB, Chen W, Gold GE, King KF. Magnetic resonance imaging near metal implants. Journal of Magnetic Resonance Imaging 2010;32:773–87.

[84] Matusiewicz H. Potential release of in vivo trace metals from metallic medical implants in the human body: from ions to nanoparticles – a systematic analytical review. Acta Biomaterialia 2014;10:2379–403.

[85] Ragamouni S, Kumar JM, Mushahary D, Nemani H, Pande G. Histological analysis of cells and matrix mineralization of new bone tissue induced in rabbit femur bones by Mg-Zr based biodegradable implants. Acta Histochemica 2013;115:748–56.

[86] Bartsch I, Willbold E, Yarmolenko S, Witte F. In vivo fluorescence imaging of apoptosis during foreign body response. Biomaterials 2012;33:6926–32.

[87] Thrall DE. Textbook of veterinary diagnostic radiology. Elsevier Health Sciences; 2013.

[88] Fazel R, Krumholz HM, Wang Y, Ross JS, Chen J, Ting HH, et al. Exposure to low-dose ionizing radiation from medical imaging procedures. New England Journal of Medicine 2009;361:849–57.

[89] Liu Y, Herman BA, Soneson JE, Harris GR. Thermal safety simulations of transient temperature rise during acoustic radiation force-based ultrasound elastography. Ultrasound in Medicine & Biology 2014;40:1001–14.

[90] Kapnisis KK, Pitsillides CM, Prokopi MS, Lapathitis G, Karaiskos C, Eleftheriou PC, et al. In vivo monitoring of the inflammatory response in a stented mouse aorta model. Journal of Biomedical Materials Research Part A 2016;104:227–38.

[91] Boutry CM, Chandrahalim H, Streit P, Schinhammer M, Hanzi AC, Hierold C. Towards biodegradable wireless implants. Philosophical Transactions of the Royal Society A: Mathematical Physical and Engineering Sciences 2012;370:2418–32.

[92] Boutry CM, Chandrahalim H, Streit P, Schinhammer M, Hänzi AC, Hierold C. Characterization of miniaturized RLC resonators made of biodegradable materials for wireless implant applications. Sensors and Actuators A: Physical 2013;189:344–55.

[93] Schumacher S, Stahl J, Baumer W, Seitz JM, Bach FW, Petersen LJ, et al. Ex vivo examination of the biocompatibility of biodegradable magnesium via microdialysis in the isolated perfused bovine udder model. International Journal of Artificial Organs 2011;34:34–43.

[94] Ulrich A, Ott N, Tournier-Fillon A, Homazava N, Schmutz P. Investigation of corrosion behavior of biodegradable magnesium alloys using an online-micro-flow capillary flow injection inductively coupled plasma mass spectrometry setup with electrochemical control. Spectrochimica Acta – Part B Atomic Spectroscopy 2011;66:536–45.

[95] Natasha S, Malon R, Wicaksono D, Córcoles E, Hermawan H. Electrochemical detection of magnesium ions using magnesium biosensor. European Cells and Materials 2013;26:S27.

[96] Frosch K-H, Stürmer KM. Metallic biomaterials in skeletal repair. European Journal of Trauma 2006;32:149–59.
[97] Peichl P, Holzer LA, Maier R, Holzer G. Parathyroid hormone 1–84 accelerates fracture-healing in pubic bones of elderly osteoporotic women. Journal of Bone and Joint Surgery. American Volume 2011;93:1583–7.
[98] Jehle PM, Schulten K, Schulz W, Jehle DR, Stracke S, Manfras B, et al. Serum levels of insulin-like growth factor (IGF)-I and IGF binding protein (IGFBP)-1 to -6 and their relationship to bone metabolism in osteoporosis patients. European Journal of Internal Medicine 2003;14:32–8.
[99] Good DM, Thongboonkerd V, Novak J, Bascands J-L, Schanstra JP, Coon JJ, et al. Body fluid proteomics for biomarker discovery: lessons from the past hold the key to success in the future. Journal of Proteome Research 2007;6:4549–55.
[100] Herr AE, Hatch AV, Throckmorton DJ, Tran HM, Brennan JS, Giannobile WV, et al. Microfluidic immunoassays as rapid saliva-based clinical diagnostics. Proceedings of the National Academy of Sciences 2007;104:5268–73.

Part two

Monitoring and evaluation of the biological response to biomaterials in vivo

Imaging biomaterial-associated inflammation

3

S. Selvam
Sree Chitra Tirunal Institute for Medical Sciences and Technology, Thiruvananthapuram, Kerala, India

3.1 Introduction

Tens of millions of people across the world live with implanted medical devices, with an estimated 25 million people living in the United States alone (Hanna et al., 2001). Furthermore, the US demand for such devices is estimated to grow 7.7% annually to $52 billion in 2015 (The Freedonia Group, 2012). These implantable medical devices primarily include reconstructive joint replacements, cardiac pacemakers, defibrillators, stents, valves, electrical leads/batteries, tissue-engineered constructs, and drug delivery systems (Domb and Khan, 2014). Although most implanted devices function optimally for years, implantation of biomaterials in general elicits a strong host inflammatory response that severely affects long-term performance and lifetime of the device in vivo (Anderson et al., 2008). Moreover, implant-associated inflammation is assessed using conventional histological methods and biochemical assays, which are all end-point measurements that involve repeated invasive surgical procedures for obtaining tissue biopsies for analysis. In addition, these methods are labor-intensive, time-consuming, and cost-prohibitive, which seriously affect the quality of lives of millions of patients each year. Furthermore, from a clinical perspective, conventional methods also deter noninvasive longitudinal monitoring of biomaterial-associated inflammation due to its inherent tissue-destructive characteristics. Hence, there is a compelling need for developing strategies to noninvasively monitor implant-associated aseptic inflammation. Such methodologies will allow for a simple, fast, reliable, accurate, and real-time assessment of device-related inflammation, which is crucial for initiating anti-inflammatory therapies to modulate the inflammatory response in a clinical scenario. This chapter reviews the different preclinical imaging modalities that are currently being explored for monitoring and assessing implant-associated inflammation in vivo.

3.2 Near-infrared fluorescence imaging

Near-infrared fluorescence (NIRF) imaging is an emerging technology that uses light in the NIR region, typically between 700–900 nm, for deep tissue imaging (Aswathy et al., 2010). This "optical window" offers several centimeters of tissue penetration with minimal autofluorescence interference that is inherent to biological tissues (Frangioni, 2003). Moreover, this technique possesses high sensitivity, less scatter,

Monitoring and Evaluation of Biomaterials and their Performance in vivo. http://dx.doi.org/10.1016/B978-0-08-100603-0.00003-1

and high optical contrast, all of which are obvious advantageous for the noninvasive real-time imaging of deep tissues in vivo (Frangioni, 2003). To this end, numerous fluorescent imaging probes have been designed and developed, and they are commercially available for clinical applications such as vascular mapping, cancer imaging, medical diagnostics, and image-guided surgery (Frangioni, 2003; Kobayashi et al., 2010; Gibbs, 2012). In addition, NIRF imaging offers three-dimensional (3-D) image reconstruction, whose spatial resolution can be augmented with higher resolution modalities such as magnetic resonance imaging (MRI) and X-ray computed tomography (CT) through multimodal imaging (Talanov et al., 2006; Guo et al., 2010). Furthermore, as this imaging modality is compatible with existing fluorescence imaging instrumentations, it is cost-effective and requires minimal infrastructural investment or regulatory compliance. Due to the aforementioned considerations, NIRF imaging has been exploited for noninvasive real-time imaging of aseptic inflammation around implanted devices and can be classified into the following three groups.

3.2.1 Inflammatory cell imaging

Implantation of a biomaterial elicits a dynamic foreign body reaction (FBR) at the implant site (Anderson et al., 2008). The recruitment of macrophages and neutrophils at the implant site is the hallmark of host inflammatory responses to implanted biomaterials (Anderson et al., 2008). Activated macrophages and neutrophils are widely implicated in the degradation of polymeric implants, which subsequently leads to increased fibrotic reactions, tissue damage, and delayed tissue regeneration (Hoemann et al., 2010). Evidently, the number of recruited macrophages and neutrophils at an implant site directly relates to the severity of implant-associated inflammation (Anderson et al., 2008). Consequently, direct imaging of these inflammatory cells around implanted biomaterials presents a clear and viable option to noninvasively assess the degree of biomaterial-associated inflammation. To this end, targeted cell imaging of activated macrophages and neutrophils near the vicinity of an implant via receptor-targeting NIR nanoprobes (NIR NPRs) has been successfully employed.

It is well established that activated monocytes/macrophages overexpress the folate receptor (FR) (Turk et al., 2004; Puig-Kroger et al., 2009). Interestingly, an FR-targeting fluorescein isothiocyanate (FITC)-conjugated macrophage antibody was used to evaluate the extent of FBR to implanted biomaterials in vivo (Bratlie et al., 2010). However, low tissue penetration and high autofluorescence limits the use of FITC-conjugated probes for optical imaging applications in vivo. Polymer nanoparticles encapsulated with NIR dye were synthesized and conjugated with folate peptides (Zhou et al., 2011). IR750 dye encapsulated poly(N-isopropyl acrylamide-co-styrene) nanoparticles (PNIPAM-co-St NPs) with an average diameter of 100 nm, and emission wavelength of 760 nm was synthesized by emulsion polymerization. Folate peptides were conjugated to the dye entrapped PNIPAM-co-St NPs using carbodiimide-coupling protocols. The FR-targeting NIR PNIPAM-co-St NPs demonstrated a high affinity for lipopolysaccharide (LPS)-activated macrophages with fluorescence intensities, correlating linearly with a number of activated macrophages in vitro (Fig. 3.1(a) and (b)). Furthermore, FR-targeting NIR PNIPAM-co-St NPs were able to quantify FBR around

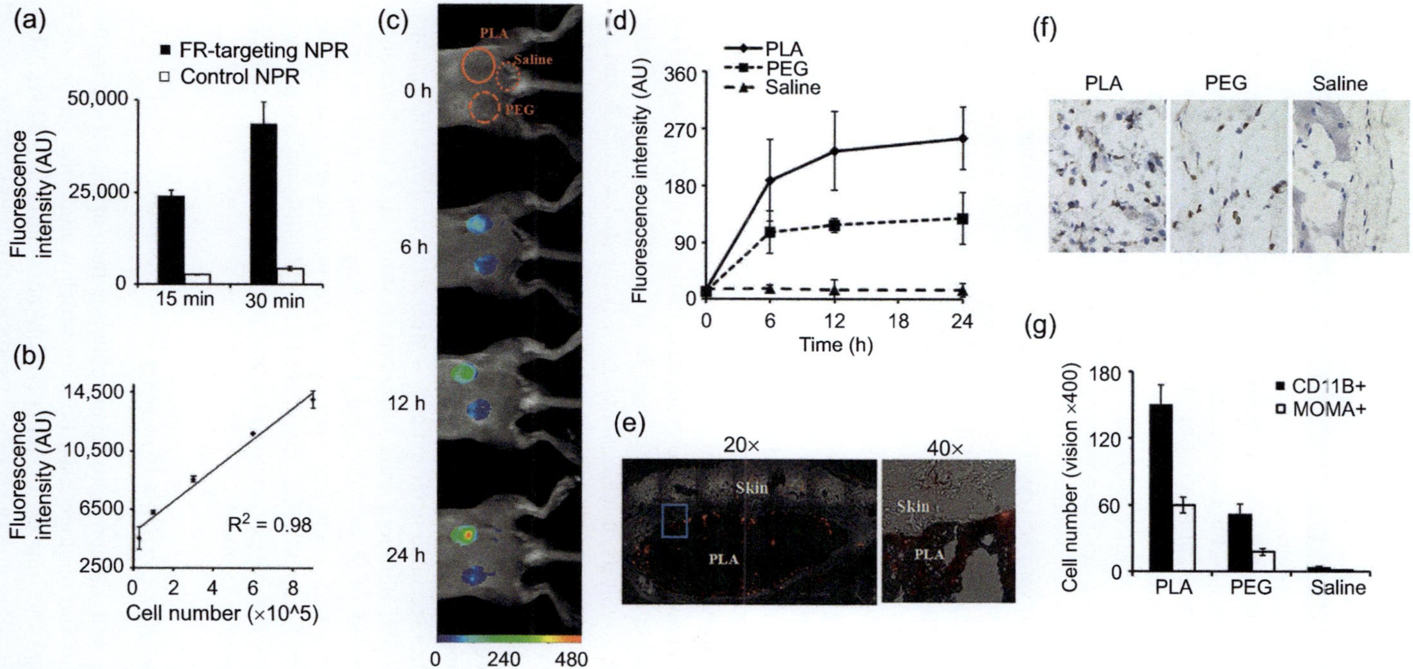

Figure 3.1 Near-infrared fluorescence (NIRF) imaging of activated macrophages around injected biomaterials using poly(N-isopropyl acrylamide-co-styrene) nanoparticles. (a) Effect of incubation time on the accumulation of folate receptor (FR)–targeting and control nanoparticles (NPs) onto lipopolysaccharide (LPS)-activated macrophages in vitro. (b) Correlation between LPS-activated macrophage number and NP fluorescence intensity in vitro. (c) Representative image of the bioimaging data obtained from live animals following intravenous administration of FR-targeting NPs in poly(L-lactic acid) (PLA), saline, and polyethylene glycol (PEG)–injected groups at different time points. (d) Fluorescence intensities from tissues surrounding PLA, PEG, and saline injection sites at different time points (mean ± standard error (SE), n = 4). (e) NIRF signals (red) acquired from unstained and unfixed tissue sections at 20× and 40× magnification. (f) Representative histological tissue sections. (g) Quantification of CD11B+ inflammatory cells and monocytes/macrophages (MOMA+) in tissues surrounding PLA, PEG, and saline-injected sites (mean ± SE, n = 4).

subcutaneously injected poly(L-lactic acid) (PLA) and polyethylene glycol (PEG) particle implants in the dorsal regions of mice. Of note, PLA and PEG were chosen as model materials for their ability to elicit mild and weak inflammatory responses, respectively (Weng et al., 2004; Ruan and Feng, 2003). Bioimaging results showed that fluorescence intensities at PLA-injected sites were consistently higher than PEG sites, while saline-injected controls had low or no fluorescence during the same time points (Fig. 3.1(c) and (d)). In addition, fluorescent images of unstained and unfixed tissue sections confirmed significant accumulation of FR-targeting NIR PNIPAM-co-St NPs surrounding PLA sites compared to normal tissue (Fig. 3.1(e)). Immunohistological analysis also revealed that PLA microparticles recruited three times higher CD11B+ inflammatory cells and monocytes/macrophages (MOMA+) compared to PEG NPs (Fig. 3.1(f) and (g)). Overall, the synthesized FR-targeting NIR PNIPAM-co-St NPs demonstrated high affinity toward activated macrophages and shows great promise for detecting inflammatory responses to subcutaneously implanted biomaterials.

A similar strategy was employed to target neutrophils at the site of FBR (Zhou et al., 2012a). The peptide, cinnamoyl-Phe-(D)Leu-Phe-(D)Leu-Phe (cFLFLF), has been shown to have a high affinity to formyl peptide receptors (FPR) of activated neutrophils (Locke et al., 2009). This peptide was conjugated to an Oyster 800 (O800) dye-incorporated, eight-arm PEG amine through carbodiimide-coupling reaction. Characterization studies showed that the FPR-targeting PEG-O800 NPR had an absorbance peak at 280 nm, corresponding to that of cFLFLF peptide and a fluorescence spectral emission at 800 nm, matching that of free Oyster 800 dye. In vitro studies showed that PEG-O800-cFLFLF NPRs were specific to activated neutrophils with fluorescence intensities in direct correlation with neutrophil numbers. Next, to evaluate the ability of PEG-O800-cFLFLF NPRs to detect localized inflammatory responses in vivo, FPR-targeting PEG-O800 NPRs were delivered intravenously in mice subcutaneously injected with PLA and PEG particle implants. Results demonstrated that fluorescence signals were significantly higher in PLA injected sites compared to PEG sites and saline-injected controls. Furthermore, fluorescent images of tissue sections around PLA and PEG implant sites revealed significantly higher concentrations of FPR-targeting PEG-O800 NPRs in PLA compared to PEG implants. This observation was further confirmed by histological analysis, which showed that PLA particles recruited neutrophils to a greater extent than PEG implants, while negligible neutrophil numbers were observed in saline-injected controls. In contrast, neutrophil-depleted mice demonstrated a substantial reduction in neutrophil recruitment (~75%) around PLA implant sites compared to controls. Cumulatively, these results prove that FPR-targetingPEG-O800-cFLFLF NIR NPRs are promising for quantitatively assessing inflammatory responses associated with activated neutrophils around implanted biomaterials in vivo.

3.2.2 Macromolecular protein imaging

Adherent macrophages and foreign body giant cells on the surface of an implant trigger fibroproliferation and angiogenesis, both of which prelude the formation of a fibrous capsule around the implanted biomaterial (Anderson et al., 2008). These inflammatory cells also differentially secrete degradative proteolytic enzymes, such as cathepsins and matrix metalloproteases, and extracellular matrix (ECM) proteins, such as fibronectin, that influence ECM remodeling/fibrosis during the wound-healing process (Anderson et al., 2008). Quite notably, the degradative protease cathepsin released by activated inflammatory cells at the site of FBR has been exploited for noninvasive monitoring of biomaterial-associated inflammation in vivo (Bratlie et al., 2010). The NIR dye, ProSense 680, was used for imaging cathepsin activity around subcutaneously injected alginate and polystyrene microparticles in mice (Fig. 3.2(a)–(c)). Alginate was chosen for its bioinert characteristics (de Vos et al., 2006), whereas polystyrene was used as a positive control for its ability to induce strong inflammatory responses (Makino et al., 2003). Imaging data showed that saline-injected controls demonstrated very low fluorescent signals compared to injected alginate and polystyrene throughout the four-week time period (Fig. 3.2(a)). Fluorescence intensities for polystyrene increased steadily from day 1, peaked at day 21, and declined by day 28 (Fig. 3.2(c) and (d)). On the other hand, fluorescent signals for alginate remained constant from day 1 to day 28 (Fig. 3.2(b) and (e)). Validation through histological analysis showed very similar trends for infiltrating neutrophils surrounding alginate and polystyrene injection sites (Fig. 3.2(f)). Macrophage recruitment was more pronounced for polystyrene, which plateaued 7 days postinjection, while alginate leveled out at day 3 (Fig. 3.2(g)). Taken together, these results show that imaging for cathepsin activity around implanted biomaterials could serve as a reliable indicator for assessing the severity of implant-associated inflammation in vivo.

Biomaterial surface chemistry has been shown to influence both cell adhesion and apoptosis in vivo (Brodbeck et al., 2001, 2002). Disruption of cell adhesion signals has been shown to activate the apoptotic pathway (Brodbeck et al., 2001). In the context of implanted-associated FBR, detachment of biomaterial-adherent macrophages and neutrophils under shear stress activates apoptosis signaling (Anderson et al., 2008). Seemingly, the imaging of apoptotic process around implanted devices is yet another promising approach to noninvasively evaluate inflammatory responses to implanted biomaterials. A cell-permeable, noncytotoxic, red fluorescent dye, SR-FLIVO, which acts as a covalent-binding inhibitor of apoptosis-specific caspases (Cursio et al., 2008; Riol-Blanco et al., 2009), was employed to image apoptotic processes around subcutaneously implanted titanium and copper-coated titanium discs in vivo (Bartsch et al., 2012). Copper served as apoptosis-inducing positive controls, whereas pure titanium discs were used as negative controls (Zhai et al., 2000; Suska et al., 2003). Clinical observation revealed swelling and low-grade redness of mouse skin around copper implants during the first few days, while titanium discs showed no visible signs of inflammation at any time during the 23-day time period. SR-FLIVO fluorescent measurements showed that the intensity of the apoptosis signal around copper implants was increased compared to signals around titanium implants throughout the study period (Fig. 3.3(a)–(e)). Furthermore, histological analysis demonstrated that inflammation-related apoptosis signals were significantly higher around copper implants compared to pure implants at any time postimplantation (Fig. 3.3(f)–(l)). This study demonstrates that monitoring apoptotic processes around implanted biomaterials is a viable option for estimating implant biocompatibility as well as device-associated inflammation.

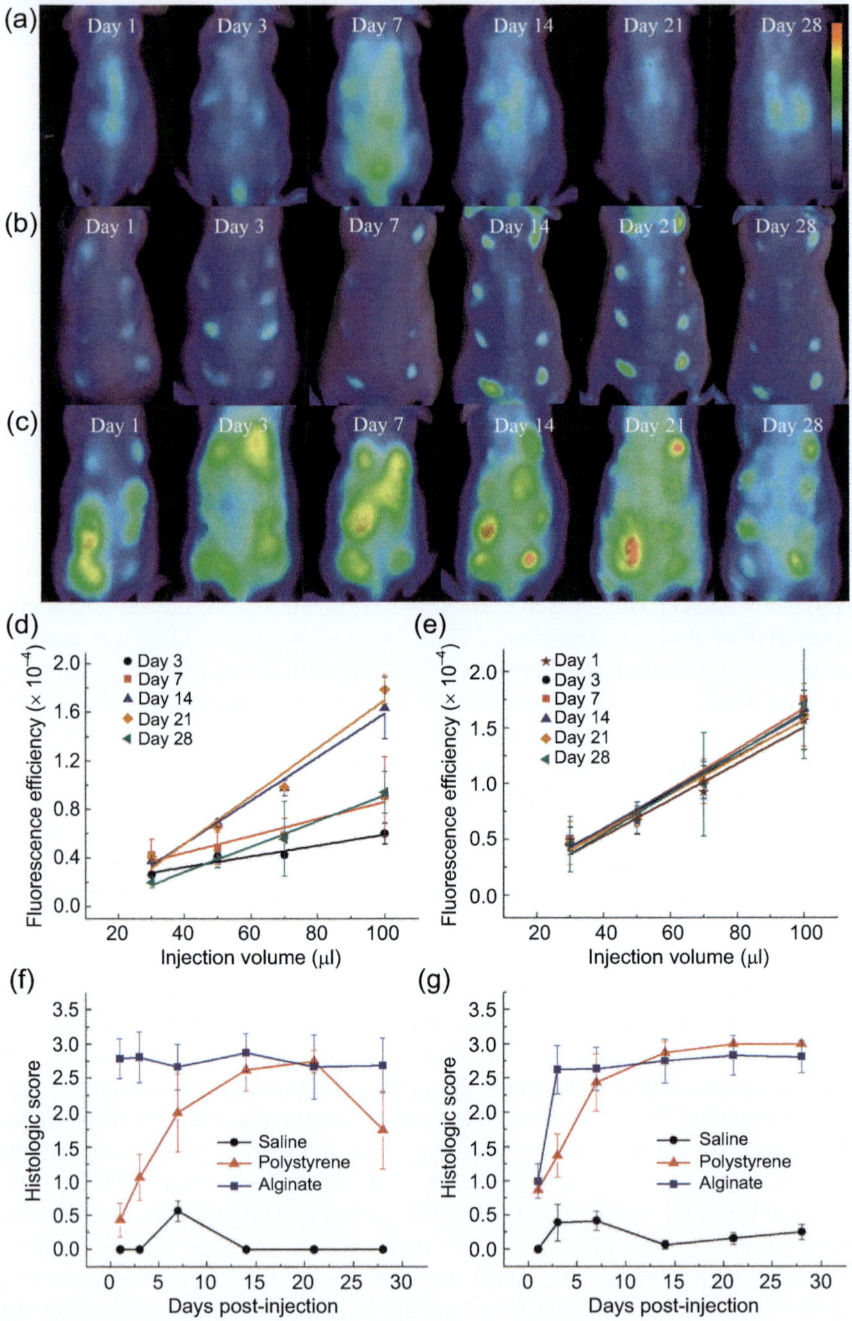

Figure 3.2 NIRF imaging of cathepsin activity around injected biomaterials using ProSense 680 dye. Representative image of cathepsin activity around (a) saline, (b) alginate, and (c) polystyrene injection sites at different time points in live animals. Quantification of fluorescence signals of cathepsin activities (mean ± standard deviation (SD), n = 4) in (d) polystyrene and (e) alginate-injected groups. Histological scores (mean ± SD, n = 4) from tissues surrounding (f) polystyrene and (g) alginate injection sites.

Cited from, Bratlie, K.M., Dang, T.T., Lyle, S., Nahrendorf, M., Weissleder, R., et al., 2010. Rapid biocompatibility analysis of materials via in vivo fluorescence imaging of mouse models. PLoS One 5 (4), e10032.

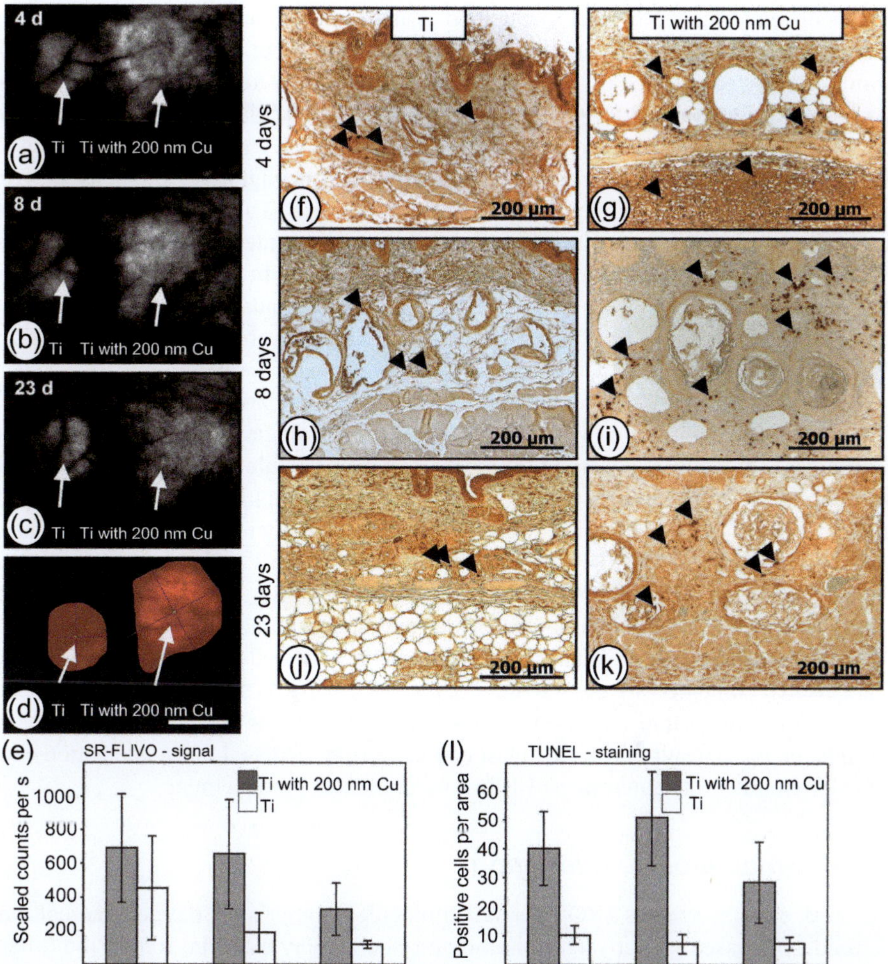

Figure 3.3 NIRF imaging of apoptosis signal around implanted biomaterials using ProSense 680 SR-FLIVO dye. (a–c) Fluorescent intensities of apoptotic signal surrounding titanium and copper-coated implants at 4, 8, and 23 days postimplantation. (d) Regions of interest created around the two implants for quantification of apoptosis signal. Scale bar = 8 mm. Apoptotic cell-specific terminal deoxynucleotidyl transferase dUTP nick end labeling (TUNEL) staining in tissues surrounding titanium (f, h, j) and copper-coated implants (g, i, k) at 4, 8, and 23 days postimplantation. *Black arrowheads* indicate apoptotic cells. (e) Quantification of SR-FLIVO apoptotic signals around implanted titanium and copper-coated implants (mean ± SD, n = 5). (f) The number of TUNEL-staining positive apoptotic cells around implanted titanium and copper-coated implants (mean ± SD, n = 5).

Mast cell activation has been associated with substantially increased localized deposition of fibrin in many inflammatory diseases (Ramos et al., 1992). Evidently, activated mast cells at implant sites mediate fibrin deposition in the pathogenesis of implant-associated FBR (Tang and Eaton, 1993; Tang et al., 1998). Hence, noninvasive imaging of mast cell-mediated fibrin deposition has emerged as an alternate strategy to detect and monitor inflammation around implanted biomaterials in vivo (Tsai et al., 2014). To this end, a fibrin-targeting peptide, GPRPPGGSKGC, with high avidity to fibrin and high resistance to proteolysis (Aruva et al., 2006; Thakur et al., 2000), was conjugated to fluorescent red O800 dye to design NIR fibrin-affinity (FA) NPRs. The FA NPRs demonstrated good fluorescence spectral characteristics (Fig. 3.4(a)) with negligible cytotoxicity in vitro. In addition, FA NPRs exhibited high fibrin avidity (Fig. 3.4(b)) and established a good linear relationship between fibrin-associated fluorescence intensities and fibrin amount compared to dye-only control NPRs in vitro (Fig. 3.4(c)). In vivo studies showed that the prepared FA NPRs were able to detect fibrin accumulation within 30 min after subcutaneous injection of thrombin, which catalyzes the conversion of fibrinogen to fibrin (Fig. 3.4(d)). To evaluate whether FA NPRs can detect fibrin accumulation around implanted materials, FA NPRs were administered intravascularly in mice subcutaneously injected with titanium oxide (TiO_2) particle implants. Imaging data revealed a significant increase in fibrin-associated fluorescence intensities within 10 min following probe injection in the TiO_2 group compared to saline-injected controls (Fig. 3.4(e)). Furthermore, fluorescence intensities of FA NPRs were substantially reduced in mice implanted with heparin-treated TiO_2 NPs compared to TiO_2 alone (Fig. 3.4(f)). Next, to confirm the role of mast cells in implant-mediated fibrin deposition, TiO_2, PLA and silicon dioxide NPs were injected in mast cell-deficient mice and their normal littermates. Interestingly, fluorescence intensities of different particles in the mast cell-deficient mice decreased dramatically compared to normal littermates (Fig. 3.4(g)), supporting that mast cell activation is responsible for fibrin accumulation surrounding biomaterial implants. In conclusion, these results show that mast cell activation-mediated fibrin deposition could serve as a marker for monitoring FBR toward implanted biomaterials.

3.2.3 Small molecule imaging

Reactive oxygen species (ROS), small molecules comprising oxygen radicals and peroxides, released by activated inflammatory cells, play a crucial role in the inflammatory response to implanted biomaterials (Hooper et al., 2000; Tsaryk et al., 2007). Numerous biomaterials induce activated macrophages and neutrophils to produce ROS (Tsaryk et al., 2007; Karlsson and Tang, 2006; Serrano et al., 2005). Elevated levels of ROS induce stress cracking and oxidative damage that alter the microarchitecture of the implant surface, ultimately leading to implant failure (Anderson et al., 2008). Consequently, methods to image ROS near the vicinity of an implant could greatly improve the diagnosis of inflammatory responses to implanted biomaterials.

Small molecule ROS imaging probes, termed the hydrocyanines, were synthesized via a one-step reduction of commercially available cyanine dyes, such as indocyanine green (ICG), Cy5, and Cy7, with sodium borohydride (Kundu et al., 2009). The hydrocyanines demonstrated excellent stability to auto-oxidation, tunable emission wavelengths, and most importantly, displayed high selectivity, specificity, and nanomolar sensitivity to ROS (Kundu et al., 2009). To evaluate the ability of hydrocyanines to detect ROS in vivo, hydro-ICG was used to detect extracellular ROS released in response to PET disks implanted under the skin in the back of mice (Selvam et al., 2011) (Fig. 3.5(a)). Fluorescence data showed that signals from PET implants were

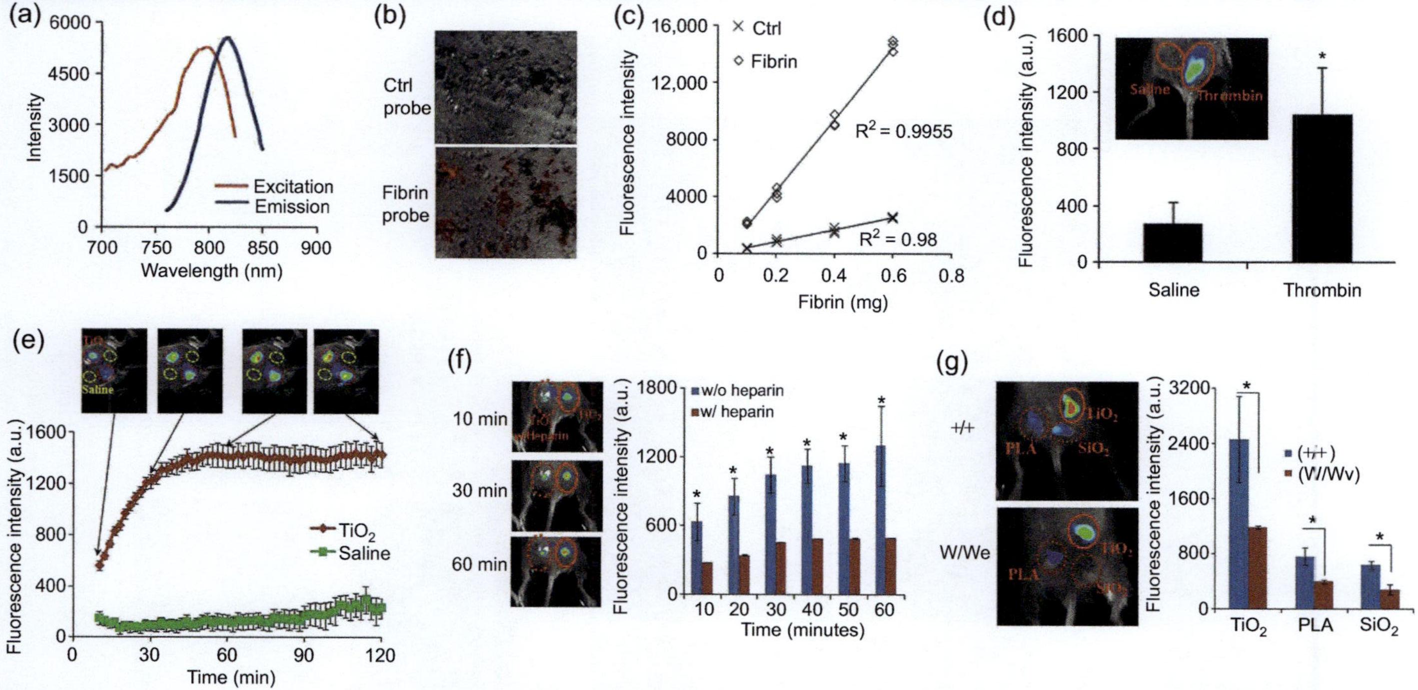

Figure 3.4 NIRF imaging of mast cell-mediated fibrin deposition around injected biomaterials using fibrin-affinity nanoprobes (FA NPRs). (a) Excitation and emission spectra of FA NPRs. (b) Red fluorescent signal of fibrin clots on glass beads incubated in fibrin-affinity (FA) and control nanoprobes (NPRs) in vitro. (c) Correlation between fibrin amounts and flucrescence intensities of FR and control NPRs in vitro. (d) Representative bioimaging scan of live animal showing accumulation of FA NPRs at saline and thrombin-injected sites. Mean fluorescence intensities at saline and thrombin-injected sites (mean ± SD, n = 4). * denotes $p < .05$, significant differences in fluorescence intensities between saline and thrombin groups. (e) Merged fluorescence and white light images of animals with TiO_2 and saline-injected sites after intravascular administration of FA NPRs and mean fluorescence intensities at TiO_2 and saline-injected sites. (f) Fluorescence imaging of animals injected with TiO_2 and with or without heparin treatment at three different time points. Bar graph shows the quantification of fluorescence intensities (mean ± SD, n = 4) of heparin-treated TiO_2 and TiO_2 injection sites within 1 h of probe administration. * denotes $p < .05$, significant differences in fluorescence intensities between heparin-treated TiO_2 and TiO_2 control groups. (g) Fluorescence intensities (mean ± SD, n = 3) of TiO_2, PLA, and SiO_2 injection sites in wild-type and mast cell deficiency mice (W/Wv). * denotes $p < .05$, significant differences in fluorescence intensities between wild-type and mast cell deficiency mice in all three groups.

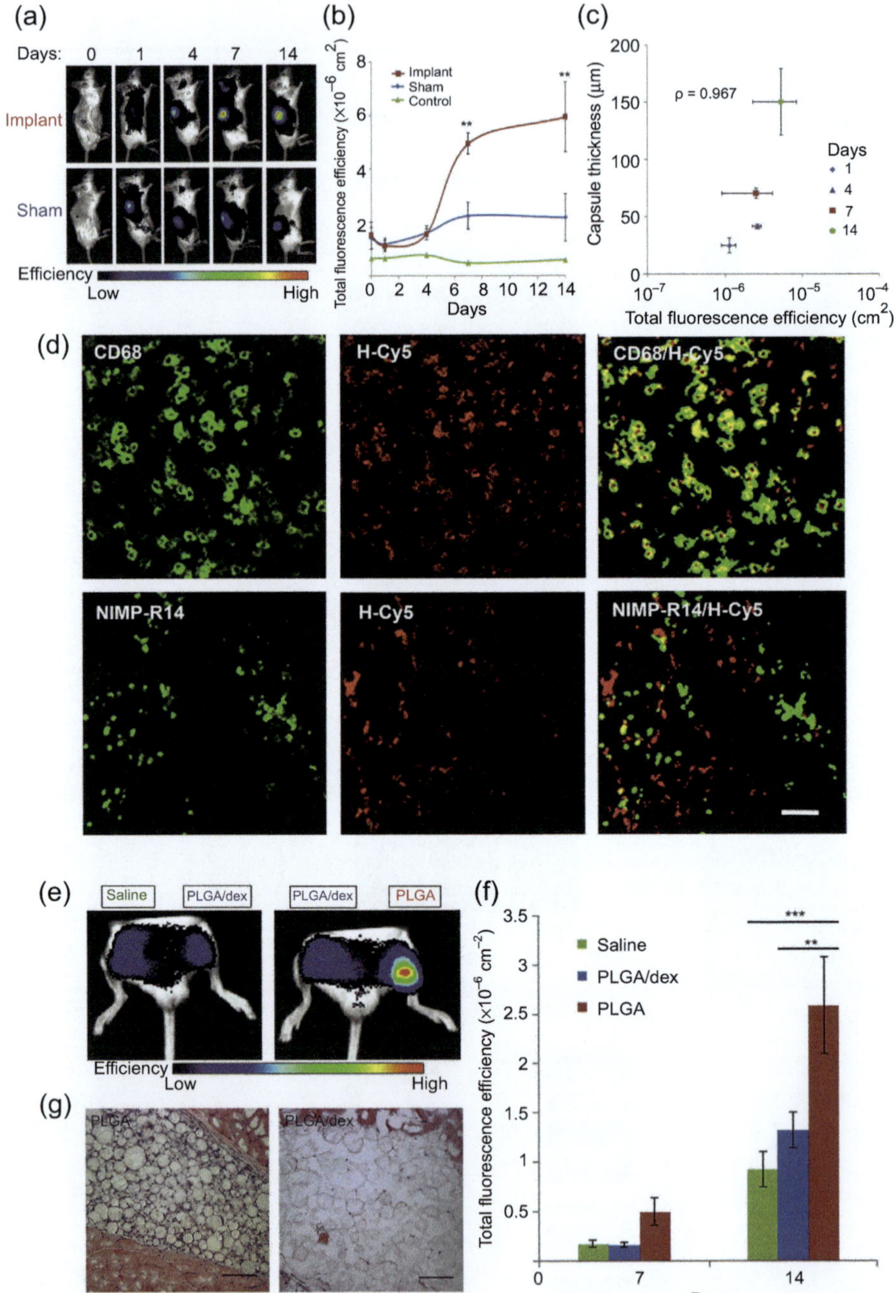
(a)
Days: 0 1 4 7 14
Implant
Sham
Efficiency
Low
High
(b)
Total fluorescence efficiency (×10^-6 cm^2)
Implant
Sham
Control
Days
(c)
Capsule thickness (μm)
ρ = 0.967
Days
1
4
7
14
Total fluorescence efficiency (cm^2)
(d)
CD68
H-Cy5
CD68/H-Cy5
NIMP-R14
H-Cy5
NIMP-R14/H-Cy5
(e)
Saline
PLGA/dex
PLGA/dex
PLGA
Efficiency
Low
High
(f)
Saline
PLGA/dex
PLGA
Total fluorescence efficiency (×10^-6 cm^-2)
Days
(g)
PLGA
PLGA/dex

2.5-fold greater than surgical sham controls at days 7 and 14 postimplantation, while nonsurgical dye-only controls demonstrated two-fold lower signal intensities compared to surgical sham controls at all time points during the two-week time period (Fig. 3.5(b)). Histological analysis on implant-associated tissues revealed that the thickness of collagenous fibrous capsules formed around implants correlated strongly with corresponding ROS fluorescence values (Fig. 3.5(c)). Furthermore, costaining analysis for inflammatory cell markers and ROS activity demonstrated that activated macrophages and neutrophils were primarily responsible for the upregulation of ROS at PET implant sites (Fig. 3.5(d)). This imaging strategy was also able to detect attenuation in inflammatory responses in response to delivery of anti-inflammatory agents (Fig. 3.5(e)). Intravenous injections of hydro-Cy7 showed a significant decrease in fluorescence intensities around dexamethasone-loaded poly(lactic-co-glycolyic acid) (PLGA) microparticles compared to blank PLGA microparticles at day 14 postimplantation (Fig. 3.5(f)). These results correlated directly with significant presence of inflammatory cells around empty PLGA compared to PLGA microparticles releasing dexamethasone (Fig. 3.5(g)). Viewed comprehensively, these results prove that ROS is a reliable indicator and an excellent diagnostic marker for evaluating biomaterial-related inflammation around implanted devices.

3.3 Chemiluminescence imaging

Chemiluminescence is the production of light without heat from a chemical reaction. The emitted light is a transient product that ceases to exist after termination of the chemical reaction. The small molecule, luminol (5-amino-2,3-dihydro-1,4-phthalazinedione), is one of the most widely used chemiluminescent probes for biomedical applications (DeChatelet et al., 1982; Hallett et al., 2003). It is relatively nontoxic and possesses good absorption and excretory characteristics upon systemic administration in the body (Sanders et al., 2000). Luminol reacts with peroxides to emit light photons at 425 nm, which can be detected noninvasively in vivo (Gross et al., 2009).

Figure 3.5 Reactive oxygen species (ROS) imaging of implant-associated inflammation using hydrocyanine dyes. (a) In vivo fluorescence imaging of ROS in surgical sham and PET implant groups after subcutaneous delivery of H-ICG. (b) Quantification of fluorescence signals (mean ± SE, n ≥ 5) of implant, sham, and dye-only control groups over a period of two weeks. ** denotes $p < .01$, significant difference in fluorescence signals between implant and sham groups. (c) Correlation of implant fibrous capsule thickness to corresponding implant-associated ROS fluorescence values (mean ± SE, n = 3). (d) Representative colocalization images of macrophages (CD68+, green) and neutrophils (NIMP-R14+, green) with intracellular ROS (H-Cy5+, red) in 14-day implants. Scale bar, 50 μm. (e) Representative images of the ROS imaging of animals injected with saline, empty poly(lactic-co-glycolyic acid) (PLGA), and dexamethasone-loaded PLGA microparticles using H-Cy7. (f) Quantification of ROS signals (mean ± SE, n ≥ 5) from saline, empty PLGA, and dexamethasone-loaded PLGA injected groups on days 7 and 14 postinjection. (g) Histological tissue sections from mice injected with empty PLGA and dexamethasone-loaded PLGA microparticles in 14-day explants. Scale bars, 100 μm.

As light is produced inherently, this imaging methodology does not require the use of excitation or emission filters, and hence light can be captured directly using a super-cooled charge-coupled device camera. However, the blue luminescence of luminol lacks tissue penetration and depth resolution, thereby severely limiting its application to 2-D imaging of only a few millimeters of tissue. Nevertheless, chemiluminescence imaging (CLI) has been successfully employed for real-time assessment of biomaterial-related inflammation around subcutaneously implanted biomaterials in vivo (Liu et al., 2011). Specifically, luminol was used to detect and assess ROS generation around implanted biomaterials (Liu et al., 2011). In vitro studies demonstrated that luminol could detect ROS released by stimulated phagocytic cells cultured on polystyrene and alginate surfaces (Fig. 3.6(a)) and that a two-fold increase in bioluminescence signals was observed on polystyrene compared to alginate (Fig. 3.6(b)). Next, polystyrene and alginate beads were subcutaneously injected in the back of mice, and luminol-induced luminescence was tracked for a four-week time period (Fig. 3.6(c)). Quantification of luminescence showed that polystyrene beads elicited higher levels of ROS at all time points examined, while alginate beads exhibited substantially lower ROS levels, similar to that of saline-only controls (Fig. 3.6(d)). The imaging data was corroborated by histological analysis, which revealed that polystyrene beads recruited more inflammatory cells compared to alginate beads throughout the four-week study interval (Fig. 3.6(e)). More broadly, these studies show that luminol can be used to monitor biomaterial-induced inflammation near the vicinity of subcutaneously implanted devices.

In an effort to improve the detection limits of luminol, a luminol derivative, L-012 (8-amino-5-chloro-7-phenylpyridol[3,4-d]pyridazine-1,4(2H,3H) dione), which has higher sensitivity to ROS, was employed to monitor localized inflammatory responses to implanted biomaterials (Zhou et al., 2012b). In vitro studies showed that protein kinase C activated polymorphonuclear neutrophils (PMNs) emitted 900-fold higher CL intensities with L-012 compared to luminol (Fig. 3.7(a)), while signal intensities reduced drastically in the presence of a superoxide dismutase mimetic, Tempol (Fig. 3.7(b)). Furthermore, CL signal intensities shared a linear relationship with increasing neutrophil cell numbers in vitro. In vivo studies demonstrated that L-012 was able to detect ROS released in response to subcutaneously injected PLA particle implants with CL signals significantly higher than saline-only controls (Fig. 3.7(c)). In addition, signal intensities around PLA implant sites were reduced by ~70% in neutropenic mice pretreated with anti-PMN antibodies, suggesting that PMN-induced ROS play a major role in implant-associated FBR (Fig. 3.7(d)). Moreover, L-012 was able to discriminate inflammatory responses to different biomaterials, including poly(N-isopropylacrylamide-co-N-(3-aminopropyl) methacrylamide) (PNIPAM-NH_2), PLA, and PEG with CL intensities increasing in the following order: PNIPAM-NH_2 > PLA > PEG > saline control (Fig. 3.7(e)). Histological analyses of implant-associated tissues also revealed similar trends in PMN and phagocyte cell recruitments with signal intensities linearly correlating to PMN cell numbers (Fig. 3.7(f)). In conclusion, these studies show that the extent of FBR to implanted biomaterials can be detected and assessed through CLI.

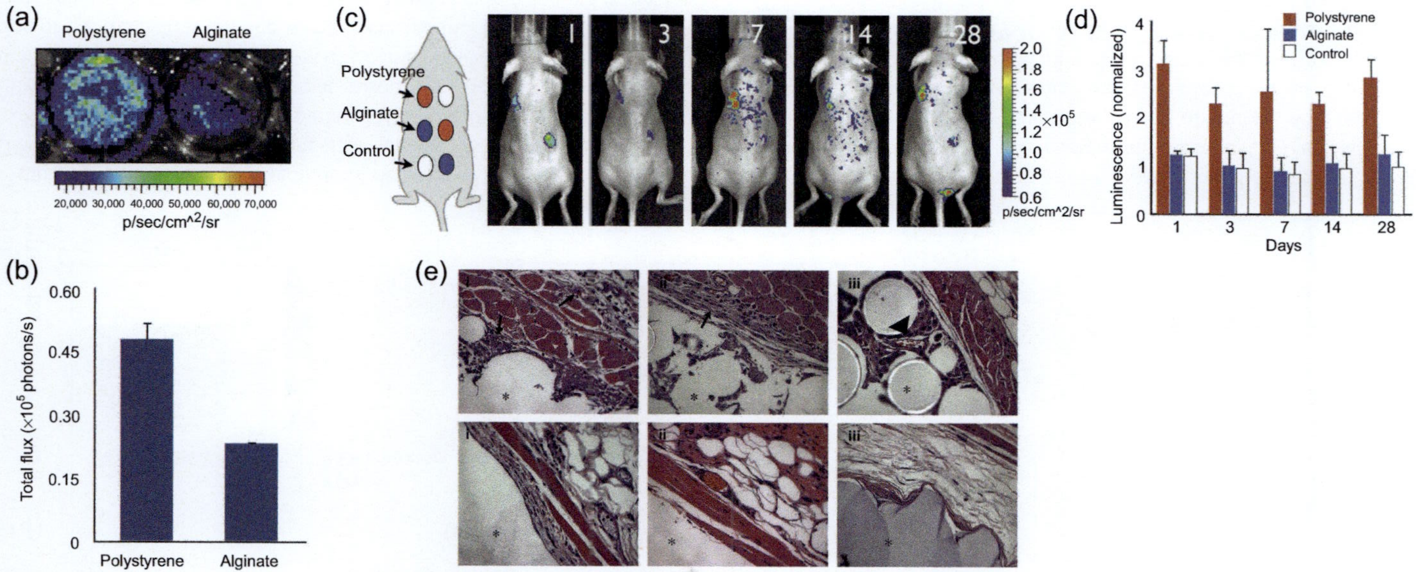

Figure 3.6 Chemiluminescence imaging (CLI) of ROS using luminol. (a). Luminol-based CLI of ROS released by stimulated phagocytes cultured on polystyrene and alginate surfaces in vitro. (b) Quantification of ROS released from stimulated phagocytes cultured on polystyrene and alginate surfaces using luminol in vitro (mean ± SE, n = 5). (c) In vivo CLI of ROS using luminol in animals with polystyrene and alginate implants. (d) Quantification of ROS released around polystyrene and alginate implant sites using luminol in vivo (mean ± SE, n = 6). (e) Histological sections of tissues around injected polystyrene and alginate particle implants on days 1 (i), 7 (ii), and 28 (iii) postimplantation. Arrows indicate the presence of phagocytic cells (i and ii), and arrowheads indicate the presence of fibroblasts (iii). * denotes the region within the material. Scale bar, 100 μm.

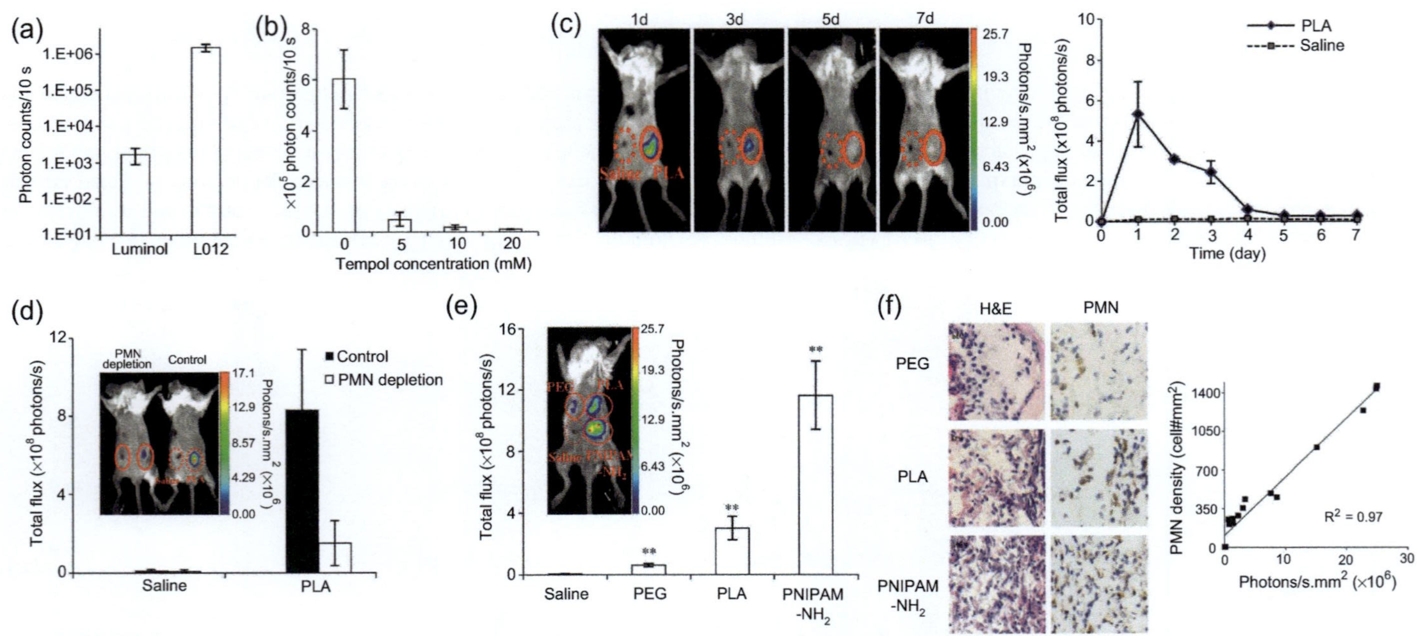

Figure 3.7 CLI of ROS using luminol derivative L-012. (a) In vitro measurements of ROS released from phorbol 12-myristate 13-acetate (PMA)-stimulated polymorphonuclear neutrophils (PMNs) incubated in luminol and L-012. (b) Mean L-012 chemiluminescence (CL) intensities of ROS released from PMA-stimulated PMNs in the presence of varying concentrations of Tempol. (c) Representative CLI of animals with injected PLA particle implants and saline at various time points. Quantification of L-012 CL intensities at PLA and saline injection sites at various time points. (d) CLI and quantification of CL intensities around PLA injection sites in control and PMN-depleted mice. (e) CL imaging and quantification of CL intensities in mice with injected saline, PEG, PLA, and poly(N-isopropyl acrylamide)-NH_2 (PNIPAM-NH_2) particles. ** denotes $p \leq .05$, significant differences in CL intensities between saline and other three groups. (f) Representative histological and neutrophil staining of tissues surrounding PEG, PLA, and PNIPAM-NH_2 injection sites and correlation between PMN number and CL intensity at various injection sites.

3.4 Bioluminescence imaging

Bioluminescence imaging (BLI) is based on the detection and quantification of light emitted from enzyme-catalyzed luminescence in living cells or tissues (Gross et al., 2009). For example, enzyme-catalyzed luminescence of luminol has been used to evaluate eosinophil peroxidase and myeloperoxidase activities through BLI (Haqqani et al., 1999; Gross et al., 2009). Furthermore, luciferase-labeled cells, cells genetically modified to stably express the enzyme luciferase, which catalyzes the oxidation of substrate luciferrin to produce light, have been used for the noninvasive monitoring of cell proliferation on biomaterial scaffolds in vivo (Blum et al., 2004; Roman et al., 2007). As the peak emission of firefly luciferase is ~600nm, it is beneficial for noninvasive imaging, as orange-red wavelengths are less prone to tissue scatter and absorption compared to bluer wavelengths (<500nm). However, the sensitivity of BLI depends greatly on the expression levels of luciferase in the target cells or tissues in vivo. Transgenic mice with luciferase reporter genes driven by a promoter of interest have also been developed for BLI (Hsieh et al., 2005; Roth et al., 2006; Sadikot et al., 2003). Particularly, reporter mice carrying firefly luciferase genes regulated by nuclear factor kappa B (NF-κB) promoters were employed to investigate host inflammatory responses to implanted biomaterials (Ho et al., 2007).

NF-κB is a nuclear transcription factor protein that plays a key role in the regulation of proinflammatory signaling pathways (Lawrence, 2009). Activated NF-κB induces the secretion of various proinflammatory cytokines such as interleukin-1 (IL-1), IL-6, and tumor necrosis factor α (TNF-α), whose levels in turn reflect the extent of biomaterial-associated inflammation around implanted devices in vivo. To this end, inflammatory responses to subcutaneously implanted genipin-crosslinked gelatin conduits (GCC) were investigated in reporter mice driven by NF-κB response elements (Ho et al., 2007). BLI showed that these transgenic mice demonstrated constitutive NF-κB activity after intraperitoneal injection of the substrate D-luciferin with diffuse luminescence detected in the whole body of mice (Fig. 3.8(a)). In addition, intraperitoneal injection of LPS further increased NF-κB-dependent BL signals throughout the body, with intense signals primarily observed in the abdominal region (Fig. 3.8(a)). BLI of inflammatory responses around implanted GCC or LPS-immersed GCC demonstrated that LPS-immersed GCC induced a stronger NF-κB-dependent BL compared to GCC implants throughout the 7-day time period (Fig. 3.8(b)). Furthermore, immunohistochemical analyses revealed the presence of both NF-κB- and luciferase protein-positive cells at the implant site, with NF-κB-driven BL signal intensities correlating directly with host inflammatory responses (Fig. 3.8(c)). Collectively, these results demonstrate that BLI is yet another imaging modality that has been successfully employed to investigate host inflammatory responses associated with implanted devices in vivo.

3.5 Magnetic resonance imaging

MRI is an imaging modality that uses nonionizing electromagnetic radiation to generate cross-sectional images of the body in any plane (Haralampieva et al., 2014). It offers excellent soft tissue contrast with high spatial and temporal resolution

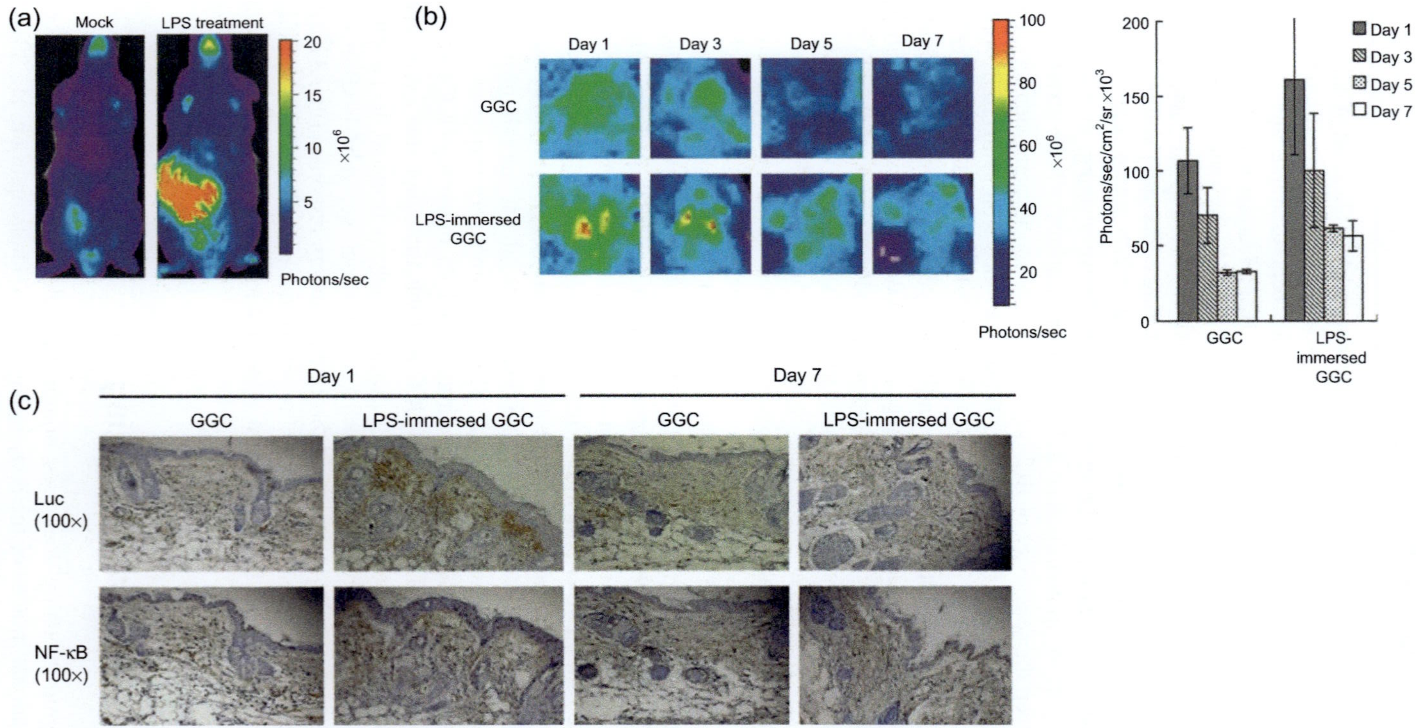

Figure 3.8 Bioluminescence imaging (BLI) of NF-κB activity around implanted biomaterials in vivo. (a) BLI NF-κB activity in transgenic mice with D-luciferin after intraperitoneal injection of saline (mock) and LPS. (b) In vivo BLI and quantification of bioluminescence signals in transgenic animals implanted with genipin-crosslinked gelatin conduits (GGC) and LPS-immersed GGC on days 1, 3, 5, and 7 postimplantation. (c) Immunohistochemical examinations of tissues surrounding GGC or LPS-immersed GGC implants using antibody for luciferase (Luc) or NF-κB (100× magnification) on days 1 and 7 postimplantation.

(Haralampieva et al., 2014) that has been exploited for noninvasive assessment of biomaterial-related FBR. As MR relaxation times of water protons are inconsistent within an implant compared to its surrounding tissues, MRI offers a unique solution for monitoring tissue/material interactions and consequently, inflammatory responses to implanted biomaterials (Alikacem et al., 1999). For example, inflammatory responses to implanted PLA scaffolds (Stroman et al., 1999) and polymeric bulk hydrogels (Traore et al., 2000) studied over a period of 6 months in rabbits showed that MR relaxometry studies and histological observations correlated well with each other. In these studies the transversal relaxation time, T_2, progressively increased and peaked 15 days following biomaterial implantation. Histological examinations of implants during this time period revealed the infiltration of inflammatory cells, such as PMNs, lymphocytes, and fibroblasts, indicating an acute inflammatory reaction. However, 3 weeks postimplantation, T_2 signals diminished rapidly, while histological observations pointed toward an intense chronic inflammation characterized by massive inflammatory cell infiltration, the presence of foreign body giant cells (FBGCs), and fibrous matrix encapsulation of the implant. This inverse trend observed in T_2 values is attributed to the accumulation of fluid at the implant site during acute inflammation, while the significant reduction of fluid is associated with increased inflammatory cell infiltration and the onset of chronic inflammation at the implant site. In contrast, T_2 signals from healthy tissues surrounding the implant remained unchanged throughout the study period.

Recently, protein polymer contrast agents (PPCAs) were developed to increase contrast-to-noise ratio (CNR) between an implant and its surroundings for MRI applications (Karfeld-Sulzer et al., 2011). PPCA was synthesized by conjugating the protein polymer K8-120 with an amino acid sequence of GH10SSGHIDDDDKHM(GKAGTGSA)$_{120}$G to gandolinium(III) chelators using carbodiimide-coupling chemistry. The PPCAs were then covalently incorporated into bulk polymeric hydrogels, which were in turn subcutaneously implanted in mice for noninvasive monitoring of host inflammatory responses to the hydrogels via MRI. Results showed that PPCA-incorporated hydrogels demonstrated at least 1.5-fold increase in CNR compared to non-PPCA hydrogels during the 22-day study period. Furthermore, PPCAs were able to distinguish the implant from surrounding inflammatory tissue with histological observations, confirming inflammatory cell recruitment, fibrinous exudate, and formation of a collagen capsule surrounding the implant 22 days postimplantation. All in all, these studies show that MR tomography is a sensitive approach for noninvasive longitudinal monitoring of tissue physiochemical changes following the implantation of biomaterials.

3.6 Conclusions and future perspectives

It is well established that material surface chemistry influences the FBR toward implanted biomaterials. The surface chemistry of an implanted device dictates the behavior of recruited macrophages, invariably affecting their adhesion, fusion, apoptosis, and cytokine secretion profiles at the site of implant (Anderson et al., 2008). A mechanistic understanding of the complex mechanisms underlying tissue/

material interactions has offered insights into the development of novel biomaterials with different surface chemistries for fabrication of implantable medical devices. As these implantable devices are developed for a multitude of clinical applications, the overall inflammatory responses evoked by these implantable devices could be highly variable and inconsistent in vivo. Presently, no single imaging modality possesses the versatility or subtlety to noninvasively image nuances in aseptic implant-associated inflammation. Such an "all-in-one" imaging solution is not possible, as all emerging imaging modalities have their own inherent limitations. For example, luminescent probes derived from luminol emit blue light, which is not quite advantageous for noninvasive deep tissue imaging applications. While NIRF imaging can overcome this shortcoming and presents unique opportunities for 3-D visualization of tissues (Bloch et al., 2005), it does not possess high spatial or temporal resolution offered by anatomical 3-D imaging modalities, such as MRI or CT, which offer unparalleled visualization of structural minutiae. To bridge the gap, imaging technologies are combined synergistically to form hybrid imaging systems, which serve as an ideal solution for addressing the limitations of each individual technique (Marti-Bonmati et al., 2010).

Multimodal technologies combine anatomical and functional imaging modalities to provide enhanced morphofunctional information in a single scan (Marti-Bonmati et al., 2010). Some of the hybrid imaging systems include positron emission tomography (PET)/CT, single-photon emission computed tomography (SPECT)/CT, and PET/MRI, of which PET/CT is a standard imaging technique available in most clinical settings. Recently, macrophage-targeting PET imaging probes have been developed for PET/CT imaging of implant-mediated inflammation (Zhou et al., 2013). PET/CT imaging was also successfully employed to detect catheter-induced aseptic inflammation and bacterial infection in vivo (Ahtinen et al., 2014). Similarly, bioluminescent and fluorescent optical imaging was combined with X-ray and micro-CT to longitudinally monitor inflammation and bone damage in an orthopedic implant infection model (Niska et al., 2012). These new developments demonstrate the great promise hybrid imaging technologies hold for the imaging of inflammatory responses around implantable medical devices. Ultimately, finding the right combination of systems for multimodal imaging will be key to the successful evaluation/diagnosis of implant-mediated inflammatory responses, as well as development of effective anti-inflammatory therapies to mitigate aseptic inflammation associated with implantable medical devices.

References

Ahtinen, H., Kulkova, J., Lindholm, L., Eerola, E., Hakanen, A.J., Moritz, N., Soderstrom, M., Saanijoki, T., Jalkanen, S., Roivainen, A., Aro, H.T., 2014. (68)Ga-DOTA-Siglec-9 PET/CT imaging of peri-implant tissue responses and staphylococcal infections. EJNMMI Res. 4, 45.

Alikacem, N., Marois, Y., Zhang, Z., Jakubiec, B., Roy, R., King, M.W., Guidoin, R., 1999. Tissue reactions to polypyrrole-coated polyesters: a magnetic resonance relaxometry study. Artif. Organs 23, 910–919.

Anderson, J.M., Rodriguez, A., Chang, D.T., 2008. Foreign body reaction to biomaterials. Semin. Immunol. 20, 86–100.

Aruva, M.R., Daviau, J., Sharma, S.S., Thakur, M.L., 2006. Imaging thromboembolism with fibrin-avid 99mTc-peptide: evaluation in swine. J. Nucl. Med. 47, 155–162.

Aswathy, R.G., Yoshida, Y., Maekawa, T., Kumar, D.S., 2010. Near-infrared quantum dots for deep tissue imaging. Anal. Bioanal. Chem. 397, 1417–1435.

Bartsch, I., Willbold, E., Yarmolenko, S., Witte, F., 2012. In vivo fluorescence imaging of apoptosis during foreign body response. Biomaterials 33, 6926–6932.

Bloch, S., Lesage, F., Mcintosh, L., Gandjbakhche, A., Liang, K., Achilefu, S., 2005. Whole-body fluorescence lifetime imaging of a tumor-targeted near-infrared molecular probe in mice. J. Biomed. Opt. 10, 054003.

Blum, J.S., Temenoff, J.S., Park, H., Jansen, J.A., Mikos, A.G., Barry, M.A., 2004. Development and characterization of enhanced green fluorescent protein and luciferase expressing cell line for non-destructive evaluation of tissue engineering constructs. Biomaterials 25, 5809–5819.

Bratlie, K.M., Dang, T.T., Lyle, S., Nahrendorf, M., Weissleder, R., Langer, R., Anderson, D.G., 2010. Rapid biocompatibility analysis of materials via in vivo fluorescence imaging of mouse models. PLoS One 5 (4), e10032.

Brodbeck, W.G., Patel, J., Voskerician, G., Christenson, E., Shive, M.S., Nakayama, Y., Matsuda, T., Ziats, N.P., Anderson, J.M., 2002. Biomaterial adherent macrophage apoptosis is increased by hydrophilic and anionic substrates in vivo. Proc. Natl. Acad. Sci. U.S.A. 99, 10287–10292.

Brodbeck, W.G., Shive, M.S., Colton, E., Nakayama, Y., Matsuda, T., Anderson, J.M., 2001. Influence of biomaterial surface chemistry on the apoptosis of adherent cells. J. Biomed. Mater. Res. 55, 661–668.

Cursio, R., Colosetti, P., Auberger, P., Gugenheim, J., 2008. Liver apoptosis following normothermic ischemia-reperfusion: in vivo evaluation of caspase activity by FLIVO assay in rats. Transplant. Proc. 40, 2038–2041.

de Vos, P., Faas, M.M., Strand, B., Calafiore, R., 2006. Alginate-based microcapsules for immunoisolation of pancreatic islets. Biomaterials 27, 5603–5617.

DeChatelet, L.R., Long, G.D., Shirley, P.S., Bass, D.A., Thomas, M.J., Henderson, F.W., Cohen, M.S., 1982. Mechanism of the luminol-dependent chemiluminescence of human neutrophils. J. Immunol. 129, 1589–1593.

Domb, A.J., Khan, W., 2014. Implantable Medical Devices. Focal Controlled Drug Delivery. Springer, US.

Frangioni, J.V., 2003. In vivo near-infrared fluorescence imaging. Curr. Opin. Chem. Biol. 7, 626–634.

The Freedonia Group, 2012. Implantable Medical Devices. Cleveland, OH.

Gibbs, S.L., 2012. Near infrared fluorescence for image-guided surgery. Quant. Imaging Med. Surg. 2, 177–187.

Gross, S., Gammon, S.T., Moss, B.L., Rauch, D., Harding, J., Heinecke, J.W., Ratner, L., Piwnica-Worms, D., 2009. Bioluminescence imaging of myeloperoxidase activity in vivo. Nat. Med. 15, 455–461.

Guo, X., Liu, X., Wang, X., Tian, F., Liu, F., Zhang, B., Hu, G., Bai, J., 2010. A combined fluorescence and microcomputed tomography system for small animal imaging. IEEE Trans. Biomed. Eng. 57, 2876–2883.

Hallett, M.B., Cole, C., Dewitt, S., 2003. Detection and visualization of oxidase activity in phagocytes. Methods Mol. Biol. 225, 61–67.

Hanna, K.E., Manning, F.J., Bouxsein, P., Pope, A., 2001. Innovation and invention. In: Medical Devices: Workshop Summary. National Academy Press, Washington, DC.

Haqqani, A.S., Sandhu, J.K., Birnboim, H.C., 1999. A myeloperoxidase-specific assay based upon bromide-dependent chemiluminescence of luminol. Anal. Biochem. 273, 126–132.

Haralampieva, D.G., Ametamey, S.M., Sulser, T., Eberli, D., 2014. Non-invasive imaging modalities for clinical investigation in regenerative medicine. In: Eberli, D. (Ed.), Cells and Biomaterials in Regenerative Medicine. InTech.

Ho, T.Y., Chen, Y.S., Hsiang, C.Y., 2007. Noninvasive nuclear factor-κB bioluminescence imaging for the assessment of host-biomaterial interaction in transgenic mice. Biomaterials 28, 4370–4377.

Hoemann, C.D., Chen, G., Marchand, C., Tran-Khanh, N., Thibault, M., Chevrier, A., Sun, J., Shive, M.S., Fernandes, M.J., Poubelle, P.E., Centola, M., El-Gabalawy, H., 2010. Scaffold-guided subchondral bone repair: implication of neutrophils and alternatively activated arginase-1+ macrophages. Am. J. Sports Med. 38, 1845–1856.

Hooper, K.A., Nickolas, T.L., Yurkow, E.J., Kohn, J., Laskin, D.L., 2000. Characterization of the inflammatory response to biomaterials using a rodent air pouch model. J. Biomed. Mater. Res. 50, 365–374.

Hsieh, C.L., Xie, Z., Liu, Z.Y., Green, J.E., Martin, W.D., Datta, M.W., Yeung, F., Pan, D., Chung, L.W., 2005. A luciferase transgenic mouse model: visualization of prostate development and its androgen responsiveness in live animals. J. Mol. Endocrinol. 35, 293–304.

Karfeld-Sulzer, L.S., Waters, E.A., Kohlmeir, E.K., Kissler, H., Zhang, X., Kaufman, D.B., Barron, A.E., Meade, T.J., 2011. Protein polymer MRI contrast agents: longitudinal analysis of biomaterials in vivo. Magn. Reson. Med. 65, 220–228.

Karlsson, M., Tang, L., 2006. Surface morphology and adsorbed proteins affect phagocyte responses to nano-porous alumina. J. Mater. Sci. Mater. Med. 17, 1101–1111.

Kobayashi, H., Ogawa, M., Alford, R., Choyke, P.L., Urano, Y., 2010. New strategies for fluorescent probe design in medical diagnostic imaging. Chem. Rev. 110, 2620–2640.

Kundu, K., Knight, S.F., Willett, N., Lee, S., Taylor, W.R., Murthy, N., 2009. Hydrocyanines: a class of fluorescent sensors that can image reactive oxygen species in cell culture, tissue, and in vivo. Angew. Chem. Int. Ed. Engl. 48, 299–303.

Lawrence, T., 2009. The nuclear factor NF-κB pathway in inflammation. Cold Spring Harb. Perspect. Biol. 1, a001651.

Liu, W.F., Ma, M., Bratlie, K.M., Dang, T.T., Langer, R., Anderson, D.G., 2011. Real-time in vivo detection of biomaterial-induced reactive oxygen species. Biomaterials 32, 1796–1801.

Locke, L.W., Chordia, M.D., Zhang, Y., Kundu, B., Kennedy, D., Landseadel, J., Xiao, L., Fairchild, K.D., Berr, S.S., Linden, J., Pan, D., 2009. A novel neutrophil-specific PET imaging agent: cFLFLFK-PEG-64Cu. J. Nucl. Med. 50, 790–797.

Makino, K., Yamamoto, N., Higuchi, K., Harada, N., Ohshima, H., Terada, H., 2003. Phagocytic uptake of polystyrene microspheres by alveolar macrophages: effects of the size and surface properties of the microspheres. Colloids Surf. B: Biointerfaces 27, 33–39.

Marti-Bonmati, L., Sopena, R., Bartumeus, P., Sopena, P., 2010. Multimodality imaging techniques. Contrast Media Mol. Imaging 5, 180–189.

Niska, J.A., Meganck, J.A., Pribaz, J.R., Shahbazian, J.H., Lim, E., Zhang, N., Rice, B.W., Akin, A., Ramos, R.I., Bernthal, N.M., Francis, K.P., Miller, L.S., 2012. Monitoring bacterial burden, inflammation and bone damage longitudinally using optical and muCT imaging in an orthopaedic implant infection in mice. PLoS One 7, e47397.

Puig-Kroger, A., Sierra-Filardi, E., Dominguez-Soto, A., Samaniego, R., Corcuera, M.T., Gomez-Aguado, F., Ratnam, M., Sanchez-Mateos, P., Corbi, A.L., 2009. Folate receptor beta is expressed by tumor-associated macrophages and constitutes a marker for M2 anti-inflammatory/regulatory macrophages. Cancer Res. 69, 9395–9403.

Ramos, B.F., Zhang, Y., Jakschik, B.A., 1992. Mast cells contribute to fibrin deposition in reverse passive Arthus reaction in mouse skin. Eur. J. Immunol. 22, 2381–2385.

Riol-Blanco, L., Delgado-Martin, C., Sanchez-Sanchez, N., Alonso, C.L., Gutierrez-Lopez, M.D., Del Hoyo, G.M., Navarro, J., Sanchez-Madrid, F., Cabanas, C., Sanchez-Mateos, P., Rodriguez-Fernandez, J.L., 2009. Immunological synapse formation inhibits, via NF-κB and FOXO1, the apoptosis of dendritic cells. Nat. Immunol. 10, 753–760.

Roman, I., Vilalta, M., Rodriguez, J., Matthies, A.M., Srouji, S., Livne, E., Hubbell, J.A., Rubio, N., Blanco, J., 2007. Analysis of progenitor cell-scaffold combinations by in vivo non-invasive photonic imaging. Biomaterials 28, 2718–2728.

Roth, D.J., Jansen, E.D., Powers, A.C., Wang, T.G., 2006. A novel method of monitoring response to islet transplantation: bioluminescent imaging of an NF-κB transgenic mouse model. Transplantation 81, 1185–1190.

Ruan, G., Feng, S.S., 2003. Preparation and characterization of poly(lactic acid)-poly(ethylene glycol)-poly(lactic acid) (PLA-PEG-PLA) microspheres for controlled release of paclitaxel. Biomaterials 24, 5037–5044.

Sadikot, R.T., Han, W., Everhart, M.B., Zoia, O., Peebles, R.S., Jansen, E.D., Yull, F.E., Christman, J.W., Blackwell, T.S., 2003. Selective I kappa B kinase expression in airway epithelium generates neutrophilic lung inflammation. J. Immunol. 170, 1091–1098.

Sanders, J.M., Chen, L.J., Burka, L.T., Matthews, H.B., 2000. Metabolism and disposition of luminol in the rat. Xenobiotica 30, 263–272.

Selvam, S., Kundu, K., Templeman, K.L., Murthy, N., Garcia, A.J., 2011. Minimally invasive, longitudinal monitoring of biomaterial-associated inflammation by fluorescence imaging. Biomaterials 32, 7785–7792.

Serrano, M.C., Pagani, R., Pena, J., Portoles, M.T., 2005. Transitory oxidative stress in L929 fibroblasts cultured on poly(epsilon-caprolactone) films. Biomaterials 26, 5827–5834.

Stroman, P.W., Dorvil, J.C., Marois, Y., Poddevin, N., Guidoin, R., 1999. In vivo time course studies of the tissue responses to resorbable polylactic acid implants by means of MRI. Magn. Reson. Med. 42, 210–214.

Suska, F., Esposito, M., Gretzer, C., Kalltorp, M., Tengvall, P., Thomsen, P., 2003. IL-1alpha, IL-1beta and TNF-alpha secretion during in vivo/ex vivo cellular interactions with titanium and copper. Biomaterials 24, 461–468.

Talanov, V.S., Regino, C.A., Kobayashi, H., Bernardo, M., Choyke, P.L., Brechbiel, M.W., 2006. Dendrimer-based nanoprobe for dual modality magnetic resonance and fluorescence imaging. Nano Lett. 6, 1459–1463.

Tang, L., Eaton, J.W., 1993. Fibrin(ogen) mediates acute inflammatory responses to biomaterials. J. Exp. Med. 178, 2147–2156.

Tang, L., Jennings, T.A., Eaton, J.W., 1998. Mast cells mediate acute inflammatory responses to implanted biomaterials. Proc. Natl. Acad. Sci. U.S.A. 95, 8841–8846.

Thakur, M.L., Pallela, V.R., Consigny, P.M., Rao, P.S., Vessileva-Belnikolovska, D., Shi, R., 2000. Imaging vascular thrombosis with 99mTc-labeled fibrin alpha-chain peptide. J. Nucl. Med. 41, 161–168.

Traore, A.S., Woerly, S., Doan, V.D., Marois, Y., Guidoin, R., 2000. In vivo magnetic resonance imaging and relaxometry study of a porous hydrogel implanted in the trapezius muscle of rabbits. Tissue Eng. 6, 265–278.

Tsai, Y.T., Zhou, J., Weng, H., Tang, E.N., Baker, D.W., Tang, L., 2014. Optical imaging of fibrin deposition to elucidate participation of mast cells in foreign body responses. Biomaterials 35, 2089–2096.

Tsaryk, R., Kalbacova, M., Hempel, U., Scharnweber, D., Unger, R.E., Dieter, P., Kirkpatrick, C.J., Peters, K., 2007. Response of human endothelial cells to oxidative stress on Ti6Al4V alloy. Biomaterials 28, 806–813.

Turk, M.J., Waters, D.J., Low, P.S., 2004. Folate-conjugated liposomes preferentially target macrophages associated with ovarian carcinoma. Cancer Lett. 213, 165–172.

Weng, H., Zhou, J., Tang, L., Hu, Z., 2004. Tissue responses to thermally-responsive hydrogel nanoparticles. J. Biomater. Sci. Polym. Ed. 15, 1167–1180.

Zhai, Q., Ji, H., Zheng, Z., Yu, X., Sun, L., Liu, X., 2000. Copper induces apoptosis in BA/F3beta cells: Bax, reactive oxygen species, and NFkappaB are involved. J. Cell Physiol. 184, 161–170.

Zhou, J., Hao, G., Weng, H., Tsai, Y., Baker, D.W., Sun, X., Tang, L., 2013. In vivo evaluation of device-associated inflammation using positron emission tomography imaging. Soc. Biomater. Boston, MA.

Zhou, J., Tsai, Y.T., Weng, H., Baker, D.W., Tang, L., 2011. Real time monitoring of biomaterial-mediated inflammatory responses via macrophage-targeting NIR nanoprobes. Biomaterials 32, 9383–9390.

Zhou, J., Tsai, Y.T., Weng, H., Tang, E.N., Nair, A., Dave, D.P., Tang, L., 2012a. Real-time detection of implant-associated neutrophil responses using a formyl peptide receptor-targeting NIR nanoprobe. Int. J. Nanomed. 7, 2057–2068.

Zhou, J., Tsai, Y.T., Weng, H., Tang, L., 2012b. Noninvasive assessment of localized inflammatory responses. Free Radic. Biol. Med. 52, 218–226.

Monitoring fibrous capsule formation

4

S. Maity, A. Sarkar
National Institute of Technology, Yupia, Papum Pare, Arunachal Pradesh, India

4.1 Introduction

The fibrous capsule completely encloses the joint. Its anterior and posterior parts are thin and weak, but collateral ligaments strengthen its sides. The fibrous capsule is attached to the proximal margins of the coronoid and radial fosse anteriorly, but not quite to the superior limit of the olecranon fossa posteriorly. Distally the fibrous capsule is attached to the margins of the trochlear notch, the anterior border of the coronoid process, and the annular ligament. The fibrous capsule of most joints is hyaline in structure, except in those bones that are ossified in membrane where it is composed of fibrocartilage. Hyaline fibrous capsule is vascular, nonnervous, and elastic. On the convex articular surface (male) the cartilage is thickest in the center and thinnest at the periphery. On the concave surface (female), however, it is thinnest in the center and thickest at the periphery. The articular cartilage/fibrous capsule, once damaged, cannot be replaced by hyaline tissue. Replacement is done by fibrous tissue; hence fibrous capsule is indispensable.

4.2 Functions

1. It provides a smooth gliding surface and reduces forces of compression during weight-bearing or muscle action. The coefficient of friction is equal to "ice on ice". The surface of the cartilage is not perfectly smooth and shows fine undulations, which are filled with synovial fluid. In fact, the fibrous capsule is extremely porous and absorbs synovial fluid in the resting condition. When the joint is compressed, the fluid is squeezed out of the cartilage [wiki].
2. It regulates the growth of epiphysis.

4.3 Structure

The fibrous capsule consists of cells and an interlacement of collagen fibers. The surface is cell free and composed essentially of a network of fine fibers. The cells are arranged in three layers, from superficial to deep:

1. Superficial layer: it consists of flattened cells, placed parallel with the articular surface.
2. Intermediate layer: the cartilage cells are rounded and arranged in longitudinal rows.
3. Deep layer: it consists of calcified matrix. Here cartilage cells die and are replaced by bones.

Monitoring and Evaluation of Biomaterials and their Performance in vivo. http://dx.doi.org/10.1016/B978-0-08-100603-0.00004-3

During growth the cartilage cells of the intermediate layer proliferate by mitosis and grow away from the advancing bones. Once growth is over, the number of cells in the fibrous capsule slowly decreases throughout life in relation to the amount of intercellular substance.

4.4 Joint classification

Joints are the weakest parts of the skeleton. Nonetheless, their structure resists various forces, such as crushing or tearing, that threaten to force them out of alignment. Generally, joints can be classified based on two things: (1) the amount of movement at the joint and (2) the type of tissue at the joint. The amount of movement at the joint can be classified in three ways:

1. synarthrotic joint: immovable joint
2. amphiarthrotic joint: immovable joint
3. diarthrotic joint: freely movable joint

The types of tissue at the joint can be classified in the following ways:

1. **Synovial joint**: most joints are synovial joints, and they are usually freely movable (diarthrotic). The ends of bones contain articular cartilage, joint capsule-like fibrous connective tissue surrounding the joint, and the synovial membrane is at the inner lining of the joint capsule. It allows back and forth movement as carpals sliding into one another during wrist movements, folding movement (e.g. elbow joint) and rotation around an axis (e.g. between atlas and axis in the odontoid process). It also acknowledges all movements such as shoulder joint and hip joint except rotation (e.g. between metacarpals amid proximal phalanges, carpals and metacarpals). It is also subdivided into gliding, hinge, pivot, condyloid, saddle, ball, and socket. Synovial joints have five distinguishing features. (1) Articular cartilage: glassy, smooth articular cartilage covers the opposing bone surface. It resists wear and minimizes friction. (2) Joint cavity: the space that is filled with synovial fluid. The synovial membrane covers the surface within the joint capsule and secretes synovial fluid. (3) Articular capsule: the joint cavity is enclosed by a double-layered articular capsule. (4) Synovial fluid: a slippery fluid that occupies all free space within the joint capsule. (5) Reinforcing ligaments are reinforced by a number of ligaments. Some synovial joints, such as hip and knee joints, have fatty pads between the fibrous capsule and the bone. Some have discs or wedges of fibrocartilage separating the articular surface of bones (e.g., menisci of the knee). Some synovial joints have bursa, which is a fluid-filled sac containing the synovial fluid. Ligament: a sheet of strong fibrous connective tissue connecting the articular ends of bones, binding them together and facilitating or limiting motion. Tendon: fibrous connective tissue that attaches muscle to bone.
2. **Cartilaginous joints**: Cartilaginous joints are entirely connected by hyaline cartilage or fibrocartilage cartilage. This type of joint is less movable (amphiarthrotic) but very strong. It is also subdivided into two catagories namely Synchondrosis and Symphysis. When hyaline cartilage (synarthrotic) is used for joint between the first rib and manubrium is known as synchondrosis. Similarly when hyaline cartilage is used at the ends of bones, and a layer of fibrocartilage at the center (amphiarthrotic) is called symphysis (e.g. intervertebraldisk).

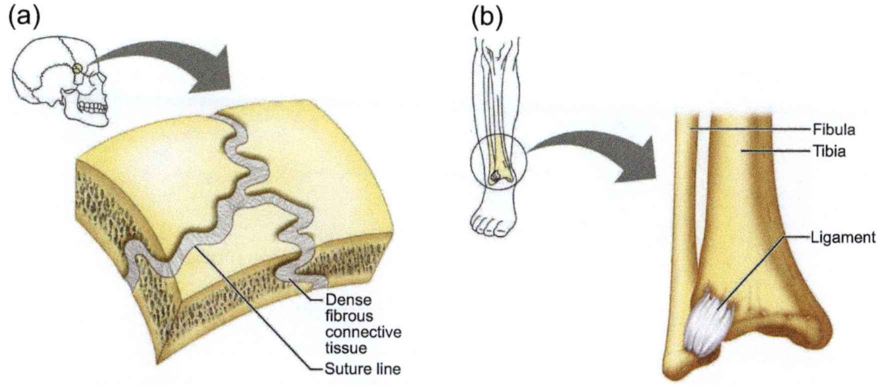

Figure 4.1 Fibrous joint: (a) suture and (b) syndesmosis.
Copyright © 2006 Pearson Education, Inc., publishing as Benjamin Cummings.

3. **Fibrous joints**: It is formed between different bones like cranial bones, tibia and fibula, ulna and radius that have close case contact. The connective tissue of fibrous fastens the mentioned bones tightly. In case of fibrous joint small amount of movement, known as amphiarthrosis or no movements, known as synarthrosis are possible. Fibrous joint are subdevided into the three catagories, as syndesmosis, suture and gomphosis. Among them Fig. 4.1 shows two catagories such as syndesmosis and suture. In fibrous joints syndesmosis is used for interosseous ligaments (amphiarthrotic), suture is used for sutural ligaments (synarthrotic) and gomphosis is used for periodontal ligaments (synarthrotic).

Disorders of joints: the displacement of articulating bones of a joint, as a result of a fall or unusual body movements, is called dislocation. Dislocation results from overstretching or tearing of the connective tissue ligament. Inflammation of the bursa (a sac filled with synovial fluid at the synovial joint) caused by excessive use of a joint is called bursitis. Inflammation of a joint that causes swelling and pain is called arthritis. Rheumatoid arthritis is an autoimmune disease where white blood cells attack the joint tissues, while osteoarthritis is a natural degeneration of joint tissues.

4.5 Fibrous capsule formation

The fibrous membrane of the joint capsule is attached to the circumference of the articular end of each bone entering into the joint and thus entirely surrounds the articulation. It is made up of dense irregular connective tissue [wiki].

There are some fundamental aspects of fibrous capsule formation:

1. **Injury** includes multiple factors, such as the extent of injury, the loss of basement membrane structures, blood–material interactions, provisional matrix formation, the extent or degree of cellular necrosis, and the extent of the inflammatory response. These events, in turn, may affect the extent or degree of granulation tissue formation, foreign body reaction, and fibrosis or fibrous capsule development. With implants, the process of organization with the development of fibrous tissue leads to the well-known fibrous capsule formation at the tissue/material interface. The proliferative capacity of cells within the tissue or organ also plays a role in determining whether resolution or organization occurs. In general, the process of implantation in vascularized tissues leads to organization with fibrous tissue development and fibrous encapsulation.

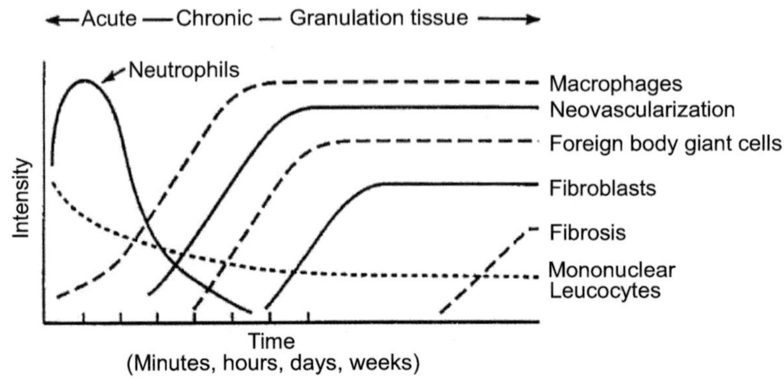

Figure 4.2 The temporal variation in the acute inflammatory response, chronic inflammatory response, granulation tissue development, and foreign body reaction to implanted biomaterials. The intensity and time variables are dependent upon the extent of injury created in the implantation and the size, shape, topography, and chemical and physical properties of the biomaterial.

2. **Temporal sequence of inflammation and wound healing**: In general, the biocompatibility of a material with tissue has been described in terms of the acute and chronic inflammatory responses and of the fibrous capsule formation that is seen over various time periods following implantation [1,2]. The sequence of events following the implantation of a biomaterial is illustrated in Fig. 4.2.
3. **Granulation tissue**: The new, small blood vessels are formed by budding or sprouting of preexisting vessels in a process known as neovascularization or angiogenesis [3–5]. This process involves proliferation, maturation, and organization of endothelial cells into capillary tubes. Fibroblasts also proliferate in developing granulation tissue and are active in synthesizing collagen and proteoglycans. In the early stages of granulation tissue development, proteoglycans predominate; later, however, collagen, especially type I collagen, predominates and forms the fibrous capsule. Some fibroblasts in developing granulation tissue may have features of smooth muscle cells. These cells are called myofibroblasts and are considered to be responsible for the wound contraction seen during the development of granulation tissue.
4. **Fibrosis and fibrous encapsulation**: The end-stage healing response to biomaterials is generally fibrosis or fibrous encapsulation. However, there may be exceptions to this general statement (e.g., porous materials inoculated with parenchymal cells or porous materials implanted into bone). The repair of implant sites involves two distinct processes: regeneration, which is the replacement of injured tissue by parenchymal cells of the same type, or replacement by connective tissue that constitutes the fibrous capsule [6–8]. These processes are generally controlled by either (1) the proliferative capacity of the cells in the tissue or the organ receiving the implant and the extent of injury as it relates to the destruction or (2) persistence of the tissue framework of the implant site. The regenerative capacity of cells permits classification into three groups: labile, stable (or expanding), and permanent (or static) cells. Labile cells continue to proliferate throughout life, stable cells retain this capacity but do not normally replicate, and permanent cells cannot reproduce themselves after birth. Perfect repair with restitution of normal structure theoretically occurs only in tissues consisting of stable and labile cells, whereas all injuries to tissues composed of permanent cells may give rise to fibrosis and fibrous capsule formation, with very little restitution of the normal tissue or organ structure. Tissues composed of permanent cells

(e.g., nerve cells, skeletal muscle cells, and cardiac muscle cells) most commonly undergo an organization of the inflammatory exudate, leading to fibrosis. Tissues composed of stable cells (e.g., parenchymal cells of the liver, kidney, and pancreas), mesenchymal cells (e.g., fibroblasts, smooth muscle cells, osteoblasts, and chrondroblasts), and vascular endothelial and labile cells (e.g., epithelial cells and lymphoid and hematopoietic cells) may also follow this pathway to fibrosis or may undergo resolution of the inflammatory exudate, leading to restitution of the normal tissue structure. The condition of the underlying framework or supporting stroma of the parenchymal cells following an injury plays an important role in the restoration of normal tissue structure. Retention of the framework may lead to restitution of the normal tissue structure, whereas destruction of the framework most commonly leads to fibrosis. It is important to consider the species-dependent nature of the regenerative capacity of cells. For example, cells from the same organ or tissue but from different species may exhibit different regenerative capacities and/or connective tissue repair. Following injury, cells may undergo adaptations of growth and differentiation. Important cellular adaptations are atrophy (decrease in cell size or function), hypertrophy (increase in cell size), hyperplasia (increase in cell number), and metaplasia (change in cell type). Other adaptations include a change in which cells stop producing one family of proteins and start producing another (phenotypic change) or begin a marked overproduction of protein. This may be the case in cells producing various types of collagens and extracellular matrix proteins in chronic inflammation and fibrosis. Causes of atrophy may include decreased workload (e.g., stress-shielding by implants), as well as diminished blood supply and inadequate nutrition (e.g., fibrous capsules surrounding implants). Local and systemic factors may play a role in the wound-healing response to biomaterials or implants. Local factors include the site (tissue or organ) of implantation, the adequacy of blood supply, and the potential for infection. Systemic factors may include nutrition, hematological and immunological derangements, glucocortical steroids, and preexisting diseases such as atherosclerosis, diabetes, and infection.

4.6 Diameters of single-polymer fibers and tissue response

An in vivo study is necessary to assess the sensitivity of fibrous capsule thickness and macrophage density to polymer fiber diameter. Implantation results of single polypropylene fibers of diameters ranging from 2.1 to 26.7 μm in the subcutaneous dorsum of Sprague–Dawley rats at 5 weeks demonstrated reduced fibrous capsule thickness for small fibers. Capsule thickness is 0.6 (±1.8) mm, 11.7 (±12.0) μm, 20.3 (±11.6) μm, and 25.5 (±10.0) μm for fibers in the ranges of 2.1–5.9, 6.5–10.6, 11.1–15.8, and 16.7–26.7 μm, respectively. Fibers very near to blood vessels have smaller capsules [9]. The macrophage density in tissue with fiber diameters 2.1–5.9 μm (23.03 ± 8.67%) is comparable to that of unoperated contralateral control skin (18.72 ± 10.06%). For fibers with diameters in the ranges of 6.5–10.6, 11.1–15.8, and 16.7–26.7 μm, macrophage densities are 33.90 ± 13.08%, 34.40 ± 15.77%, and 41.68 ± 13.98%, respectively, all of which were significantly larger ($p < .002$) than that for the control [10]. The reduced fibrous capsule thickness and macrophage density for small fibers (<6 mm), compared with large fibers, could be due to the reduced cell–material contact surface area or to a curvature threshold effect that triggers cell signaling. The analysis to meshes to evaluate fiber-spacing effects on small fiber biomaterials is important in this regard [11].

4.7 Monitor capsule formation around soft tissue

Piezoelectric sensors have been shown to respond reproducibly to changes in tissue mechanical properties surrounding an implant over a four-month period. A statistically significant change in vibrational amplitude at a frequency corresponding to the radial resonance is seen over time. The significant reduction in amplitude implies the initial period of inflammation, which indicates an increase in viscous dissipation of the tissue. As collagen effects the cellular response, the amplitude starts decreasing. Finally, as the tissue matures, the capsule becomes stiffer, and the viscous dissipation lessens. These results are consistent with qualitative assessments of explanted capsules.

Piezoelectric materials show piezoelectric effect. The piezoelectric effect is a reversible process in that materials exhibiting the direct piezoelectric effect (the internal generation of electrical charge resulting from an applied mechanical force) also exhibit the reverse piezoelectric effect (the internal generation of a mechanical strain resulting from an applied electrical field) [12]. When AC electric field is applied, devices such as the piezoelectric wafer active sensors (PWAS) are oscillated over a spectrum of frequencies[13]. The devices will resonate at a certain frequency and will have a high amplitude of motion. They can be made to possess characteristic motions (resonances) at specific frequencies, as there is a control over the structure of the piezomaterial. The sensor expands at a lower frequency resonance and contracts radially at a higher frequency thickness vibration. The amplitude of vibration changes over the frequency domain when the piezosensor is mechanically coupled with the medium, such as attachment to a rigid object or implantation in soft tissue, and the resonating frequencies of the sensor change as well. Thus both the phenomena constitute an electromechanical impedance shift, which is measured by an impedance analyzer. The impedance changes as the mechanical properties of the tissue surrounding the sensor change. Shear waves are generated when PWAS starts oscillating. And it propagates away from the surface in an exponentially decaying magnitude on the viscosity of the medium and the frequency of oscillation. The viscosity of the medium and the frequency of oscillation are the main factors affecting the rate of decay. For these sensors the interaction depth is calculated to be of order 50 μm at 100 kHz, assuming the viscosity of water. Thus the sensitivity of PWAS is much higher with respect to the variations in mechanical properties of materials to this distance. The amplitude of the radial resonance changes with the change in the viscoelasticity of the tissue surrounding the implant. As the tissue becomes more viscous, it dissipates more of the energy of the PWAS, leading to a damp PWAS amplitude of vibration. In this sense, the PWAS can quantify the relative viscous nature of the tissue during the process of wound healing.

4.7.1 Strain gauges

Strain gauges are complementary to the PWAS sensor, where the contractile force generated by the surrounding tissue is directly measured. The change in resistance of a thin metallic circuit is seen considerably as the circuit is compressed, expanded, or bent and is directly related to the compressive or bending force [14].

4.8 Glucose monitoring in vivo through fluorescent hydrogel fibers

The use of fluorescence-based sensors holds great promise for continuous glucose monitoring in vivo, allowing wireless transdermal transmission and long-lasting functionality in vivo. Here a long-term in vivo glucose monitoring method using glucose-responsive fluorescent hydrogel fibers is discussed. The glucose-responsive fluorescent hydrogel in a fibrous structure is acceptable because this structure enables the sensors to remain at the implantation site for a long period. Moreover, these fibers allow easy control of the number of fluorescent sensors implanted, simply by cutting the fibers to the desired length, and facilitate sensor removal from the implantation site after use. In this particular case the polyethylene glycol-bonded polyacrylamide (PAM) hydrogel fibers reduce inflammation compared with PAM hydrogel fibers, transdermally glowed, and continuously respond to blood glucose concentration changes for up to 140 days, showing their potential application for long-term in vivo continuous glucose monitoring.

The fluorescent hydrogel microfibers can be fabricated using adhesion-resistant polyolefin microcapillaries. After the analysis of the fluorescence intensity in vitro and in vivo the inflammation evaluation and transdermal detection over an extended period is done [15].

4.9 Cellular and molecular composition of fibrous capsules formed around silicone breast implants

Since 1985, much debate has centered around the side effects of silicone breast implants. Therefore the cellular and molecular composition of the fibrous capsule is important. If it has side effects, then the detection is also required. The cellular and molecular composition of fibrous capsules are analyzed when it is removed from patients at various times after surgery for diagnostic purposes (breast cancer relapse) or to relieve painful constrictive fibrosis. Frozen sections of capsule tissue are immunohistochemically stained for subsets of lymphocytes, macrophages, dendritic cells, fibroblasts, and smooth muscle cells, for collagenous and noncollagenous extracellular matrix proteins, for heat shock protein 60 (HSP60), and for adhesion molecules. A massive deposition of fibronectin and tenascin is adjacent to the implant surface. A palisade-like single or multilayered cell accumulation consisting of HSP60+macrophages and HSP60+fibroblasts is there to characterize the capsule/silicone implant contact zone. Mononuclear cell infiltrates consist of activated CD4+T-cells, expressing CD25 and CD45RO, as well as macrophages, which are seen beneath the contact zone and perivascularly. Importantly, many Langerhans-cell-like dendritic cells are found with a predilection at the frontier layer zone abutting the silicone implant. Also, at this site, a massive expression of ICAM-1, but not VCAM-1 or ELAM-1, emerges. Endothelial cells of the intracapsular neovasculature are P-Selectin+. Experiments show that silicone induces a strong local T-cell immune response, and the specificity and function of these T-lymphocytes is a good topic for research.

Histologically, the fibrous capsules (Fig. 4.3) from the above-noted patients showed a three-layered composition:

1. The internal layer abutting the silicone surface appeared to be single/or multilayered. It was previously considered to be exclusively formed by macrophages, but it is now shown to also contain abundant fibroblasts;
2. The layer of loosely arranged connective tissue including the internal vascular supply; and
3. The outer layer of dense connective tissue with the external vascular supply.

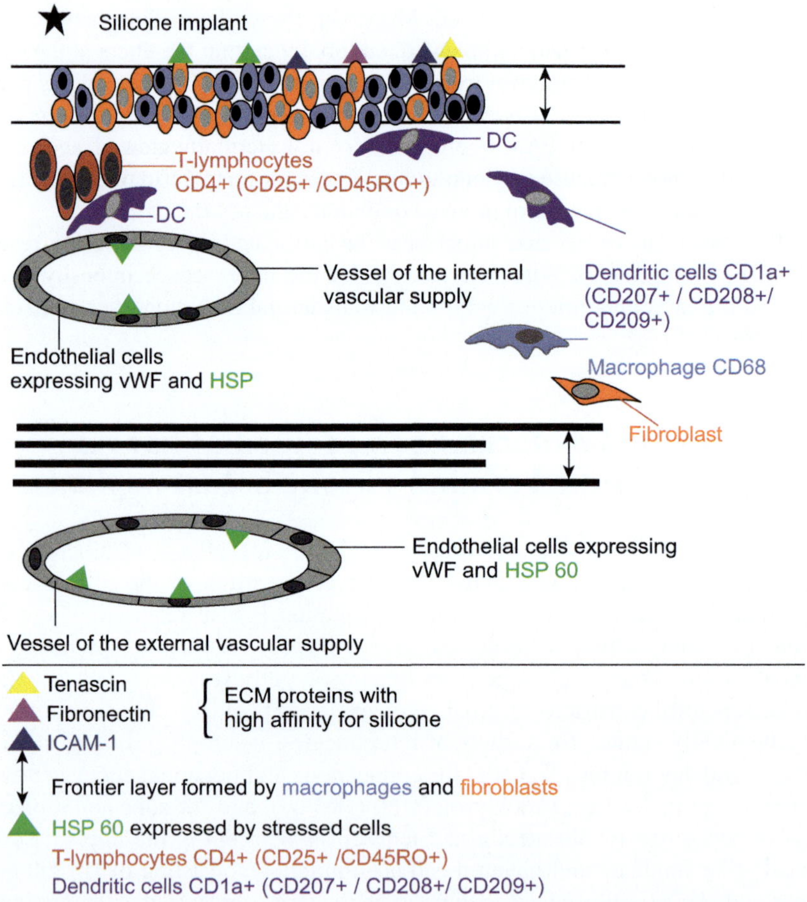

Figure 4.3 The fibrous capsules show a three-layered composition: (a) The internal layer abutting the silicone surface formed by macrophages and fibroblasts, (b) the layer of loosely arranged connective tissue including the internal vascular supply, and (c) the outer layer of dense connective tissue with the external vascular supply. Pronounced infiltration of activated CD4+cells can be documented directly beneath the frontier layer as well as around vessels. Also, constant presence of CD1a+cells in the frontier zone adjacent to the silicone implant as well as next to the accumulations of activated CD4+cells can be shown [16]. The extracellular matrix (ECM) proteins tenascin, fibronectin, as well as the adhesion molecule ICAM-1, and HSP60 are massively expressed by the cells of the frontier layer [17].

4.10 Capsular contracture after two-stage breast reconstruction

Fibrous contracture of the prosthesis capsule is a relatively common complication following breast reconstruction. Etiologic theories have considered periprosthetic infection, hematoma, and a host implant response as possible causes. The occurrence of unilateral capsular contracture contradicts the theory that a host implant reaction is responsible, and many studies have failed to show hematoma as a direct etiologic factor. Several studies suggest that bacterial contamination of the periprosthetic capsule may play a role in causing contracture of permanent breast implants. The subject of microbial growth, both within the saline medium and the periprosthetic tissue around breast implants, has been addressed by a number of authors. Burkhardt et al. cultured a series of capsules at the time of capsulectomy for capsular contracture of breast implants used in augmentation mammoplasty. This group found a positive culture rate of 71%, and an 87% incidence of *Staphylococcus epidermidis*. They suggested that the cause of fibrous capsular contracture is most likely a subacute periprosthetic infection. They also hypothesized that the source of the pathogen may be from the breast ducts, a claim that has been substantiated by studies examining the bacteriology of nipple secretions. Another possible source of capsular colonization is the translocation of bacteria introduced to the lumen from skin during the expansion phase of two-stage reconstruction. A number of authors have reported the viability of bacteria within the intraluminal saline of explanted devices [18,19]. Truppman et al. cultured *S. epidermidis* in the saline of an implant in place for five years. Nordstrom described growth of *Serratia marcescens* in the saline of tissue expanders. Liang et al. described a patient in which cultures from within and external to a tissue expander grew *Pseudomonas aeruginosa*. Peters et al. described cultures from the saline within Simaplast implants which grew *Staphylococcus cohnii*, *Proprionibacacterium acnes*, and *Diphtheroid* species. The possibility of transmigration of pathogens from the lumen to the periprosthetic environment has also been addressed. Periprosthetic capsular contracture continues to be a difficult problem associated with breast reconstruction. A number of etiologic theories have been studied in an effort to prove factors such as infection, premastectomy irradiation, duration of the prosthesis operation, the patient's menopausal state, and the presence of hematoma as causal to capsular contracture. To prevent this complication, it is necessary to identify the primary mechanism responsible. This study examined periprosthetic colonization of the tissue expander and its possible role in contributing to capsular contracture of the permanent implant placed at the second stage of breast reconstruction [20].

4.11 Graphene-based biosensor for future perspectives

Graphene nano structure (GN) and its related derivatives have attracted the interest of bioscience/biotechnologies [21–24] because of their physiochemical and electric–electronic properties. Particularly, these exceptional values include high surface area (2630 m2/g)

Table 4.1 Properties of graphene compared with other carbonaceous materials

	Graphene	Carbon nanotube	Fullerene	Graphite
Dimensions	2	1	0	3
Hybridization	sp^2	Mostly sp^2	Mostly sp^2	sp^2
Tenacity	Flexible, elastic	Flexible, elastic	Elastic	Flexible, nonelastic
Hardness	Highest (for single layer)	High	High	High
Electrical conductivity (S/cm)	~2000	Structure-dependent	10^{-10}	Anisotropic: $2–3 \times 10^4$
Experimental SSA (m^2/g)	~1500	~1300	80–90	~10–20
Thermal conductivity (W/m/K)	4840–5300	3500	0.4	Anisotropic: 1500–2000

[25], excellent electrical conductivity (1738 S/m) [26], strong mechanical strength (about 1100 GPa) [27], good thermal conductivity (5000 W/m/K) [28], high charge carrier mobility (about 10,000 cm2 V—1 s—1) [29], good optical transparency (~97.7%) [30], and ease of biological as well as chemical functioning of graphene [31]. It is really a great opportunity to design a graphene-based sensor for wide application in the biomedical field due to its physiochemical properties [32]. A summary of the key properties of GN compared to its related carbon materials has been provided in Table 4.1 [33].

Herein, the overview of the applications of GN in biomedical fields are briefed, and it is an updated comprehensive work to those described in the reviews mentioned earlier, rather than an attempt to give a systematic and detailed review of this field. Graphene is accepted for different biosensing applications including DNA, glucose, hemoglobin (Hb), and cholesterol biosensors, drug and gene delivery, and cancer therapy. So graphene has potential applications in tissue engineering and fibrous capsule monitoring [34].

References

[1] Spector M, Cease C, Tong-Li X. Crit Rev Biocompat 1989;5:269–95.

[2] Wokalek H, Ruh H. J Biomater Appl 1991;5:337–62.

[3] Maciag T. In: DeVita VT, Hellman S, Rosenberg S, editors. Important advances in oncology. Philadelphia: Lippincott; 1990. p. 85.

[4] Thompson JA, Anderson KD, DiPetro JM, Zweibel JA, Zmaetta M, et al. Science 1988;241:1349–52.

[5] Ziats NP, Miller KM, Anderson JM. Biomaterials 1988;9:5–13.
[6] Cotran RZ, Kumar V, Robbins SL. In: Pathologic basis of disease. 6th. ed Philadelphia: Saunders; 1999. p. 50–112.
[7] Clark RAF, Henson PM. In: The molecular and cellular biology of wound repair. New York: Plenum Publishing; 1988.
[8] Hunt TK, Heppenstall RB, Pines E, Rovee D. In: Soft and hard tissue repair. New York: Praeger Scientific; 1984.
[9] Karp RD, Johnson KH, Buoen LC, Ghobrial HKG, Brand I, Brand KG. Tumorigenesis by Millipore filters in mice: histology and ultrastructure of tissue reactions as related to pore size. J Natl Cancer Inst 1973;51:1275–85.
[10] Campbell CE, Von Recum AF. Microtopography and soft tissue response. J Invest Surg 1989;2:51–74.
[11] Sanders JE, Stiles CE, Hayes CL. Tissue response to single-polymer fibers of varying diameters: evaluation of fibrous encapsulation and macrophage density. © 2000 John Wiley & Sons, Inc J Biomed Mater Res 2000;52:231–7.
[12] Wiki. https://en.wikipedia.org/wiki/Piezoelectricity.
[13] Giurgintiu V, Zagrai A. Characterization of piezoelectric wafer active sensors. J Intell Mater Syst Struct 2000;11:959–76.
[14] Bender JW, Friedman HI, Giurgiutiu V, Watson C, Fitzmaurice M, Yost ML. The use of biomedical sensors to monitor capsule formation around soft tissue implants. Ann Plast Surg January 2006;56(1):72–7. 2005 Lippincott Williams & Wilkins.
[15] Heo YJ, Shibata H, Okitsu T, Kawanishi T, Takeuchi S. Long-term in vivo glucose monitoring using fluorescent hydrogel fibers. PNAS August 16, 2011;108(33):13399–403.
[16] Wolfram D, Rainer C, Niederegger H, Piza H, Wick G. Cellular and molecular composition of fibrous capsules formed around silicone breast implants with special focus on local immune reactions. W. Dolores et al J Autoimmun 2004;23:81–91.
[17] Dolores W, et al. J Autoimmun 2004;23:81–91.
[18] Holmes JD. Capsular contracture after breast reconstruction with tissue expansion. Br J Plast Surg 1989;42:591–4.
[19] Shah Z, Lehman JA, Tan J. Does infection play a role in breast capsular contracture? Plast Reconstr Surg 1981;68:34–42.
[20] Macadam SA, Clugston PA, Germann ET. Retrospective case review of capsular contracture after two-stage breast reconstruction. Ann Plast Surg 2004;53:420–4.
[21] Wang Y, Li Z, Wang J, Li J, Lin Y. Graphene and graphene oxide: biofunctionalization and applications in biotechnology. Trends Biotechnol 2011;29(5):205–12.
[22] Avouris P, Dimitrakopoulos C. Graphene: synthesis and applications. Mater Today 2012;15(3):86–97.
[23] Chen CH, Lin CT, Hsu WL, Chang YC, Yeh SR, Li LJ, et al. A flexible hydrophilic-modified graphene microprobe for neural and cardiac recording. Nanomed Nanotechnol Biol Med 2013;9(5):600–4.
[24] Zhu Y, Murali S, Cai W, Li X, Suk JW, Potts JR, et al. Graphene and graphene oxide: synthesis, properties, and applications. Adv Mater 2010;22(35):3906–24.
[25] Weiss NO, Zhou H, Liao L, Liu Y, Jiang S, Huang Y, et al. Graphene: an emerging electronic material. Adv Mater 2012;24(43):5782–825.
[26] An X, Butler TW, Washington M, Nayak SK, Kar S. Optical and sensing properties of 1 pyrenecarboxylic acid-functionalized graphene films laminated on polydimethylsiloxane membranes. ACS Nano 2011;5(2):1003–11.
[27] Balandin AA, Ghosh S, Bao W, Calizo I, Teweldebrhan D, Miao F, et al. Superior thermal conductivity of single-layer graphene. Nano Lett 2008;8(3):902–7.

[28] Bolotin KI, Sikes KJ, Jiang Z, Klima M, Fudenberg G, Hone J, et al. Ultrahigh electron mobility in suspended graphene. Solid State Commun 2008;146(9):351–5.
[29] Bonaccorso F, Sun Z, Hasan T, Ferrari AC. Graphene photonics and optoelectronics. Nat Photonics 2010;4(9):611–22.
[30] Georgakilas V, Otyepka M, Bourlinos AB, Chandra V, Kim N, Kemp KC, et al. Functionalization of graphene: covalent and non-covalent approaches, derivatives and applications. Chem Rev 2012;112(11):6156–214.
[31] Chung C, Kim YK, Shin D, Ryoo S-R, Hong BH, Min D-H. Biomedical applications of graphene and graphene oxide. Acc Chem Res 2013;46(10):2211–24.
[32] Li H, Xu C, Srivastava N, Banerjee K. Carbon nanomaterials for next-generation interconnects and passives: physics, status, and prospects. IEEE Trans Electron Devices 2009;56(9):1799–821.
[33] Raccichini R, Varzi A, Passerini S, Scrosati B. The role of graphene for electrochemical energy storage. Nat Mater 2015;14:271–9.
[34] Celik N, Balachandran W, Manivannan N. Graphene-based biosensors: methods, analysis and future perspective. IET Circuits Devices Syst 2015;9(6):434–45.

Monitoring biomineralization of biomaterials in vivo

5

N. Mehrban[1], J. Bowen[2]
[1]University College London, London, United Kingdom; [2]The Open University, Walton Hall, Milton Keynes, United Kingdom

5.1 Introduction

Changes in physiological chemistry and morphology are caused by a number of factors including pH, mechanical stresses induced by the natural movement of tissue, and proteins excreted by surrounding cells and tissues, all of which can lead to mineralization. While healthy tissue follow a specific mineralization process, diseased and damaged tissue often require external intervention. For mineralized tissue, often this intervention is in the form of surgery and when this fails, biomaterials can be introduced to the wound site in the hope that the materials will integrate with surrounding healthy tissue and provide mechanical stability, thus restoring the patient's health.

Biomineralization is a dynamic process with distinct phases, and the monitoring techniques for these events must be able to detect the chemical and physical changes occurring. Although in vitro experiments can supply us with a wealth of knowledge on how these conditions may affect the biomaterial, both individually and in combination, it is difficult to translate these data to in vivo environments due to the increased chemical and mechanical complexity.

In this chapter, we describe the biomineralization process and explain how in vitro research can help us to identify the natural repair process of damaged mineralized tissue. We also describe how technological advancements have improved our ability to probe deeper into understanding this repair process and how noninvasive clinical technologies have become faster, safer, and cheaper to use, while also providing more accurate data. These data can be directly translated into creating better materials for repairing damaged tissue and improving patient care with minimal discomfort.

It should be noted that the field of in vivo biomaterial monitoring is one that is rapidly changing with existing technologies being merged and new analysis methods created at a very fast pace. Readers should therefore not treat the technologies described herein as an exhaustive list of those currently available. This chapter is intended to provide a taste of the range of techniques in use today.

5.2 Biomineralization

Biomineralization is the formation of inorganic solid materials from an ionic source in biology. This can occur in two ways: crystal growth on an organic matrix, as is

Monitoring and Evaluation of Biomaterials and their Performance in vivo. http://dx.doi.org/10.1016/B978-0-08-100603-0.00005-5

the case for many animals, or extracellular/intercellular mineral aggregate formation, as in certain algae and bacteria (Lowenstam, 1981). While mineral aggregation in the aforementioned algae and bacterial examples lead to random crystal orientation, the skeletons of mammals, for example, exhibit an ordered crystal structure, with some or total alignment (Lowenstam, 1981). Biomineralization also occurs in marine organisms such as diatoms (Poulsen et al., 2003), corals (Silva et al., 2012), and echinoderms (Vidavsky et al., 2015); its role ranging from protection to buoyancy and directing movement (Addadi et al., 2012). The precise structural organization, i.e., crystal orientation, spacing, and size, depends on the chemical and physical environment surrounding the site of initial crystal growth.

The human skeleton is an intricate network of moving parts, which come together to form complex machinery. Bone is composed of inorganic apatite, of which hydroxyapatite is the main form, as well as type I collagen, osteoblasts, osteoclasts, osteocytes, and a small percentage of other proteins, including proteoglycans, glycoproteins, osteocalcin, and osteonectin (Florencio-Silva et al., 2015).

In the formation of bone the process begins with the release of minerals by osteoblasts and their anionic–cationic pair bonding. These ions form aggregates, which condense and form an amorphous phase. Guided by their chemical and physical surroundings, for example, protein interactions and pH, these structures then align and order to produce lattices within a crystal. The first crystal formed in this way provides a nucleation point for other crystals to grow and form biomineralized tissue. Osteoclasts are responsible for bone resorption while osteocytes form a connective lattice throughout the structure, although their role also includes the production of nerve growth factors post bone trauma, i.e., the generation of chemical signals to start the bone formation process and as general phosphate metabolism regulators (Sims and Gooi, 2008). The resorption of minerals occurs via multinucleated osteoclasts (Baslé et al., 1993). Once attached, osteoclasts surround themselves with a clear/sealing zone of actin where they release protons and acid hydrolases to digest the bone (Chambers and Fuller, 2011). The human body is constantly remodeling the hard tissue through osteoclast resorption and osteoblast deposition in a process known as ossification (Vanden Bossche and Vanderstraeten, 2005). In contrast, human oral biomaterials form via dentinogenesis (Linde and Goldberg, 1993), the production of dentine, and amelogenesis (Rönnholm, 1962), the production of enamel. Dentine development can continue throughout life, similar to bone, whereas enamel development only occurs prior to the emergence of a tooth.

5.3 Disruption to the biomineralization process and tissue engineering

Ossification can occur in two ways: either intramembranous, through mesenchyme replacement, or endochondral, from the growth of a cartilage model. When bone undergoes slight damage, such as a hairline fracture, a slow healing process is started. This begins as an inflammatory response consisting of an influx of inflammatory cells, formation of granular tissue, and the migration of mesenchymal stem cells and vascular tissue growth. This is followed by repair, which entails the enhancement of vascular ingrowth, collagen formation, and mineralization into a callus, and finally remodeling, incorporating resorption and deposition processes (Minkin and Marinho, 1999). Natural healing can take months to years to complete (Sims, 2008), although when the trauma is significant, either due to disease (such as bone metastasis, i.e., malignant bone tumor) or blunt force, this may not occur at all and the tissue is considered to be damaged beyond repair.

Surgery attempts to address some of the issues, for example, the use of prosthetic titanium replacements to provide mechanical strength at the site of injury and the use of cement, fixation pins, and screws to hold the tissue together (Bonfante and Ceolho, 2016). However, these materials lack cellular compatibility and do not aid the formation of new, healthy mineralized tissue (Bonfante and Ceolho, 2016). Furthermore, some of the surgical repair methods create further problems, such as ectopic bone formation following total hip replacement, and require more surgery and patient discomfort.

None of the current prevention and repair methods are adequate, and patients often suffer from severely reduced mobility (Boeckstyns, 2014). It is at this point, where existing gold-standard methods fail, that tissue engineering offers an alternative. Here cells/materials/drugs may be introduced to the wound site and, unlike titanium implants, they integrate with the surrounding tissue promoting the formation of new healthy tissue (Naderi et al., 2011). While many cells, materials, drugs, or combinations of all of these are researched heavily for the formation of mineralized tissue, the key to successful tissue engineering is providing a nontoxic environment to serve as a bridge between the native tissue and the damaged areas.

5.4 Biomaterials for the repair of mineralized tissue

For better integration, i.e., to support the growth of healthy cells, which integrate with the surrounding environment and restore the original functional role of the tissue without inducing cytotoxic effects on the body, it is necessary to use biomaterials that actively promote the formation of new tissue. Modification of the original titanium plates and pins led to the development of apatite-coated implants. Apatites refer to a group of phosphate minerals including hydroxyapatite, fluorapatite, and chlorapatite. As they are also the major components in bone, they are the obvious choice of replacement material and as such have been used to coat implants through techniques such as plasma spraying (Geesink et al., 1988) and selective laser melting (Mróz et al., 2015).

Another approach to repair mineralized tissue is to develop biodegradable materials, which break down into harmless constituents as healthy cells grow and populate the surrounding space. For this purpose hard scaffolds, based on calcium phosphate and apatite, have been used to provide a bone-like substitute, as well as soft materials, such as hydrogels, for their well-known cellular compatibility characteristics.

The engineering, or regenerative, approach is heavily reliant on understanding how native bones develop over time, their nanocomposite nature, their role in the body, and how their movement and chemistry is both affected by, and equally affects, the surrounding tissue. Once this is understood, the biomaterial can be chemically and physically adapted to suit the requirement. Passive biomaterials are designed to ensure that the natural mineralization process in the body is not disrupted upon implantation (i.e., biomaterials that are not functionalized with chemical cues). In contrast, active biomaterials promote the formation of mineral crystals by promoting attachment and differentiation in bone cells. However, one of the main problems in introducing bone-like scaffolds into the body is the production of fibrous tissue through scar formation (fibrosis), which inhibits integration between the native tissue and the implant material, leading to inflammation. It is therefore necessary to not only create a biomaterial which mimics mineralized tissue and promotes new tissue formation but also to monitor the integration of the material with the surrounding tissue.

5.5 In vitro characterization of biomineralization

The analysis of biomaterials must begin at an in vitro level to better understand material characteristics, how they will behave in an in vivo-like environment, and minimize the use of animals. Often these techniques are employed as end-point analyses. For this reason, many in vitro methods for assessing biomineralization are destructive. A brief overview of these techniques has been provided in the following section. It should be noted that these techniques can all be applied to ex vivo samples also. The techniques are presented in order of increasing spatial resolution. The actual spatial resolution for each technique is not quoted, as this will vary with the configuration of a particular instrument, e.g., lens magnification, detector pixel density, as well as the refractive index of the media with which it interacts.

5.5.1 Histology

Histology is one of the oldest and most popular means of assessing biomineralization and a perfect example of a qualitative but destructive in vitro technique for the identification of biomineralized tissue. Extensive sample manipulation through chemical fixation and processing (from embedding through to sectioning) before staining and imaging is required (Carleton et al., 1980), which can be time-consuming. Although sample preparation is extensive and laborious, requiring some level of experience, it is cheap and therefore popular among researchers. The dyes used in histology are either acidic or basic, and their use depends on the chemistry of the target tissue. Thus they can be used to highlight specific regions within tissues, i.e., intra- or extracellular components. Once dyed, high magnification images are taken using traditional bright-field microscopy techniques.

Specifically for biomineralization a further limitation of histology is that, depending on the stain used, a demineralizing step may also be required which defeats the purpose of staining for mineral content (Carleton et al., 1980). The most common biomineralization stains are Von Kossa, Alizarin Red, Safranin O, Picrosirius Red, Aniline Blue, Masson's Trichrome, and Sanderson's Bone Stain (Horobin and Kiernan, 2002).

5.5.2 Microradiography

Using X-rays absorbed by dense bone, high-resolution radiographic images can be generated of mineralized tissue slices (Darling et al., 2009). First used to histomorphometrically study bone in the 1950s the technique allowed quantification of mineral tissue. Since then microradiography (MR) has been successfully used to identify specific minerals in teeth (de Josselin de Jong et al., 1987) and to detect mineralized tissue boundaries (Schortinghuis et al., 2003).

Typically for MR the excised samples to be analyzed must be between 150 μm and 180 μm thick (Donath and Breuner, 1982), which are achieved through sectioning. X-rays directed toward the sample are absorbed at varying rates depending on the density of the different areas within the tissue. The transmitted radiation intensities are imaged in black and white on photographic film, producing a micrograph. Advances in technology have superseded the use of radiographic emulsions, and now images are captured digitally and projected directly onto screens. MR is a quick analysis method producing images at high resolution (micron-level) and is ideal for identifying the different mineral states that occur during biomineralization.

5.5.3 Fluorescent microscopy

To observe changes in biomineralization, other imaging techniques may also be used, such as fluorescent microscopy. Here samples are irradiated at a specific wavelength (excitation), and while some radiation is absorbed by the sample, some is reflected/emitted back toward a detector (emission) (van Gaalen et al., 2010). Some tissues autofluoresce (such as the weak autofluorescence of tooth enamel, Pautke et al., 2007), while others require the attachment of specific markers (fluorochromes/fluorophores), which bind to the target and emit fluorescence at a specific wavelength (Lee et al., 2003). For the visualization of biological species, fluorochromes exist as fluorescing antibodies, which bind to the target. By targeting specific proteins or minerals via fluorochrome labeling, individual biomineralization events may be observed over time. Fluorochromes used for bone studies include tetracycline (Canalis and Lechago, 1982; Pautke et al., 2010a,b), xylenol orange (Wang et al., 2006), alizarin red (Moester et al., 2014), and calcein green (Fu et al., 2012). The main disadvantage of using fluorescent dyes is that the colors observed may overlap, making it difficult to discriminate between the different targeted sites (Pautke et al., 2005). Furthermore, photobleaching, the fading or photochemical alteration of the fluorescence, leads to signals getting weaker over time.

5.5.4 Infrared spectrometry and Raman spectroscopy

Infrared (IR) spectroscopy uses IR light to provide information regarding the chemical composition of materials and material surfaces (Banwell and McCash, 1994). Chemical bonds absorb IR light at specific frequencies if there is a change in the dipole moment of the bond due to a positional or conformational change, i.e., a vibration. Each vibration is associated with a specific frequency in the IR spectrum, which depends on the masses and bonding between the two atoms that form the chemical bond. These frequencies are used for the identification of specific chemical bonds. IR spectroscopy has been used extensively in the characterization of biomineralization involving calcium species (Addadi et al., 1987, 2003). In contrast to IR spectroscopy, Raman spectroscopy is concerned with the polarizability of molecules. Here chemical bond information is obtained without undergoing a change in dipole moment. Raman spectroscopy utilizes the phenomenon of light scattering to provide information regarding the chemical composition of materials and material surfaces (Smith and Dent, 2005), producing a chemical "fingerprint" of the sample. Both IR and Raman spectroscopy can be combined with optical microscopy to permit two-dimensional (2-D) and three-dimensional (3-D) imaging of a sample, providing a spatially resolved grid of spectra with location-specific fingerprinting of chemical bonds (Carden and Morris, 2000).

5.5.5 X-ray diffraction

X-ray diffraction (XRD) utilizes electromagnetic radiation with wavelengths comparable to the interatomic spacing of atoms in crystal lattices on the order 10^{-10} m (Elliott and Gibson, 1974). X-rays interact with atomic nuclei, creating a diffraction pattern, which can be recorded and analyzed to determine the spatial distribution of atoms in the crystal from which the diffraction occurred. Three-dimensional information is obtained by rotating the sample relative to the incident electron beam. Hence XRD is used for the identification of the atomic and molecular structures of crystals.

XRD has been used extensively for the characterization of crystalline biomaterials, including calcium carbonates, silica, and apatites (Königsberger and Königsberger, 2006; Naka and Carney, 2006; DiMasi and Gower, 2014; Aparicio and Ginebra, 2015). Studies of collagen and apatite have proven particularly useful, revealing structural information regarding the interactions between these two key constituents of bone during the mineralization process (Drouet, 2013; Matsugaki and Nakano, 2014; Tao et al., 2015; Tomoaia and Pasca, 2015).

5.5.6 Transmission and scanning electron microscopy

Electron microscopes (EMs) use beams of electrons, exhibiting shorter wavelengths than visible light, for visualizing surfaces. The two types of EM are scanning electron microscopy (SEM) and transmission electron microscopy (TEM). Both SEM and TEM require sample preparation, including immobilization. SEM has a much better depth of focus than light microscopy, with images formed by scanning the electron beam across the sample surface. For this technique, it is common to coat the sample surface with a thin metal film, which acts as an electron reflector and provides a path to the ground. In TEM a beam of electrons is passed through a very thin section of material, typically hundreds of nanometers in thickness. The detector displays where the electrons passed through the sample and where they did not. TEM sample preparation procedures can be time-consuming and highly specific for certain material types.

For example, organic materials require metallic stains such as uranyl acetate/lead citrate or potassium permanganate (Lewis and Knight, 1992). Alternative forms of EM have been developed to overcome issues related to sample preparation, such as dehydration. Cryogenic EM allows the samples to be frozen in a hydrated environment, thus mimicking the in vivo environment more closely (Carragher et al., 2015). Using this technique, Hendley et al. (2015) describe crystal formation and development of the different apatitic phases. However, freezing can also cause sample damage and therefore methods that avoid the freezing technique altogether have been developed. AirSEM allows samples to be imaged in air and does not require them to be coated (Han et al., 2015), while liquid-phase TEM allows imaging in a cell filled with liquid (Nielsen et al., 2014). Other advances in EM technology have led to the use of immunogold labeling, which allows specific proteins within the sample to be targeted (Mass et al., 2014) and the stitching of sequential TEM slices to render a 3-D image of the sample (Midgley and Weyland, 2003).

Selected-area electron diffraction (SAED) provides localized crystallographic information at high resolution and is performed inside EMs (Williams and Carter, 2009). Electrons pass through thin sample sections, their trajectories being altered by interactions with the atomic structure of the sample. The resultant diffraction pattern can be analyzed to determine the structure of the sample material. In conjunction with Raman spectroscopy, SAED has been used for the identification of calcite crystals isolated from the pineal gland (Baconnier et al., 2002).

5.5.7 Energy dispersive X-ray spectrometry and electron energy-loss spectroscopy

Energy-dispersive X-ray spectroscopy (EDX) is used to analyze the elemental composition of solid surfaces. X-ray emission is stimulated by the irradiation of the surface with a high energy beam of charged particles or a focused X-ray beam. Excitation of the electronic structure of an atom can produce an X-ray emission, the energy signature of which is a unique characteristic of each element. Therefore a "fingerprint" or "signature" spectrum can be obtained allowing element identification via comparison with reference spectra. Electron microscopes often contain the instrumentation to perform EDX analysis, as the technology required to generate a high energy beam of charged particles, i.e., electrons, is already present. Electron energy-loss spectroscopy (EELS) requires the use of electrons with much lower energies than EDX, typically a beam of 100–1000 eV energy. These electrons are detected upon their reflection from a surface, and the loss of energy due to their interaction with the surface material is used to determine information regarding its chemical structure. Similarly to XRD, EDX and EELS are used extensively for the characterization of crystalline biomaterials (Königsberger and Königsberger, 2006; Naka and Carney, 2006; DiMasi and Gower, 2014; Aparicio and Ginebra, 2015).

5.5.8 Atomic force microscopy

Atomic force microscopy (AFM) is a technique which maps the surface of a material using a microfabricated cantilever as a scanning probe. A piezoelectric scanner is used to create precision nanoscale displacements of the sample and cantilever. A laser beam, typically a red or infrared laser, is used to monitor the cantilever movement as the cantilever and sample are scanned relative to each other. Laser light is reflected off the flexible, free end of the cantilever, onto a position-sensitive photodetector. The feedback system is used to maintain the cantilever's vertical motion at a set point value, permitting the acquisition of surface topography during scanning. The sensitivity afforded by this technique provides imaging resolution at the nanometer scale. As well as the resolution this technique allows, the samples may be analyzed in both dried and hydrated conditions, and therefore offers a significant advantage over techniques such as histology and EM. Sample preparation for AFM is mostly associated with reducing the possibility for mechanical motion. For biomineralization, this technology can potentially capture the different phases of mineralization over time (Habraken et al., 2013; Hamm et al., 2014). A variation in this technique is dynamic force microscopy, whereby the cantilever tip can be functionalized to interact with the sample surface and provide force and chemical bond information. Collectively these data may provide information on chemical moieties and functional groups present on the sample and how they change over time.

5.5.9 Atom probe tomography

Atom probe tomography (APT) requires samples to be milled to a sharp point before using a pulsed laser to induce atom evaporation, and therefore sample preparation is extensive. However, the imaging resolution is less than 1 nm and the technique offers atomic level information to be obtained (Miller et al., 2012). Other than sample preparation, the main limitations of this technique are (1) the small size of sample that can be analyzed and (2) that the technique is destructive. APT utilizes a position-sensitive detector to reconstruct the location of atoms, affording 3-D structural information. Apatites (Gordon et al., 2012) and the organic/inorganic interface (Gordon and Joester, 2011) are common topics for study using APT.

5.6 In vivo characterization of biomineralization

While these techniques provide a wealth of information about biomaterials, often both in vitro and in vivo techniques are employed to better understand the changes biomaterials undergo in different environments (Mehrban et al., 2013). In vivo experiments are further complicated by the lack of control of the surrounding environment. Implanted biomaterials may be affected by changes in pH, temperature, mechanical stresses (Ananth et al., 2015), proteins deposited by the surrounding cells (Mehrban et al., 2013), and enzymes (Zelzer et al., 2013). The immune response of the host organism when a foreign body is implanted is also a factor for consideration (Major et al., 2015). Furthermore, reducing the need for repeated surgery and patient discomfort and increasing safety are priorities in selecting appropriate analysis techniques. Advances in technology have greatly expanded the number of techniques that now meet these requirements. An overview of these techniques, although not an exhaustive list, has been provided. Once again, the techniques are presented in order of increasing spatial resolution.

5.6.1 Radiography

Radiography is an X-ray-based technique. Initial film-based radiography used layered film cassettes to detect X-rays attenuated by absorption and scattering effects on the target tissue, depending on the tissue's density, thickness, and composition. The film cassettes contain a screen consisting of a fluorescent coating, which emits light as X-rays pass through the tissue and interact with it. These rays then expose areas on the photographic layer of the cassette, which is developed by automated chemical photograph processing techniques. Thus radiography is a 2-D imaging technique. The development of computed radiography, and a phosphor-coated imaging plate (Moore, 1980), eliminated the use of films and allowed the production of digital radiographs. Once X-rays are captured on the plate it is then "read" using a helium–neon laser which emits lights. Emitted light is captured by a photomultiplier tube and a digital image is produced (Fig. 5.1). The main advantage of computed radiography over the initial film-based system is that the receptor may be erased and used repeatedly. Current radiographic imaging systems are purely digital, i.e., no cassette or plate is required. The X-rays are detected electronically and an image is produced by direct read-out detectors, making the technique faster and less costly. To produce live images fluoroscopy may also be employed, wherein X-rays are continuously detected by a fluorescing screen, which amplifies the signal and produces an image on a monitor (Körner et al., 2007).

Images produced through radiography are black, white, and gray with everything appearing black where little of the X-ray beam is attenuated. Thus dense tissues, such as bone, appear white on the final image. With such high contrast, the availability of radiography, its cheap running costs, the speed at which a scan may be made, and the relatively simple equipment used, it remains a popular technique for examining bone damage and defects (Geusens et al., 2014). For the analysis of biomaterials and biomineralization, it is possible radiography may serve as an initial screening test for radio-dense areas but may be better coupled to more sensitive techniques, such as X-ray computed tomography (Wojtowicz et al., 2010; Seto et al., 2012). Furthermore, as an X-ray-based technique the ionizing radiation poses a health risk to patients and as such the X-ray beam and duration of test must be tightly controlled (Einstein et al., 2016).

5.6.2 Ultrasound

For this imaging technique, ultrasonic waves are produced by stimulating a piezoelectric crystal: the transducer (Ventura et al., 2014). These waves are pulsed toward the target area and while some of the waves will be absorbed or refracted, some are backscattered and received as an echo by the transducer. The echoes are converted to electrical impulses, which are then shown as an image on an oscilloscope (Appel et al., 2013).

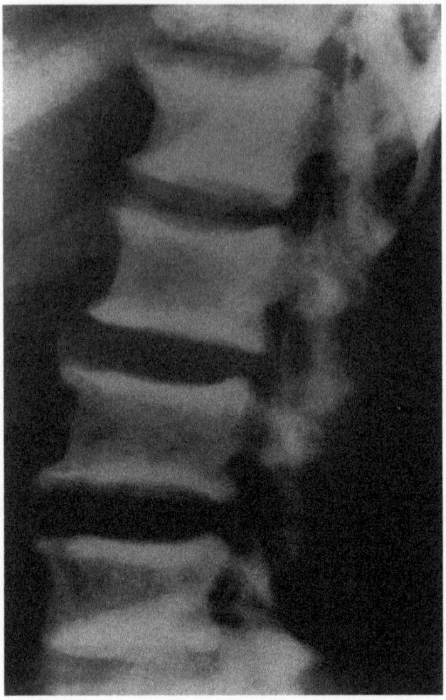

Figure 5.1 X-ray of lumbar spine illustrating the osteosclerosis of fluoritic patients. Reproduced from Boivin, G., Chavassieux, P., Chapuy, M.C., Baud, C.A., Meunier, P.J. 1989. Skeletal fluorosis: histomorphometric analysis of bone changes and bone fluoride content in 29 patients. Bone 10, 89–99, Fig. 1.

The time taken for an echo to be detected and the signal strength (known collectively as the A-mode) can be used to develop 2-D images (B-mode), which can then be stacked to produce 3-D images. By using higher frequencies (20–60 MHz), high-resolution images may be produced (Deng et al., 2016), while by using a number of detectors to increase the capture rate, "real-time" images can be created (Chan et al., 2016). Grayscale ultrasound displays the echo amplitude or signal intensity as different shades of gray in the captured frame and has been used to image extracellular matrix proteins in a range of biomaterials (Chapman-Jones et al., 1998; Kreitz et al., 2011), including mineral formation (Karjalainen et al., 2009; Hoffmeister et al., 2002; Gudur et al., 2012) (Fig. 5.2). The success of grayscale ultrasonography is highly dependent on the system used and the operator as both the setup and analysis can vary (Lizzi et al., 1997).

Quantitative ultrasound techniques also exist (based on the analysis of the initial radio frequency data collected), allowing researchers to acquire more data fast, safely, and cheaply. In a similar way, ultrasound technology has also been used to acquire mechanical data. This form is often referred to as ultrasound elasticity imaging or elastography (Chung et al., 2015; Greenleaf et al., 2003) and involves imaging before and after a compressive load has been applied to the region of interest (Bilgen and Insana, 1996). This is particularly useful for imaging areas of hard tissue

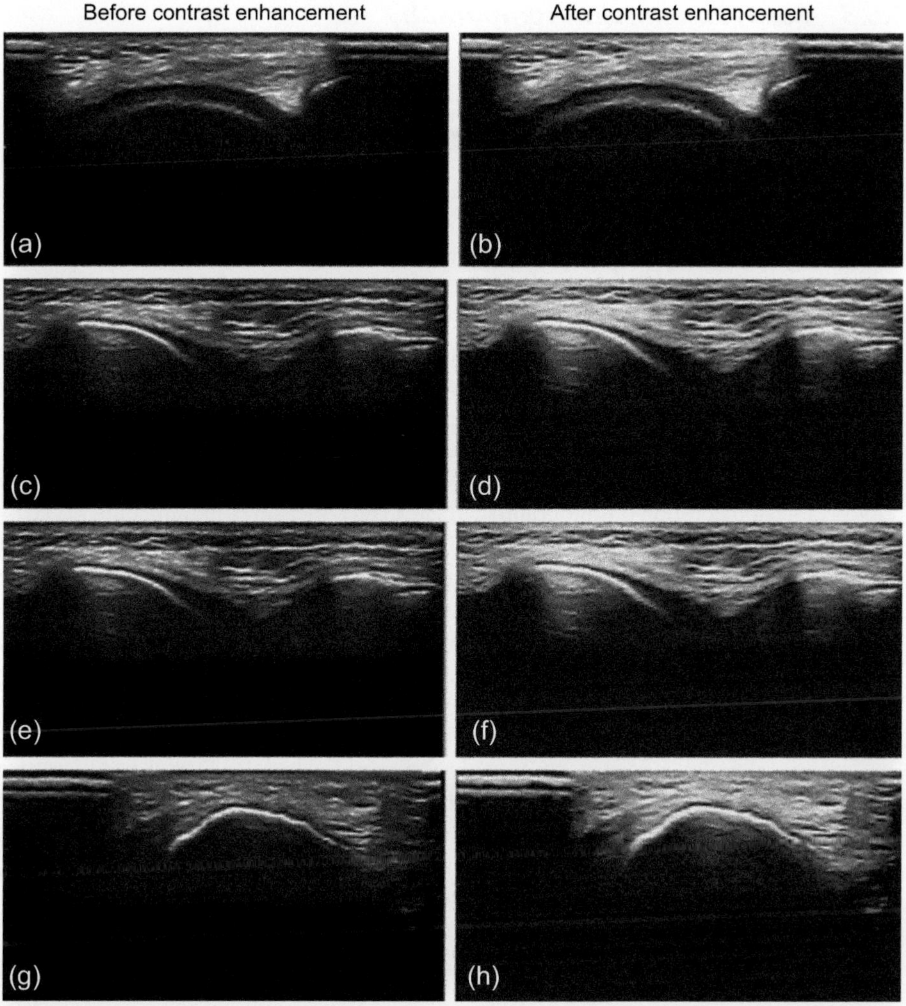

Figure 5.2 Ultrasound images of cartilage of knee joint for different subjects before (a, c, e, g) and after (b, d, f, h) contrast enhancement.
Reproduced from Hossain, M.B., Lai, K.W., Pingguan-Murphy, B., Hum, Y.C., Salim, M.I.M., Liew, Y.M., 2014. Contrast enhancement of ultrasound imaging of the knee joint cartilage for early detection of knee osteoarthritis. Biomedical Signal Processing and Control 13, 157–167, Fig. 3.

formation which are likely to deform less under load than the surrounding soft tissue (Aglyamov et al., 2007), and can be used to provide quantitative data (Jurvelin et al., 2008). Elastography imaging should always be interpreted with caution as stress distribution within the tissue will also be influenced by the surrounding tissues to which it is attached. However, as ultrasound technologies are not reliant on ionizing radiation they are considered safe. Furthermore, the equipment is cheap to run and readily available. For these reasons ultrasound remains a popular in vivo imaging tool.

5.6.3 Positron emission tomography

Positron emission tomography (PET) is a nuclear medicine technique and, like CT imaging, uses radiotracers to emit positrons which, when meeting electrons, create gamma rays. Mapping the gamma rays allows an image to be created (Fig. 5.3). For hard tissue sodium fluoride ^{18}F is often used as the tracing agent (Kao et al., 2010). The $^{18}F^{-}$ ion is known to selectively bind to hydroxyapatite, forming fluorapatite (Hsu et al., 2007) and therefore enhance image contrast.

Recently there has been a drive to combine technologies to create systems that offer the benefits of the individual techniques in one measurement. In this way PET and CT have also been combined (Townsend et al., 2003). The particular advantage of this hybrid is imaging accuracy, via fluoride PET, combined with the rotational scanning features offered by CT. PET-CT hybridization has already been used to show mineralization in tissue surrounding hip implants (Ullmark et al., 2013) and is likely to be a powerful biomineralization analysis tool for studying scaffold integration with native tissue.

Other examples of PET hybrid technologies include PET-SPECT. Like PET, single photon emission computed tomography (SPECT) also measures gamma emission from tracers. However, where PET uses ^{15}O, ^{11}C, ^{18}F, ^{76}Br isotopes, i.e., short half-life emitters, SPECT uses lower energy γ-emitting isotopes (^{123}I, ^{99m}T), and while PET is more sensitive, SPECT is cheaper and the isotopes are more readily available (Brooks, 2005). Two of these tracer isotopes, biphosphonate and fluoride, have been used to monitor bone formation in vivo at high resolution (Lienemann et al., 2015). Furthermore, whole-body scans may also be acquired through PET-SPECT (Tremoleda et al., 2011).

Exploitation of PET technology shows that it is a versatile yet important technique. Research is already underway to develop the world's first PET total-body scanner, termed Explorer, with better resolution than the previously mentioned whole-body systems (Poon et al., 2012) and requiring lower radiation doses (~100 μSv). Radiation is the biggest concern with PET and while combinatorial approaches to technology allow high-resolution images to be produced at quicker scanning times, patient safety is also something that must be addressed (Huang et al., 2009).

5.6.4 X-ray computed tomography

Much like traditional radiography, X-ray computed tomography fires an X-ray beam at the sample from various angles, and the decrease in intensity is measured along linear paths, defined by Beer's Law. The attenuation of X-rays can be correlated to the tissue through which they are traveling. This data is then computed to produce a 3-D image, layer by layer, as the patient is scanned (Fig. 5.4).

The first CT system was created by Hounsfield in 1972 (Lusic and Grinstaff, 2013), and since then it has become the gold-standard for imaging bone architecture in animals and humans. Advantages of using CT are that it is nondestructive, fast, and provides high-resolution images (Tremoleda et al., 2011). At less than $10\,\mu m^3$ resolution, micro-CT is a popular form of this technology (Jones et al., 2007). Variations in micro-CT methods include scanning magnification either by rotating the X-ray source and detector or by rotating the specimen and the beam geometry to speed up the acquisition process,

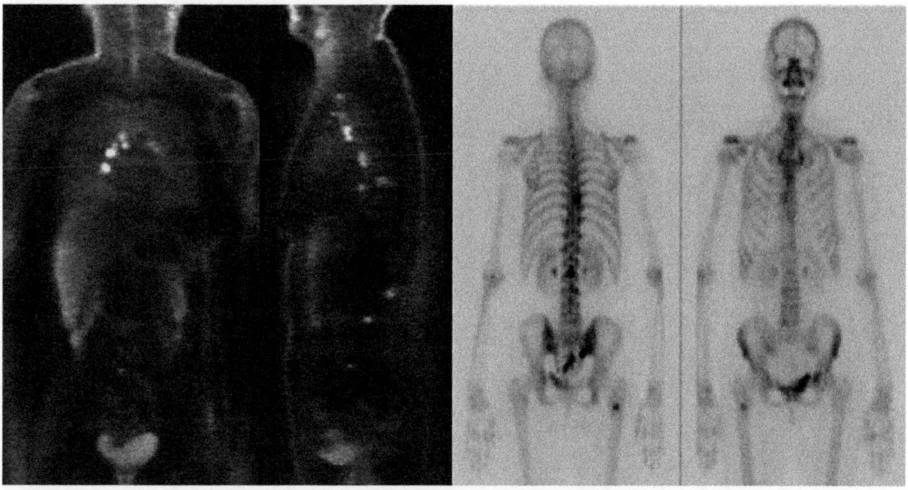

Figure 5.3 Positron emission tomography (left) and bone scintigraphy (right) showing lymph node and bone metastases.
Reproduced from Schirrmeister, H., 2007. Detection of bone metastases in breast cancer by positron emission tomography. Radiologic Clinics of North America 45, 669–676, Fig. 7.

although the latter results in lower resolution (Tremoleda et al., 2011). CT offers high contrast with mineralized crystals, such as hydroxyapatite and calcium phosphate, and is therefore routinely used for in vivo research based on animal models (Freeman et al., 2009; Johnson et al., 2011; Gauthier et al., 2005; von Doernberg et al., 2006). Researchers report at least 100 μm isotropic resolution (Kristensen et al., 2008) with some reporting 15 μm (Ritman, 2007). It is currently only possible to achieve this high resolution by increasing the number of scans, although this also results in dangerous levels of ionizing radiation (Klinck et al., 2008). The use of ionizing radiation is one of the biggest downfalls of CT imaging, especially when techniques such as MRI require no radiation and are therefore deemed safer than CT and PET scanning methods (Lusic and Grinstaff, 2013). Even so, the data obtained through CT imaging has allowed researchers to understand important biomineralization events such as bone mineral density, ossification, and general bone morphology in animals (Botter et al., 2006). Precise imaging of events at high resolution is marred by the lack of sensitivity micro-CT has for soft tissue. Therefore integration of newly developed bone, with existing healthy tissue at the junction where hard tissues and soft tissues meet, is difficult (Tremoleda et al., 2011). Contrast agents, such as those that chelate Ca^{2+} ions, may be used to overcome these issues (Lusic and Grinstaff, 2013; Müller et al., 1997).

5.6.5 Magnetic resonance imaging

Magnetic resonance imaging (MRI) is a nondestructive technique based on proton charge and spin. In a magnetic field, protons align with respect to the field, and at a specific resonance frequency, they can change their direction. As their absorbed

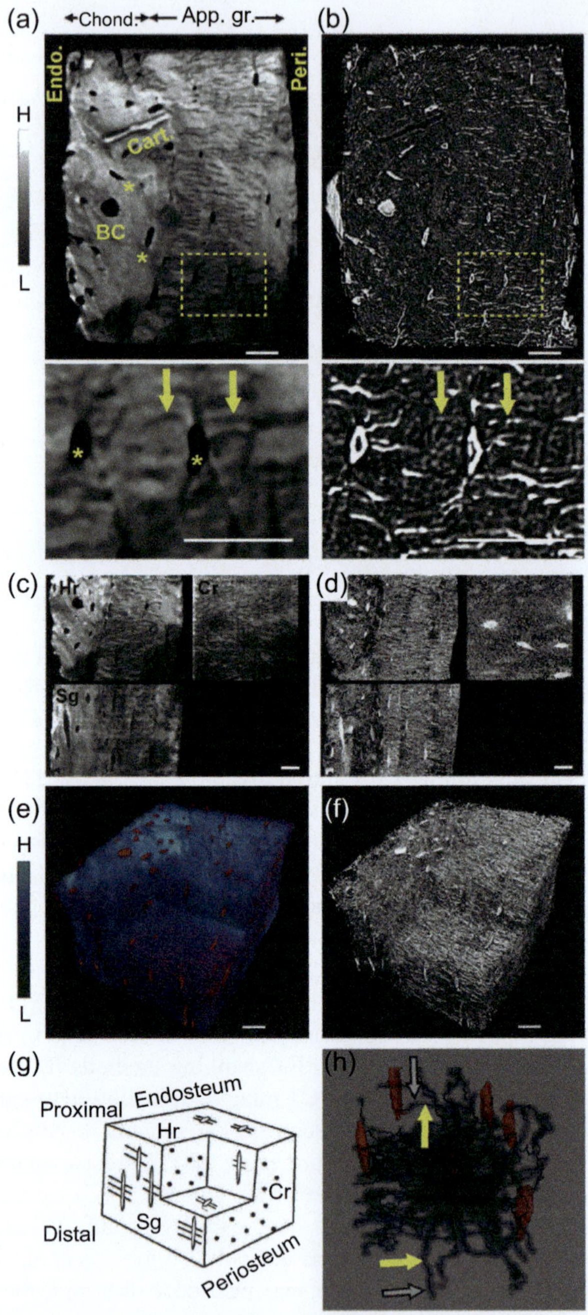

Figure 5.4 X-ray tomographic images of tibial diaphyseal cortex in four-week-old wild-type mice. (a) Degree of mineralization depicted as grayscale (H, high mineralization; L, low mineralization) obtained by Talbot phase-contrast imaging. Endo., endosteum. Peri., periosteum. Chond., endochondral ossification. App. gr., appositional growth. Cart. Cartilage. BC, bone canal. Boxed region is enlarged in the bottom panel. Asterisks, osteocyte lacuna. Arrows, osteocyte canaliculus. (b) Osteocytic lacunae and canaliculi observed by defocus phase-contrast. Boxed region is enlarged in the bottom panel. (c,d) Multiplanar images (Hr, horizontal, Cr, coronal, Sg, sagittal) for Talbot (c) and defocus (d) phase-contrast. (e) 3D overlay image

energy is released the protons are able to relax back to their original alignment. The rate at which this occurs is termed relaxation times, which together with the voltage produced by the protons during the relaxation process (magnetic resonance signal) can be translated to physical and chemical states within the sample. By varying the gradient of the magnetic field the proton resonance frequencies can be tuned through each slice to form a 3-D data set (Edeleman and Warach, 1993). Images produced from an MRI scan are composed of bright and dark areas (Fig. 5.5). The contrast between the two may be improved by using chemical agents, such as iron oxide nanocrystals (Starmans et al., 2013).

MRI scanning of bone is difficult. As bone mineral has a low number of hydrogen atoms, cortical bone is not easily imaged via MRI. To improve the imaging, a faster capture rate may be used, but this requires specialized equipment. Instead bone marrow is often scanned, although data interpretation between the marrow and the solid tissue is difficult, as magnetic field artefacts can distort the final image (Xu et al., 2008). Even so, the general sensitivity of MRI has allowed researchers to observe bone development in vivo (Hartman et al., 2002; Potter et al., 2006), although, as previously discussed, the introduction of biomaterials into the body can cause an inflammatory response and some researchers have noted that the intensity of MRI signals characteristic of mineralization are similar to those observed for infections and abscesses (Shirkhoda et al., 1995). To overcome this, it is possible to use contrast agents, which also act as specific bone biomarkers such as gadolinium phosphonate conjugate markers, which bind with hydroxyapapatite (Adzamli et al., 1989). Furthermore, some studies suggest that MRI does not represent the true density of mineralized tissue in the body. Biomarkers could potentially resolve these issues too (Einstein et al., 2016). MRI is a safe, noninvasive, and sensitive technique but other limiting factors include running costs and long scanning times.

5.6.6 Optical coherence tomography

Optical coherence tomography (OCT) is a technique for obtaining subsurface images of translucent or opaque materials with similarities to ultrasound, using light of typically infrared wavelengths rather than sound. Minimal sample preparation is required for OCT, and there is no use of ionizing radiation. Most of the incident light is not reflected but is scattered, and therefore an interferometer is used to preferentially collect only the directly reflected light, permitting the construction of clear 3-D images at high resolution (Li et al., 2005).

showing degree of mineralization (Blue scale: H, high mineralization; L, low mineralization) as revealed by Talbot phase-contrast and the lacuno–canalicular system, obtained by defocus phase-contrast (red). (f) The canalicular network corresponding to (e). (g) Schematic representation of multiplanar images. (h) Canalicular network with central canaliculi (yellow arrows) and cylindrical mineral dissolution (gray arrows) originating from one osteocyte lacuna (red, center) and five lacunae connected to it (red, in periphery). Scale bars, 20 μm.
Reproduced from Nango, N., Kubota, S., Hasegawa, T., Yashiro, W., Momose, A., Matsuo, K., 2016. Osteocyte-directed bone demineralization along canaliculi. Bone 84, 279–288, Fig. 1.

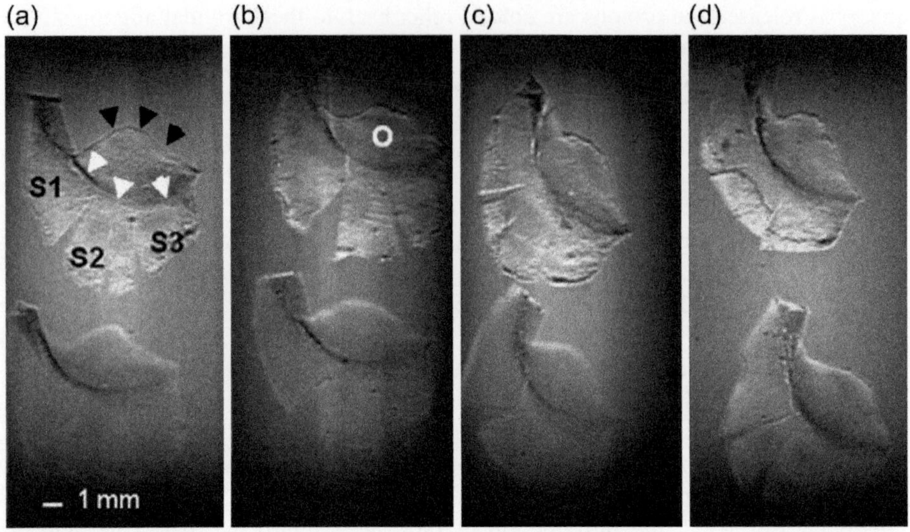

Figure 5.5 Magnetic resonance images of manganese-treated (top) and control (bottom) calvariae specimens. T1-weighted images of manganese-treated specimens exposed to culture medium containing 100 μM MnCl2 for just 24 h. MRI images of manganese-treated (top) and control (bottom) specimens after (a) 4 days in vitro (DIV), (b) 11 DIV, (c) 18 DIV, and (d) 25 DIV. Images were acquired with a nominal in-plane resolution of 117 μm, 48 h post-treatment. The calvarial ridge (white arrows), midline suture (black arrows), and the orbital (O) and superior S1, S2, and S3 zones of the calvaria are indicated. Scale bar = 1 mm.
Reproduced from Chesnick, I.E., Centeno, J.A., Todorov, T.I., Koenig, A.E., Potter, K., 2011. Spatial mapping of mineralization with manganese-enhanced magnetic resonance imaging. Bone 48, 1194–1201, Fig. 4.

Due to the high level of detail obtainable though OCT, it has been widely applied for the imaging of a variety of tissues in vitro including retinas (Fercher et al., 1988; Swanson et al., 1993; Drexler et al., 2001b), corneas (Lim et al., 2008), skin (Caspers et al., 2003), and vascular tissues (Brezinski et al., 1996). Significant research has also taken place into improving the rapidity of data acquisition and the structural resolution, so that OCT can be applied to in vivo studies (Bornemann et al., 2006). In vivo research using this technique includes the pancreas, via fiber optic needles (Hwang et al., 2005), and the gastrointestinal tract (GT), via catheter-based probes (Testoni, 2007). Particular interest has been given to studies of dysplasia and cancer in the GT and biliopancreatic ductal system (Testoni and Mangiavillano, 2008). Specifically for biomineralization, OCT has been successfully employed to study dentin and enamel (Wang et al., 1999), calcification of the cornea (Wirbelauer and Pham, 2004), and calcium-containing deposits formed during atherosclerosis (Mizukoshi et al., 2013; Ong et al., 2016; Yahagi et al., 2016).

The versatility of OCT means that it is possible to combine other analysis techniques with it. Research on combining OCT with absorption, dispersion, and polarization spectroscopy are already under way (Drexler et al., 2001a; Liu et al., 2004).

5.6.7 Fluorescent imaging

Using fluorescent tags, it is possible to observe changes in mineralization (Lambers et al., 2013). Fluorescent microscopy in vivo allows specific proteins to be detected in the near-infrared region (700–1000 nm) (Rao et al., 2007).

Nanoparticles can be used for this purpose, and their size, shape, and chemistry can be altered to bind specific targets. However, although nanoparticles have great potential in imaging biomineralization in vivo, to administer such probes routinely the costs could escalate. Furthermore, some probes, such as the Fluorescein isothiocyanate (FITC)-conjugated F4/80 antibody (which detects macrophages at biomaterial implant sites), have limitations. FITC-F4/80 has an emission wavelength close to skin autofluorescence (Bratlie et al., 2010), therefore limiting its use in vivo. Some of the more routinely used chemicals for in vivo fluorescent imaging are cyanine-biophosphonate dyes, which have a high affinity for bone (Wen et al., 2011; Kozloff et al., 2007, 2010; Bhushan et al., 2007). As well as degradation of fluorophores long-term (Kassab, 2002), there are reports that suggest that the dyes contribute to osteoclast apoptosis and therefore alter tissue physiology (Stern, 2007). Other dyes do exist that may be used to avoid these issues, such as squarine rotaxanes (Harmatys et al., 2013) and tetracyclines (Pautke et al., 2010a,b, 2005).

Quantum dots (QDs) are semiconductive and can also be used for biological tagging (Rosenthal et al., 2011). Their versatility allows them to be detected via electrical and optical methods (Walling et al., 2009) and their emission wavelength can be altered by changing the particle size. Other advantages of using QDs are that multiple targets can be imaged simultaneously and they are known to have high absorbency, high quantum yield, narrow emission bands, large Stokes shifts, and high resistance to photobleaching (Rao et al., 2007). QDs have good clinical potential (Iga et al., 2007), particularly as they may be bioconjugated to specific proteins to improve their

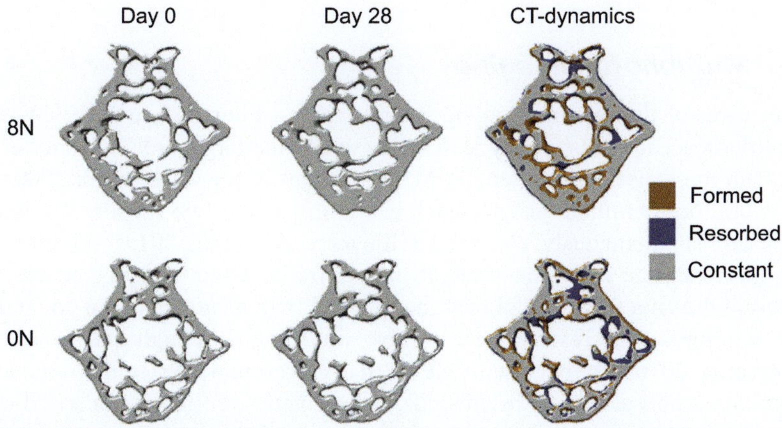

Figure 5.6 Cross sections showing bone formation in mouse vertebra obtained in vivo using fluorescent molecular tomography.
Reproduced from Lambers, F.M., Stuker, F., Weigt, C., Kuhn, G., Koch, K., Schulte, F.A., Ripoll, J., Rudin, M., Müller, R., 2013. Longitudinal in vivo imaging of bone formation and resorption using fluorescence molecular tomography. Bone 52, 587–595, Fig. 6.

specificity (Zhou et al., 2015). Zaheer et al. (2001) used these principles to conjugate pamidronate, a biophosphonate already used clinically to prevent bone loss, to a commercially available near-infrared dye to observe ossification in vivo. Although the specificity of fluorescent labeling has a lot of clinical potential, current techniques are limited to 2-D imaging and low spatial resolution (Einstein et al., 2016) (Fig. 5.6).

5.6.8 Raman spectroscopy

The development of Raman technology for in vivo studies is an area of great interest due to it being noninvasive and label-free. Akiva et al. (2015) showed that zebrafish larvae bone formation could be observed in vivo through Raman spectroscopy. Similar studies have also been performed on rats (Demers et al., 2015; Okagbare et al., 2012). Unlike infrared spectroscopy, this technique can be used for samples containing water and is therefore ideal for analyzing the chemical composition in vivo (Demers et al., 2015). While the use of Raman spectroscopy in zebrafish and rodents has been well documented, its use clinically is a more recent development. The main hurdles with the technique are background fluorescence, interference from other tissue lying above the target site, and scattering effects (Schulmerich et al., 2008). Furthermore, minerals present at lower concentrations within the tissue, such as noncollagenous proteins in bone, are difficult to isolate from signals of greater intensity, such as phosphate and collagen (Penel et al., 2005).

Advances in both the optics and spectroscopic techniques have shown that it is possible to tailor Raman spectroscopy for clinical applications (Duraipandian et al., 2012; Matousek et al., 2006). Specifically, the development of spatially offset Raman spectroscopy and transmission Raman allow patient tissues to be assessed noninvasively (Stone and Matousek, 2008; Matousek et al., 2006; Schulmerich et al., 2009). The main limitations with these techniques are the depth of penetration, signal interference and scattering (Morris and Mandair, 2011).

5.6.9 Multiphoton imaging

Another form of fluorescent imaging is multiphoton fluorescence (MF). Where traditional fluorescence microscopy techniques excite the target area at a shorter wavelength than the emission wavelength, MF excites at longer wavelengths (700 nm and above) than those emitted, and for each excitation event, two (or more) low-energy photons are simultaneously absorbed (Hoover and Squier, 2013; Williams et al., 2001). Based on the anti-Stokes effect, near-infrared lasers are used to elevate the electrons at the target site to a higher energy level than a single photon could achieve and as it returns to a resting state a short wavelength of high energy is emitted (Einstein et al., 2016). The benefits of MF are that background interference is reduced due to fluorescence only at areas of beam focus, and as scattering effects are also reduced, the depth of penetration, and therefore imaging, is two to three times deeper than confocal microscopy (Centonze and White, 1998). It is worth noting that by only fluorescing areas where the beam is targeted the detectors for MF are designed to collect the maximum amount of fluorescence and are no longer reliant on traditional confocal optics (William et al., 2001). Furthermore, photobleaching effects are also reduced, the use of infrared light reduces the toxicity of imaging for long periods (Williams et al., 2001), and with the development of ultrafast (pulsed) lasers the imaging time is improved (Liu et al., 2007). Therefore by combining advanced MF techniques with fluorescent biomarkers, it is possible to image cellular level detail, which is extremely beneficial in observing cellular changes and cell–environment interactions that occur through the biomineralization process (Kim et al., 2008; Liu et al., 2007; Villa et al., 2013). With some tissues, such as autofluorescing dentin and enamel, it is even possible to use MF to noninvasively study the development of mineralized tissue without the need for fluorochromes (Lin et al., 2011).

Although MF technology has vastly improved in vivo imaging in animal models, allowing observations to be made at high spatial resolution, the use of MF in biomineralization is still limited. Specific challenges include finding suitable nontoxic fluorescent labels, perhaps through greater use of autofluorescence (Holloschi et al., 2012), and reducing the need for secondary surgery for the insertion of probes to obtain images at greater depths.

5.7 Future trends

Biomineralization is a complex and dynamic biological process. Nature forms mineral crystals, a nucleation event, under physiological conditions using the surrounding chemistry and morphology to kick-start crystallization events and manipulate the growth and development of the crystals into functional mineralized tissue.

For decades, researchers have attempted to use nature as inspiration for the design and development of unique biomaterial-based systems that, once implanted, offer the possibility of repairing and restoring the original tissue. While these are grand ambitions, significant research has already been conducted in mimicking native biomineralization, as evidenced in this chapter. However, to produce implantable material the problem is two-fold: biomineralization mimicry and the integration of the biomaterial with host tissue. For successful mineral tissue restoration the introduced biomaterial must not only integrate well with the native environment but also induce no cytotoxic side-effects, adding further complexity to the engineering of functional tissue. Integration can be confirmed by observing and quantifying biomineralization events, which typically take place in the natural tissue-repair process. Capturing these events requires noninvasive precision equipment, and this often demands the development of highly specialized imaging and analysis techniques, some of which have been outlined in this chapter. However, the field of in vivo imaging has been developing at a dizzying rate. Techniques that were traditionally reserved for in vitro studies are rapidly finding their way to the bedside and allow real-time evaluation of implanted biomaterials. Most interestingly, many of these techniques are complementary and are therefore combined to create one-stop multianalysis equipment capable of producing data faster, in a safer way, and at higher resolution than ever before. While in vitro analysis techniques remain fairly unchanged, this progression and amalgamation of techniques is necessary in vivo for the reduction of animal/patient discomfort.

Furthermore, observing biomineralization at higher resolution allows researchers to understand changes that occur between the biomaterial and native tissue.

While this may seem like an obvious point, it must be remembered that the chemical and morphological changes that occur at this border are likely to be on the micro- and nanolevel. Some of the traditional techniques used for this purpose are likely to miss these changes due to insufficient resolution. Section 6 provides a taste of techniques designed to address this issue, among others. With ever-improving resolution, researchers are able to probe deeper and understand better not only how the materials impact on the native tissue surrounding wound sites but also how the patient's own tissue affects the biomaterial and its integration into the body. The rate at which complex biomineralized materials are being produced call for more ambitious techniques to be developed, and as the rate of noninvasive technologies available today indicates, this is an area of continuous development with endless possibilities. The future of in vivo monitoring of biomaterials for mineralization is therefore limited only by the technology we have at our disposal and our imagination.

5.8 Conclusions

In this chapter, we have sought to provide readers with an overview of in vivo techniques currently used for the imaging of biomineralization materials. To provide a background to this ambition, we have described biomineralization, the need for replacement biomaterials, and in vitro techniques used for their analysis. Rather surprisingly, there appears to be very little literature available on this subject in a concise form. We have therefore attempted to guide the reader through how the techniques work and how they are used for biomineralization monitoring. The technologies described in this chapter highlight the relationship between researchers producing ever more complex biomaterials that promote and mimic native biomineralization processes and the technological world that builds equipment suited to their analysis. We conclude this chapter by drawing the reader's attention to the fact that as soon as there is a significant change in one, the other must also adapt, and therefore although we have attempted to condense this information into a list of in vivo monitoring techniques, this is likely to require updating regularly.

References

Addadi, L., Moradian, J., Shay, E., Maroudas, N.G., Weiner, S., 1987. A chemical model for the cooperation of sulfates and carboxylates in calcite crystal nucleation: relevance to biomineralization. Proceedings of the National Academy of Sciences 84, 2732–2736.

Addadi, L., Raz, S., Weiner, S., 2003. Taking advantage of disorder: amorphous calcium carbonate and its roles in biomineralization. Advanced Materials 15, 959–970.

Addadi, L., Vidavsky, N., Weiner, S., 2012. Transient precursor amorphous phases in biomineralization. In the footsteps of Heinz A. Lowenstam. Zeitschrift für Kristallographie 227, 711–717.

Adzamli, I.K., Gries, H., Johnson, D., Blau, M., 1989. Development of phosphonate derivatives of gadolinium chelates for NMR imaging of calcified soft tissues. Journal of Medicinal Chemistry 32, 139–144.

Aglyamov, S.R., Skovoroda, A.R., Xie, H., Kim, K., Rubin, J.M., O'Donnell, M., Wakefield, T.W., Myers, D., Emelianov, S.Y., 2007. Model-based reconstructive elasticity imaging using ultrasound. International Journal of Biomedical Imaging Article ID 35830.

Akiva, A., Malkinson, G., Masic, A., Kerschnitziki, M., Bennet, M., Fratzl, P., Addadi, L., weiner, S., Yaniv, K., 2015. On the pathway of mineral deposition in larval zebrafish caudal fin bone. Bone 75, 192–200.

Ananth, H., Kundapur, V., Mohammed, H.S., Anand, M., Amarnath, G.S., Mankar, S., 2015. A review on biomaterials in dental implantology. International Journal of Biomedical Science 11, 113–120.

Aparicio, C., Ginebra, M.P., 2015. Biomineralization and Biomaterials, Fundamentals and Applications. Woodhead Publishing, Cambridge, UK.

Appel, A.A., Anastasio, M.A., Larson, J.C., Brey, E.M., 2013. Imaging challenges in biomaterials and tissue engineering. Biomaterials 34, 6615–6630.

Baconnier, S., Lang, S.B., Polomska, M., Hilczer, B., Berkovic, G., Meshulam, G., 2002. Calcite microcrystals in the pineal gland of the human brain: first physical and chemical studies. Bioelectromagnetics 23, 488–495.

Banwell, C.N., McCash, E.M., 1994. Fundamentals of Molecular Spectroscopy, fourth ed. McGraw-Hill, Maidenhead, UK.

Baslé, M.F., Chappard, D., Grizon, F., Filmon, R., Delecrin, J., Daculsi, G., Rebel, A., 1993. Osteoclastic resorption of Ca-P biomaterials implanted in rabbit bone. Calcified Tissue International 53, 348–356.

Bhushan, K.R., Tanaka, E., Frangioni, J.V., 2007. Synthesis of conjugatable bisphosphonates for molecular imaging of large animals. Angewandte Chemie International Edition 46, 7969–7971.

Bilgen, M., Insana, M.F., 1996. Deformation models and correlation analysis in elastography. Journal of the Acoustical Society of America 99, 3212–3224.

Boeckstyns, M.E., 2014. Wrist arthroplasty – a systematic review. Danish Medical Journal 61, A4834.

Boivin, G., Chavassieux, P., Chapuy, M.C., Baud, C.A., Meunier, P.J., 1989. Skeletal fluorosis: histomorphometric analysis of bone changes and bone fluoride content in 29 patients. Bone 10, 89–99.

Bonfante, E.A., Ceolho, P.G., 2016. A critical perspective on mechanical testing of implants and prostheses. Advances in Dental Research 28, 18–27.

Bornemann, J., Hagner, D., Brandenburg, R., Hauger, C., Wilkens, L., Lenarz, T., Heermann, R., 2006. In vitro measurement conditions for optical coherence tomography (OCT). Acta Oto-Laryngologica 126, 1084–1090.

Botter, S.M., van Osch, G.J., Waarsing, J.H., Day, J.S., Verhaar, J.A., Pols, H.A., van Leeuwen, J.P., Weinans, H., 2006. Quantification of subchondral bone changes in murine osteoarthritis model using micro-CT. Biorheology 43, 379–388.

Bratlie, K.M., Dang, T.T., Lyle, S., Nahrendorf, M., Weissleder, R., Langer, R., Anderson, D.G., 2010. Rapid biocompatibility analysis of materials via in vivo fluorescence imaging of mouse models. PLoS One 5, e10032.

Brezinski, M.E., Tearney, G.J., Bouma, B.E., Boppart, S.A., Hee, M.R., Swanson, E.A., Southern, J.F., Fujimoto, J.G., 1996. Imaging of coronary artery (in vitro) with optical coherence tomography. America Journal of Cardiology 77, 92–93.

Brooks, D.J., 2005. Positron emission tomography and single-photon emission computed tomography in central nervous system drug development. NeuroRx 2, 226–236.

Canalis, R.F., Lechago, J., 1982. Tetracycline bone labelling: an improved technique using incident fluorescence. Annals of Otology, Rhinology & Laryngology 91, 160–162.

Carden, A., Morris, M.D., 200 0. Application of vibrational spectroscopy to the study of mineralized tissues. Journal of Biomedical Optics 5, 259–268.

Carleton, H.M., Drury, R.A.B., Wallington, E.A., 1980. Carleton's Histological Technique, fifth ed. Oxford University Press, Oxford, UK.

Carragher, B., Schneemann, A., Sung, J.J., Mulligan, S.K., Speir, J.A., On, K., Quispe, J., Potter, C.S., 2015. Electron microscopy as an emerging analytical tool for characterizing biopharmaceuticals. Microscopy and Microanalysis 21, 65–66.

Caspers, P.J., Lucassen, G.W., Puppels, G.J., 2003. Combined in vivo confocal Raman spectroscopy and confocal microscopy of human skin. Biophysical Journal 85, 572–580.

Centonze, V.E., White, J.G., 1998. Multiphoton excitation provides optical sections from deeper within scattering specimens than confocal imaging. Biophysical Journal 75, 2015–2024.

Chambers, T.J., Fuller, K., 2011. How are osteoclasts induced to resorb bone? Annals of the New York Academy of Sciences 1240, 1–6.

Chan, H.L., Wang, H.L., Fowlkes, J.B., Giannobile, W.V., Kripfgans, O.D., 2016. Non-ionizing real-time ultrasonography in implant and oral surgery: a feasibility study. Clinical Oral Implants Research 1–7.

Chapman-Jones, D., Paterson, A., Johnston, S., 1998. Plain radiography of the knee: a useful diagnostic modality for patients with non-specific knee pain? Radiography 4, 183–187.

Chesnick, I.E., Centeno, J.A., Todorov, T.I., Koenig, A.E., Potter, K., 2011. Spatial mapping of mineralization with manganese-enhanced magnetic resonance imaging. Bone 48, 1194–1201.

Chung, C.Y., Heebner, J., Baskaran, H., Welter, J.F., Mansour, J.M., 2015. Ultrasound elastography for estimation of regional strain of multilayered hydrogels and tissue-engineered cartilage. Annals of Biomedical Engineering 43, 2991–3003.

Darling, C.L., Le, C.Q., Featherstone, J.D.B., Fried, D., 2009. An automated digital microradiography system for assessing tooth demineralization. Proceedings of the SPIE: International Society of Optical Engineers 7162, 71620T.

de Josselin de Jong, E., van der Linden, A.H., ten Bosch, J.J., 1987. Longitudinal microradiography: a non-destructive automated quantitative method to follow mineral changes in mineralised tissue slices. Physics in Medicine and Biology 32, 1209–1220.

Demers, J.-L.H., Esmonde-White, F.W.L., Esmonde-White, K.A., Morris, M.D., Pogue, B.W., 2015. Next-generation Raman tomography instrument for non-invasive in vivo bone imaging. Biomedical Optics Express 6, 793–806.

Deng, C.X., Hong, X., Stegemann, J.P., 2016. Ultrasound imaging techniques for spatiotemporal characterization of composition, microstructure, and mechanical properties in tissue engineering, Tissue Engineering Part B. Reviews 22, 311–321.

Drexler, W., Stamper, D., Jesser, C., Li, X., Pitris, C., Saunders, K., Martin, S., Lodge, M.B., Fujimoto, J.G., Brezinski, M.E., 2001a. Correlation of collagen organization with polarization sensitive imaging of in vitro cartilage: implications for osteoarthritis. Journal of Rheumatology 28, 1311–1318.

DiMasi, E., Gower, L.B., 2014. Biomineralization Sourcebook: Characterization of Biominerals and Biomimetic Materials. CRC Press, Boca Raton, USA.

Donath, K., Breuner, G., 1982. A method for the study of undecalcified bones and teeth with attached soft tissues. The Sage–Schliff (sawing and grinding) technique. Journal of Oral Pathology 11, 318–326.

Drexler, W., Morgner, U., Ghanta, R.K., Kärtner, F.X., Schuman, J.S., Fujimoto, J.G., 2001b. Ultrahigh-resolution ophthalmic optical coherence tomography. Nature Medicine 7, 502–507.

Drouet, C., 2013. Apatite formation: why it may not work as planned, and how to conclusively identify apatite compounds. BioMed Research International 2013 490946.

Duraipandian, S., Sylvest Bergholt, M., Zheng, W., Yu Ho, K., The, M., Guan Yeoh, K., Bok Yan So, J., Shabbir, A., Huang, Z., 2012. Real-time Raman spectroscopy for in vivo, online gastric cancer diagnosis during clinical endoscopic examination. Journal of Biomedical Optics 17, 081418.

Edeleman, R.R., Warach, S., 1993. Magnetic resonance imaging. The New England Journal of Medicine 708–716.

Einstein, N.M., Cox, S.C., Williams, R.L., Stapley, S.A., Grover, L.M., 2016. Bedside, benchtop, and bioengineering: physicochemical imaging techniques in biomineralisation. Advanced Healthcare Materials 5, 507–528.

Elliott, R.J., Gibson, A.F., 1974. An Introduction to Solid State Physics and Its Applications. Macmillan, London, UK.

Fercher, A.F., Mengedoht, K., Werner, W., 1988. Eye-length measurement by interferometry with partially coherent light. Optics Letters 13, 186–188.

Florencio-Silva, R., Sasso, G.R., Sasso-Cerri, E., Simões, M.J., Cerri, P.S., 2015. Biology of bone tissue: structure, function, and factors that influence bone cells. BioMed Research International 2015 421746.

Freeman, T.A., Patel, P., Parvizi, J., Antoci Jr., V., Shapiro, I.M., 2009. Micro-CT analysis with multiple thresholds allows detection of bone formation and resorption during ultrasound-treated fracture healing. Journal of Orthopaedic Research 27, 673–679.

Fu, D.-L., Jiang, Q.-H., He, F.-M., Yang, G.-L., Liu, L., 2012. Fluorescence microscopic analysis of bone osseointegration of strontium-substituted hydroxyapatite implants. Journal of Zhejiang University Science B 13, 364–371.

Gauthier, O., Müller, R., von Stechow, D., Lamy, B., Weiss, P., Bouler, J.M., Aguado, E., Daculsi, G., 2005. In vivo bone regeneration with injectable calcium phosphate biomaterial: a three-dimensional micro-computed tomographic, biomechanical and SEM study. Biomaterials 26, 5444–5453.

Geesink, R.G., de Groot, K., Klein, C.P., 1988. Bonding of bone to apatite-coated implants. Journal of Bone and Joint Surgery 70, 17–22.

Geusens, P., Chapurlat, R., Schett, G., Ghasem-Zadeh, A., Seeman, E., de Jong, J., van den Bergh, J., 2014. High-resolution in vivo imaging of bone and joints: a window to microarchitecture. Nature Reviews 10, 304–313.

Gordon, L.M., Joester, D., 2011. Nanoscale chemical tomography of buried organic–inorganic interfaces in the chiton tooth. Nature 469, 194–198.

Gordon, L.M., Tran, L., Joester, D., 2012. Atom probe tomography of apatites and bone-type mineralized tissues. ACS Nano 6, 10667–10675.

Greenleaf, J.F., Fatemi, M., Insana, M., 2003. Selected methods for imaging elastic properties of biological tissues. Annual Reviews of Biomedical Engineering 5, 57–78.

Gudur, M., Rao, R.R., Hsiao, Y.S., Peterson, A.W., Deng, C.X., Stegemann, J.P., 2012. Noninvasive, quantitative, spatiotemporal characterization of mineralization in three-dimensional collagen hydrogels using high-resolution spectral ultrasound imaging. Tissue Engineering Part C: Methods 18, 935–946.

Habraken, W.J., Tao, J., Brylka, L.J., Friedrich, H., Bertinetti, L., Schenk, A.S., Verch, A., Dmitrovic, V., Bomans, P.H., Frederik, P.M., Laven, J., van der Schoot, P., Aichmayer B, de With, G., DeYoreo, J.J., Sommerdijk, N.A., 2013. Ion-association complexes unite classical and non-classical theories for the biomimetic nucleation of calcium phosphate. Nature Communications 4, 1507.

Hamm, L.M., Giuffre, A.J., Han, N., Tao, J., Wang, D., De Yoreo, J.J., Dove, P.M., 2014. Reconciling disparate views of template-directed nucleation through measurement of calcite nucleation kinetics and binding energies. Proceedings of the National Academy of Sciences of the United States of America 111, 1304–1309.

Han, Y., Nguyen, K., Ogawa, Y., Shi, H., Park, J., Muller, D.A., 2015. Electron microscopy in air: transparent atomic membranes and imaging modes. Microscopy and Microanalysis 21, 1111–1112.

Harmatys, K.M., Cole, E.L., Smith, B.D., 2013. In vivo imaging of bone using a deep-red fluorescent molecular probe bearing multiple iminodiacetate groups. Molecular Pharmaceutics 10, 4263–4271.

Hartman, E.H.M., Pikkemmat, J.A., Vehof, J.W.M., Heerschap, A., Jansen, J.A., Spauwen, P.H.M., 2002. In vivo magnetic resonance imaging explorative study of ectopic bone formation in the rat. Tissue Engineering 8, 1029–1036.

Hendley IV, C.T., Tao, J., Kunitake, J.A.M.R., De Yoreo, J.J., Estroff, L.A., 2015. Microscopy techniques for investigating the control of organic constituents on biomineralisation. MRS Bulletin 40, 480–489.

Hoffmeister, B.K., Whitten, S.A., Kaste, S.C., Rho, J.Y., 2002. Effect of collagen and mineral content on the high-frequency ultrasonic properties of human cancellous bone. Osteoporosis International 13, 26–32.

Holloschi, A., Kuhn, H.M., Muller, C., Worf, M., Rauen, M., Roder, T., Kessler, W., Mollenhauer, J., Kioschis, P., 2012. Label-free microscopy: spectral imaging of multiphoton-excited cellular autofluorescence. In: Current Microscopy Contributions to Advances in Science and Technology, vol. 1, pp. 103–111.

Hoover, E.E., Squier, J.A., 2013. Advances in multiphoton microscopy technology. Nature Photonics 7, 93–101.

Horobin, R.W., Kiernan, J.A., 2002. Conn's Biological Stains. A Handbook of Dyes Stains and Fluorochromes for Use in Biology and Medicine, tenth ed. BIOS Scientific, Oxford, UK.

Hossain, M.B., Lai, K.W., Pingguan-Murphy, B., Hum, Y.C., Salim, M.I.M., Liew, Y.M., 2014. Contrast enhancement of ultrasound imaging of the knee joint cartilage for early detection of knee osteoarthritis. Biomedical Signal Processing and Control 13, 157–167.

Hsu, W.K., Feeley, B.T., Krenek, L., Stout, D.B., Chatziioannou, A.F., 2007. The use of ^{18}F-fluoride and ^{18}F-FDG PET scans to assess fracture healing in a rat femur model. European Journal of Nuclear Medicine and Molecular Imaging 34, 1291–1301.

Huang, B., Law, M.W.-M., Khong, P.-L., 2009. Whole-body PET/CT scanning: estimation of radiation dose and cancer risk. Radiology 251, 166–174.

Hwang, J.H., Cobb, M.J., Kimmey, M.B., Li, X., 2005. Optical coherence tomography imaging of the pancreas: a needle-based approach. Clinical Gastroenterology and Hepatology 3, S49–S52.

Iga, A.M., Robertson, J.H., Winslet, M.C., Seifalian, A.M., 2007. Clinical potential of quantum dots. Journal of Biomedicine and Biotechnology 76087.

Johnson, L.C., Johnson, R.W., Munoz, S.A., Mundy, G.R., Peterson, T.E., Sterling, J.A., 2011. Longitudinal live animal microCT allows for quantitative analysis of tumor-induced bone destruction. Bone 48, 141–151.

Jones, A.C., Arns, C.H., Sheppard, A.P., Hutmacher, D.W., Milthorpe, B.K., Knackstedt, M.A., 2007. Assessment of bone ingrowth into porous biomaterials using MICRO-CT. Biomaterials 28, 2491–2504.

Jurvelin, J.S., Kröger, H., Töyräs, J., 2008. Recent developments and future prospects in bone ultrasound diagnostics. European Musculoskeletal Review 3, 87.

Kao, C.H.K., Hsu, W.L., Kao, P.F., Lan, W.C., Xie, H.L., Lin, M.C., Chao, H.Y., 2010. An efficient and aseptic preparation of "sodium fluoride (18F) injection" in a GMP compliant facility. Annals of Nuclear Medicine 24, 149–155.

Karjalainen, J.P., Toyras, J., Riekkinen, O., Hakulinen, M., Jurvelin, J.S., 2009. Ultrasound backscatter imaging provides frequency-dependent information on structure, composition and mechanical properties of human trabecular bone. Ultrasound in Medicine & Biology 35, 1376–1384.

Kassab, K., 2002. Photophysical and photosensitizing properties of selected cyanines. Journal of Photochemistry and Photobiology B 68, 15–22.

Kim, P., Puoris'haag, M., Côté, D., Lin, C.P., Yun, S.H., 2008. In vivo confocal and multiphoton microendoscopy. Journal of Biomedical Optics 13, 010501.

Klinck, R.J., Campbell, G.M., Boyd, S.K., 2008. Radiation effects on bone architecture in mice and rats resulting from in vivo micro-computed tomography scanning. Medical Engineering & Physics 30, 888–895.

Königsberger, E., Königsberger, L., 2006. Biomineralization: Medical Aspects of Solubility. Wiley, Chichester, UK.

Körner, M., Weber, C.F., Wirth, S., Pfeifer, K.-J., Reiser, M.F., Trietl, M., 2007. Advances in digital radiography: physical principles and system overview. RadioGraphics 27, 675–686.

Kozloff, K.M., Weissleder, R., Mahmood, U., 2007. Noninvasive optical detection of bone mineral. Journal of Bone and Mineral Research 22, 1208–1216.

Kozloff, K.M., Volakis, L.I., Marini, J.C., Caird, M.S., 2010. Near-infrared fluorescent probe traces bisphosphonate delivery and retention in vivo. Journal of Bone and Mineral Research 25, 1748–1758.

Kreitz, S., Dohmen, G., Hasken, S., Schmitz-Rode, T., Mela, P., Jockenhoevel, S., 2011. Nondestructive method to evaluate the collagen content of fibrin-based tissue engineered structures via ultrasound. Tissue Engineering Part C: Methods 17, 1021–1026.

Kristensen, E., Parsons, T.E., Hallgrímsson, B., Boyd, S.K., 2008. A novel 3-D image-based morphological method for phenotypic analysis. IEEE Transactions on Biomedical Engineering 55, 2826–2831.

Lambers, F.M., Stuker, F., Weigt, C., Kuhn, G., Koch, K., Schulte, F.A., Ripoll, J., Rudin, M., Müller, R., 2013. Longitudinal in vivo imaging of bone formation and resorption using fluorescence molecular tomography. Bone 52, 587–595.

Lee, T.C., Mohsin, S., Taylor, D., PArkesh, R., Gunnlaugsson, T., O'Brien, F.J., Giehl, M., Gowin, W., 2003. Detecting microdamage in bone. Journal of Anatomy 203, 161–172.

Lewis, P.R., Knight, D.P., 1992. Cytochemical Staining Methods for Electron Microscopy. Elsevier, Amsterdam, The Netherlands.

Lienemann, P.S., Metzger, S., Kiveliö, A.-S., Blanc, A., Papageorgiou, P., Astolfo, A., Pinzer, B.R., Cinelli, P., Weber, F.E., Schibli, R., Béhé, M., Ehrbar, M., 2015. Longitudinal in vivo evaluation of bone regeneration by combined measurement of multi-pinhole SPECT and micro-CT for tissue engineering. Scientific Reports 5, 1038.

Li, X., Martin, S., Pitris, C., Ghanta, R., Stamper, D.L., Harman, M., Fujimoto, J.G., Brezinski, M.E., 2005. High-resolution optical coherence tomographic imaging of osteoarthritic cartilage during open knee surgery. Arthritis Research and Therapy 7, R318.

Lim, L.S., Aung, H.T., Aung, T., Tan, D.T.H., 2008. Corneal imaging with anterior segment optical coherence tomography for lamellar keratoplasty procedures. American Journal of Ophthalmology 145, 81–90.

Lin, P.-Y., Lyu, H.-C., Hsu, C.-Y.S., Chang, C.-S., Kao, F.-J., 2011. Imaging carious dental tissues with multiphoton fluorescence lifetime imaging microscopy. Biomedical Optics Express 2, 149–158.

Linde, A., Goldberg, M., 1993. Dentinogenesis. Critical Reviews in Oral Biology and Medicine 4, 679–728.

Liu, B., Macdonald, E.A., Stamper, D.L., Brezinski, M.E., 2004. Group velocity dispersion effects with water and lipid in 1.3 μm optical coherence tomography system. Physics in Medicine and Biology 49, 923–930.

Liu, E., Treiser, M.D., Johnson, P.A., Patel, P., Rege, A., Kohn, J., Moghe, P.V., 2007. Quantitative biorelevant profiling of material microstructure within 3D porous scaffolds via multiphoton fluorescence microscopy. Journal of Biomedical Materials Research: Part B Applied Biomaterials 82B, 284–297.

Lizzi, F.L., Astor, M., Liu, T., Deng, C., Coleman, D.J., Silverman, R.H., 1997. Ultrasonic spectrum analysis for tissue assays and therapy evaluation. International Journal of Imaging Systems and Technology 8, 3–10.

Lowenstam, H.A., 1981. Minerals formed by organisms. Science 211, 1126–1130.

Lusic, H., Grinstaff, M.W., 2013. X-ray computed tomography contrast agents. Chemical Reviews 113.

Major, M.R., Wong, V.W., Nelson, E.R., Longaker, M.T., Gurtner, G.C., 2015. The foreign body response: at the interface of surgery and bioengineering. Plastic and Reconstructive Surgery 135, 1489–1498.

Mass, T., Drake, J.L., Peters, E.C., Jiang, W., Falkowski, P.G., 2014. Immunolocalization of skeletal matrix proteins in tissue and mineral of the coral *Stylophora pistillata*. Proceedings of the National Academy of Sciences of the United States of America 111, 12728–12733.

Matousek, P., Draper, E.R., Goodship, A.E., Clark, I.P., Ronayne, K.L., Parker, A.W., 2006. Noninvasive Raman spectroscopy of human tissue in vivo. Applied Spectroscopy 60, 758–763.

Matsugaki, A., Nakano, T., 2014. Anisotropic crystallization of biominerals. Clinical Calcium 24, 193–202.

Mehrban, N., Bowen, J., Vorndran, E., Gbureck, U., Grover, L.M., 2013. Structural changes to calcium phosphate bioceramics aged in vitro. Colloids and Surfaces B: Biointerfaces 111, 469–478.

Midgley, P.A., Weyland, M., 2003. 3D electron microscopy in the physical sciences: the development of Z-contrast and EFTEM tomography. Ultramicroscopy 96, 413–431.

Miller, M.K., Kelly, T.F., Rajan, K., Ringer, S.P., 2012. The future of atom probe tomography. Materials Today 15, 158–165.

Minkin, C., Marinho, V.C., 1999. Role of the osteoclast at the bone-implant interface. Advances in Dental Research 13, 49–56.

Mizukoshi, M., Kubo, T., Takarada, S., Kitabata, H., Ino, Y., Tanimoto, T., Komukai, K., Tanaka, A., Imanishi, T., Akasaka, T., 2013. Coronary superficial and spotty calcium deposits in culprit coronary lesions of acute coronary syndrome as determined by optical coherence tomography. American Journal of Cardiology 112, 34–40.

Moester, M.J., Schoeman, M.A., Oudshoom, I.B., van Beusekom, M.M., Mol, I.M., Kaijzel, E.L., Löwik, C.W., de Rooij, K.E., 2014. Validation of a simple and fast method to quantify in vitro mineralization with fluorescent probes used in molecular imaging of bone. Biochemical and Biophysical Research Communications 443, 80–85.

Morris, M.D., Mandair, G.S., 2011. Raman assessment of bone quality. Clinical Orthopaedics and Related Research 469, 2160–2169.

Moore, R., 1980. Computed radiography. Medical Electronics 11, 78–79.

Mróz, W., Budner, B., Syroka, R., Niedzielski, K., Golański, G., Slósarczyk, A., Schwartze, D., Douglas, T.E.L., 2015. In vivo implantation of porous titanium alloy implants coated with magnesium-doped octacalcium phosphate and hydroxyapatite thin films using pulsed laser deposition. Journal of Biomedical Materials Research 103, 151–158.

Müller, R., Matter, S., Neuenschwander, P., Suter, U.W., Rüegsegger, P., 1997. 3D micro-tomographic imaging and quantitative morphometry for the nondestructive evaluation of porous biomaterials. In: Briber, R.M., Pfeiffer, D.G., Han, C.C. (Eds.), Morphological Control in Multiphase Polymer MixturesMaterials Research Society, vol. 461, pp. 217–221.

Naderi, H., Matin, M.M., Bahrami, A.R., 2011. Review paper: critical issues in tissue engineering: biomaterials, cell sources, angiogenesis, and drug delivery systems. Journal of Biomaterials Applications 26, 383–417.

Naka, K., Carney, C.K., 2006. Biomineralization I: Crystallization and Self-organization Process. Springer-Verlag, Berlin, Germany.

Nango, N., Kubota, S., Hasegawa, T., Yashiro, W., Momose, A., Matsuo, K., 2016. Osteocyte-directed bone demineralization along canaliculi. Bone 84, 279–288.

Nielsen, M.H., Aloni, S., De Yoreo, J.J., 2014. In situ TEM imaging of $CaCO_3$ nucleation reveals coexistence of direct and indirect pathways. Science 345, 1158–1162.

Okagbare, P.I., Begun, D., Tecklenburg, M., Awonusi, A., Goldstein, S.A., Morris, M.D., 2012. Noninvasive Raman spectroscopy of rat tibiae: approach to in vivo assessment of bone quality. Journal of Biomedical Optics 17, 090502-1–090502-3.

Ong, D.S., Lee, J.S., Soeda, T., Higuma, T., Minami, Y., Wang, Z., Lee, H., Yokoyama, H., Yokota, T., Okumura, K., Jang, I.K., 2016. Coronary calcification and plaque vulnerability: an optical coherence tomographic study. Circulation: Cardiovascular Imaging 9, e003929.

Pautke, C., Bauer, F., Bissinger, O., Tischer, T., Kreutzer, K., Steiner, T., Weitz, J., Otto, S., Wolff, K.D., Stürzenbaum, S.R., Kolk, A., 2010a. Tetracycline bone fluorescence: a valuable marker for osteonecrosis characterization and therapy. Journal of Oral and Maxillofacial Surgery 68, 125–129.

Pautke, C., Tischer, T., Vogt, S., Haczek, C., Deppe, H., Neff, A., Horch, H.-H., Schieker, M., Kolk, A., 2007. New advances in fluorochrome sequential labelling of teeth using seven different fluorochromes and spectral image analysis. Journal of Anatomy 210, 117–121.

Pautke, C., Vogt, S., Kreutzer, K., Haczek, C., Wexel, G., Kolk, A., Imhoff, A.B., Zitzelsberger, H., Milz, S., Tischer, T., 2010b. Characterization of eight different tetracyclines: advances in fluorescence bone labelling. Journal of Anatomy 217, 76–82.

Pautke, C., Vogt, S., Tischer, T., Wexel, G., Deppe, H., Milz, S., Schieker, M., Kolk, A., 2005. Polychrome labeling of bone with seven different fluorochromes: enhancing fluorochrome discrimination by spectral image analysis. Bone 37, 441–445.

Penel, G., Delfosse, C., Descamps, M., Leroy, G., 2005. Composition of bone and apatitic biomaterials as revealed by intravital Raman microspectroscopy. Bone 36, 893–901.

Poon, J.K., Dahlbom, M.L., Moses, W.W., Balakrishnan, K., Wang, W., Cherry, S.R., Badawi, R.D., 2012. Optimal whole-body PET scanner configurations for different volumes of LSO scintillator: a simulation study. Physics in Medicine and Biology 57, 4077–4094.

Potter, K., Sweet, D.E., Anderson, P., Davis, G.R., Isogai, N., Asamura, S., Kusuhara, H., Landis, W.J., 2006. Nondestructive studies of tissue-engineered phalanges by magnetic resonance microscopy and X-ray microtomography. Bone 38, 350–358.

Poulsen, N., Sumper, M., Kröger, N., 2003. Biosilica formation in diatoms: characterization of native silaffin-2 and its role in silica morphogenesis. Proceedings of the National Academy of Sciences 100, 12075–12080.

Rao, J., Dragulescu-Andrasi, A., Yao, H., 2007. Fluorescence imaging in vivo: recent advances. Current Opinion in Biotechnology 18, 17–25.

Ritman, E.L., 2007. Small-animal CT: its difference from, and impact on, clinical CT. Nuclear Instruments and Methods in Physics Research A 580, 968–970.

Rönnholm, E., 1962. The amelogenesis of human teeth as revealed by electron microscopy. II. The development of the enamel crystallites. Journal of Ultrastructure Research 6, 249–303.

Rosenthal, S.J., Chang, J.C., Kovtun, O., McBride, J.R., Tomlinson, I.D., 2011. Biological quantum dots for biological applications. Chemistry & Biology 18, 10–24.

Schirrmeister, H., 2007. Detection of bone metastases in breast cancer by positron emission tomography. Radiologic Clinics of North America 45, 669–676.

Schortinghuis, J., Ruben, J.L., Meijer, H.J., Bronckers, A.L., Raghoebar, G.M., Stegenga, B., 2003. Microradiography to evaluate bone growth into a rat mandibular defect. Archives of Oral Biology 48, 155–160.

Schulmerich, M.V., Cole, J.H., Dooley, K.A., Morris, M.D., Kreider, J.M., Goldstein, S.A., 2008. Optical clearing in transcutaneous Raman spectroscopy of murine cortical bone tissue. Journal of Biomedical Optics 13, 021108.

Schulmerich, M.V., Cole, J.H., Kreider, J.M., Esmonde-White, F., Dooley, K.A., Goldstein, S.A., Morris, M.D., 2009. Transcutaneous Raman spectroscopy of murine bone in vivo. Applied Spectroscopy 63, 286–295.

Seto, J., Busse, B., Gupta, H.S., Schäfer, C., Krauss, S., Dunlop, J.W.C., Masic, A., Kerschnitzki, M., Zaslansky, P., Boesecke, P., Catalá-Lehnen, P., Schinke, T., Fratzl, P., Jahnen-Dechent, W., 2012. Accelerated growth plate mineralization and foreshortened proximal limb bones in fetuin-A knockout mice. PLos One 7, e47338.

Shirkhoda, A., Armin, A.R., Bis, K.G., Makris, J., Irwin, R.B., Shetty, A.N., 1995. MR imaging of myositis ossificans: variable patterns at different stages. Journal of Magnetic Resonance Imaging 5, 287–292.

Silva, T.H., Alves, A., Ferreira, B.M., Oliveira, J.M., Reys, L.L., Ferreira, R.J.F., Sousa, R.A., Silva, S.S., Mano, J.F., Reis, R.L., 2012. Materials of marine origin: a review on polymers and ceramics of biomedical interest. International Materials Reviews 57, 276–306.

Sims, K.B., Pastores, G.M., Weinreb, N.J., Barranger, J., Rosenbloom, B.E., Packman, S., Kaplan, P., Mankin, H., Xavier, R., Angell, J., Fitzpatrick, M.A., Rosenthal, D., 2008. Improvement of bone disease by imiglucerase (Cerezyme) therapy in patients with skeletal manifestations of type 1 Gaucher disease: results of a 48-month longitudinal cohort study. Clinical Genetics 73, 430–440.

Sims, N.A., Gooi, J.H., 2008. Bone remodeling: multiple cellular interactions required for coupling of bone formation and resorption. Seminars in Cell & Developmental Biology 19, 444–451.

Smith, E., Dent, G., 2005. Modern Raman Spectroscopy: A Practical Approach. John Wiley & Sons, Chichester, UK.

Starmans, L.W., Burdinski, D., Haex, N.P., Moonen, R.P., Strijkers, G.J., Nicolay, K., Grüll, H., 2013. Iron oxide nanoparticle-micelles (ION-micelles) for sensitive (molecular) magnetic particle imaging and magnetic resonance imaging. PLoS One 8, e57335.

Stern, P.H., 2007. Antiresorptive agents and osteoclast apoptosis. Journal of Cellular Biochemistry 101, 1087–1096.

Stone, N., Matousek, P., 2008. Advanced transmission Raman spectroscopy: a promising tool for breast disease diagnosis. Cancer Research 68, 4424–4430.

Swanson, E.A., Izatt, J.A., Hee, M.R., Huang, D., Lin, C.P., Schuman, J.S., Puliafito, C.A., Fujimoto, J.G., 1993. In vivo retinal imaging by optical coherence tomography. Optics Letters 18, 1864–1866.

Tao, J., Battle, K.C., Pan, H., Salter, E.A., Chien, Y.C., Wierzbicki, J., De Yoreo, J.J., 2015. Energetic basis for the molecular-scale organization of bone. Proceedings of the National Academy of Sciences 112, 326–331.

Testoni, P.A., 2007. Optical coherence tomography. Scientific World Journal 26, 87–108.

Testoni, P.A., Mangiavillano, B., 2008. Optical coherence tomography in detection of dysplasia and cancer of the gastrointestinal tract and bilio-pancreatic ductal system. World Journal of Gastroenterology 14, 6444–6452.

Tomoaia, G., Pasca, R.D., 2015. On the collagen mineralization. A review. Clujul Medical 88, 15–22.

Townsend, D.W., Beyer, T., Blodgett, T.M., 2003. PET/CT scanners: a hardware approach to image fusion. Seminars in Nuclear Medicine 33, 193–204.

Tremoleda, J.L., Khalil, M., Gompels, L.L., Wylezinska-Arridge, M., Vincent, T., Gsell, W., 2011. Imaging technologies for preclinical models of bone and joint disorders. EJNMMI Research 1.

Ullmark, G., Nilsson, O., Maripuu, E., Sörensen, J., 2013. Analysis of bone mineralization on uncemented femoral stems by [^{18}F]-fluoride-PET. Acta Orthopaedica 84, 138–144.

van Gaalen, S.M., Kruyt, M.C., Geuze, R.E., de Bruijn, J.D., Alblas, J., Dhert, W.J.A., 2010. Use of fluorochrome labels in in vivo bone tissue engineering research. Tissue Engineering Part B: Reviews 16, 209–217.

Vanden Bossche, L., Vanderstraeten, G., 2005. Heterotopic ossification: a review. Journal of Rehabilitation Medicine 37, 129–136.

Ventura, M., Boerman, O.C., de Korte, C., Rijpkema, M., Heerschap, A., Oosterwijk, E., Jansen, J.A., Walboomers, F., 2014. Preclinical imaging in bone tissue engineering. Tissue Engineering Part B: Reviews 20, 578–595.

Vidavsky, N., Masic, A., Schertel, A., Weiner, S., Addadi, L., 2015. Mineral-bearing vesicle transport in sea urchin embryos. Journal of Structural Biology 192, 358–365.

Villa, M.M., Wang, L., Huang, J., Rowe, D.W., Wei, M., 2013. Visualizing osteogenesis in vivo within a cell-scaffold construct for bone tissue engineering using two-photon microscopy. Tissue Engineering Part C: Methods 19, 839–849.

von Doernberg, M.C., von Rechenberg, B., Bohner, M., Grunenfelder, S., van Lenthe, G.H., Müller, R., Gasser, B., Mathys, R., Baroud, G., Auer, J., 2006. In vivo behavior of calcium phosphate scaffolds with four different pore sizes. Biomaterials 27, 186–198.

Walling, M.A., Novak, J.A., Shepard, J.R.E., 2009. Quantum dots for live cell and in vivo imaging. International Journal of Molecular Sciences 10, 441–491.

Wang, X.J., Milner, T.E., de Boer, J.F., Zhang, Y., Pashley, D.H., Nelson, J.S., 1999. Characterization of dentin and enamel by use of optical coherence tomography. Applied Optics 38, 2092–2096.

Wang, Y.-H., Liu, Y., Maye, P., Rowe, D.W., 2006. Examination of mineralized nodule formation in living osteoblastic cultures using fluorescent dyes. Biotechnology Progress 22, 1697–1701.

Wen, D., Qing, L., Harrison, G., Golub, E., Akintoye, S.O., 2011. Anatomic site variability in rat skeletal uptake and desorption of fluorescently labeled bisphosphonate. Oral Diseases 17, 427–432.

Williams, D., Carter, C., 2009. Tranmission Electron Microscopy: A Textbook for Materials Science. Springer, New York, USA.

Williams, R.M., Zipfel, W.R., Webb, W.W., 2001. Multiphoton microscopy in biological research. Current Opinion in Chemical Biology 5, 603–608.

Wirbelauer, C., Pham, D.T., 2004. Imaging and quantification of calcified corneal lesions with optical coherence tomography. Cornea 23, 439–442.

Wojtowicz, A.M., Shekaran, A., Oest, M.E., Dupont, K.M., Templeman, K.L., Hutmacher, D.W., Guldberg, R.E., García, A.J., 2010. Coating of biomaterial scaffolds with the collagen-mimetic peptide GFOGER for bone defect repair. Biomaterials 31, 2574–2591.

Xu, H., Othman, S.F., Magin, R.L., 2008. Monitoring tissue engineering using magnetic resonance imaging. Journal of Bioscience and Bioengineering 106, 515–527.

Yahagi, K., Joner, M., Virmani, R., 2016. The mystery of spotty calcification: can we solve it by optical coherence tomography? Circulation: Cardiovascular Imaging 9, e004252.

Zaheer, A., Lenkinski, R.E., Mahmood, A., Jones, A.G., Cantley, L.C., Frangioni, J.V., 2001. In vivo near-infrared fluorescence imaging of osteoblastic activity. Nature Biotechnology 19, 1148–1154.

Zelzer, M., Todd, S.J., Hirst, A.R., McDonald, T.O., Ulijn, R.V., 2013. Enzyme responsive materials: design strategies and future developments. Biomaterials Science 1, 11–39.

Zhou, J., Yang, Y., Zhang, C.-Y., 2015. Toward biocompatible semiconductor quantum dots: from biosynthesis and bioconjugation to biomedical application. Chemical Reviews 115, 11669–11717.

Measuring gene expression changes on biomaterial surfaces

6

P. Morissette Martin, K. Creber, D.W. Hamilton
The University of Western Ontario, London, ON, Canada

6.1 Introduction

Assessing cell responses to biomaterials has evolved significantly through the continued development, refinement, and improvement of technologies for measuring cell response, particularly in applications of molecular biology and analysis of gene expression. When mammalian cells attach to biomaterials, it sets in motion cascades of complex molecular signals that regulate downstream processes including cell spreading, migration, proliferation, survival, and gene expression (Liu and Chen, 2005). The ability of a biomaterial to influence and regulate these types of cellular responses is essential for the functional integration of the material into the host tissue.

A commonly used method of assessing cell response to a biomaterial is measurement of gene expression (Groen et al., 2016). Understanding which genes are active in a cell gives an insight into cell phenotype, maturation state, and overall bioactivity. As will be discussed in this chapter, this is typically done in vitro, with specific cells being seeded onto, or into, a biomaterial or scaffold. In vivo assessment of a biomaterial efficacy is more complicated, as will be illustrated in Section 6.4. The continued development of techniques for assessing gene expression (quantitative PCR and microarray technology, for example) and gene localization (in situ hybridization) has permitted increased accuracy in profiling active and inactive genes. These assays also allow for a reduction in cell density required for techniques such as northern blotting, although such techniques still have validity (Roth, 2002). Technological advances in gene expression have been, and will continue to be, paramount in the development of specific biologically active materials through assessment of their functionality in biological systems (Groen et al., 2016; Hanagata, 2015).

The goal of this chapter is not to discuss the details underlying the technical aspect of each methodology for assessing gene expression, but rather to discuss the relevance and design of experiments to maximize the information that can be gained through gene expression profiling as a method of quantifying cell response to a given biomaterial. In addition, assumptions, limitations, and potential pitfalls related to the analysis of gene expression in biomaterial research will be discussed.

6.1.1 Measuring global gene expression

Development of DNA microarray technology (commonly known as microarray or DNA chip) has allowed simultaneous analysis of thousands of genes in a single sample

Monitoring and Evaluation of Biomaterials and their Performance in vivo. http://dx.doi.org/10.1016/B978-0-08-100603-0.00006-7

(Roth, 2002). Microarrays can be used to hybridize to RNA or DNA sequences; the former is used to measure the expression of multiple genes, while the latter is more commonly used to assess possible mutations in a genome (Goodkind and Edwards, 2005). It must be considered though: of the many thousands of genes contained within a genome, comparatively few of them are expressed within a cell at any given time.

Microarrays are substrates upon which oligonucleotide probes are printed and on which labeled transcriptome samples are applied. Before being applied on the microarray, the mRNA of interest is transcribed into stable complementary DNA (cDNA) and labeled with fluorescent, chemiluminescent, or radioactive tags. Subsequently, they are allowed to hybridize with the arrays where each cDNA can bind to the probes for each gene. Unbound cDNA is then discarded during the wash cycles following the hybridization, and based on the amount of hybridization that occurs, a signal is generated for each gene. There are many excellent review articles that focus on all the microarray technology available (Goodkind and Edwards, 2005; Groen et al., 2016; Hanagata, 2015; Roth, 2002).

Microarray-based gene expression profiling is often used to compare and contrast the influence of particular stimuli (e.g., growth factor, pathogen, biomaterial) on the mRNA abundance within a cell or cell population. While a powerful technique to assess thousands of mRNA transcripts simultaneously, the analysis of the generated data is complex, and the information generated can be difficult to interpret (Li and Wong, 2001). Furthermore, it is necessary to use PCR-based methods to confirm mRNA changes detected by microarrays.

6.1.2 Measuring specific gene expression patterns

While targeted arrays are now available, such arrays still probe between 50 and 500 genes depending on the array (e.g., Kim et al., 2015). When using gene expression to assess cell function, particularly phenotype, many studies tend to focus on a subset of genes that are known to be indicative of the differentiated function of that particular cell type. It typically yields important information and can significantly reduce associated costs, as the gene expression profile is typically assessed using three to five genes (e.g., Miron et al., 2010).

Measuring individual genes is based on reverse transcription polymerase chain reaction (RT-PCR) methodology. Conventional RT-PCR involves creation of a cDNA library from mRNA using reverse transcription, followed by PCR amplification, and electrophoresis of the products on gels (Roth, 2002). The bands of the amplified products are visualized with DNA-binding dyes such as ethidium bromide. By measuring the intensity of the endpoint products on the gel, this technique is only semiquantitative and is not precise enough to compare the gene expression between multiple treatment groups. The main limitation of RT-PCR is that the most accurate phase for measuring differences in mRNA copy is during the linear phase, which conventional RT-PCR does not measure (Roth, 2002).

This limitation leads to the development of another PCR-based approach that specifically measures amplification of the target during the linear phase (Wong and Medrano, 2005) (Fig. 6.1). This approach is referred to as reverse transcriptase

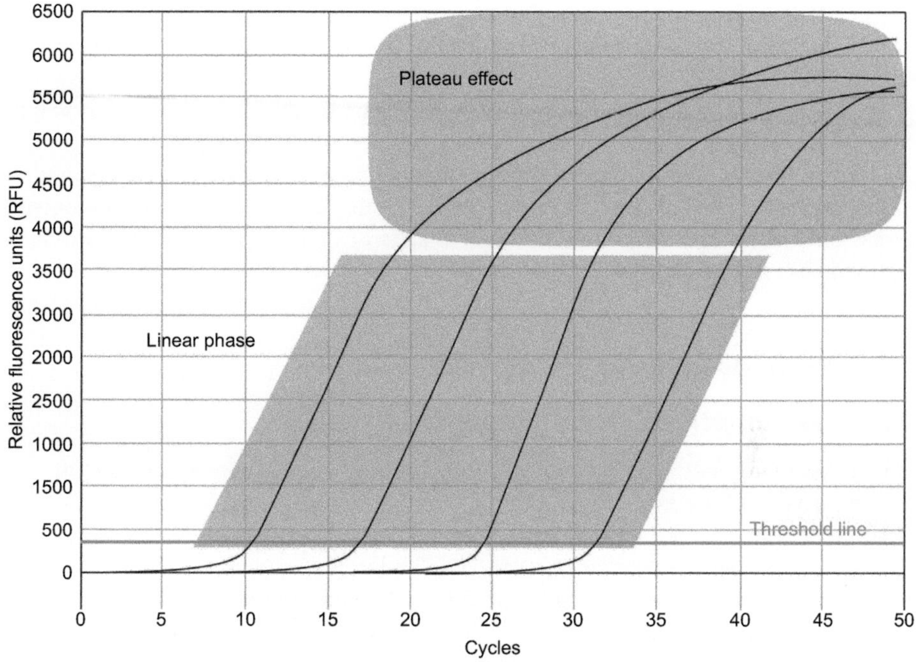

Figure 6.1 Typical RT-qPCR amplification curves. The most accurate phase for measuring a PCR product is during the linear phase of the curve, when the conditions are ideal and should result in the product doubling every cycle.

real-time PCR, or reverse transcriptase quantitative PCR. The commonly accepted abbreviation of real-time PCR is RT-qPCR, which we will use for the remainder of the chapter. Detection of amplified targets in real time is possible through the addition of a fluorescent reporter molecule in the reactions, with increased fluorescence corresponding with increased cDNA product (Heid et al., 1996). As RT-qPCR measures the amount of product in the linear phase of amplification, it becomes possible to measure the initial quantity of the template in the sample based on the knowledge that the template will double approximately every cycle.

While PCR-based methods are specific and highly appropriate for biomaterial research, they can be considered less encompassing compared to the microarray technology. With RT-PCR or RT-qPCR, the user is selecting which genes will be analyzed, and as such, important genes that maybe up- or downregulated may not be studied. However, it is important to understand that differentiation markers are well defined in many cell and tissue systems, and PCR-based methods are still a powerful method for analyzing changes in cell phenotype.

6.1.3 Localizing the expression of genes of interests

Whereas DNA microarrays and RT-qPCR are methods that measure the amount of specific mRNA levels in samples, neither allows the mRNA signal to be localized within tissues. Using fluorescent, chemi-luminescent, or radioactive-labelled nucleic acid probes, in situ hybridization allows the localisation of specific mRNA sequences on tissue cross-sections.

In situ hybridization can be seen as complementary to immunohistochemistry; both can reveal the distribution of specific mRNA (in situ hybridization) or protein (immunohistochemistry) within a tissue, although neither technique can quantify the amount of the targeted mRNA or protein present in the tissue. As it is a powerful technique to assess the distribution of specific mRNAs to specific cell populations, in situ hybridization is often used for in vivo experiments.

6.2 Considerations when measuring gene expression

6.2.1 Assumptions underlying mRNA analysis

One of the major assumptions underlying analysis of gene expression is that all cells within a given culture express similar levels of the mRNA being measured in response to a biomaterial. The possibility exists, particularly if phenotypic heterogeneity exists within a culture, such as occurs in rat calvarial cultures (Bellows et al., 1986), that the message levels may not correspond to all cells within the population. The level of complexity increases yet further if trying to measure gene expression in vivo, where multiple cell populations are in contact with the biomaterial. It then becomes extremely problematic to assign any mRNA to any particular cell population, certainly without combining gene expression analysis with methods such as immunohistochemistry (protein) and in situ hybridization (mRNA) for further analysis.

The next major assumption often made by researchers is that if a given mRNA transcript is higher in cells cultured on a biomaterial versus control cultures, then the transcript must be important or required in cell response, and further, the effects of the biomaterial cause this transcript to increase directly. Moreover, it is not always correct to conclude that mRNA levels always have to change for a protein level to change as well. It is now well established that mRNAs have different half-lives, and cells can also store mRNA without ever translating the protein (Gilbert, 2000). Because of these regulatory steps, the measured increase in mRNA is not necessarily reflected at the protein level. Measurement of gene expression represents a temporal snapshot only of what is occurring in any given cell culture or tissue, and if expression of the gene is cyclical in nature, this will not be detected unless multiple time points are analyzed. Typically, researchers in the biomaterial field will measure differentiation markers, which as a rule, are known to increase at the mRNA level as the cells adopt their differentiated function. However, this represents only one measure of cell activity and the gene level, and several other steps occur prior to the mRNA resulting in the presence of a functional protein.

6.2.2 Gene expression versus protein expression

When assessing gene expression of cells on biomaterials, either in vitro or in vivo, it is important to consider that this represents only one aspect of a complex chain of events that ultimately will give rise to a functional protein. So while gene profiling gives an insight into the cell phenotype at the mRNA level, it does not provide definitive information on whether gene expression changes actually translate through to altered functionality, which occurs at the protein level. Therefore it is necessary to consider further the steps bridging increase in transcript levels for a gene to change in cell functionality.

6.2.2.1 Alternate RNA splicing

When first produced, premessenger RNA is formed, which is complementary to the region of DNA from which it was derived. Containing introns, which are noncoding regions, and exons, the coding regions, it undergoes processing to give rise to the final mRNA from which the protein is transcribed. During the processing of mRNA, different exons can be removed, which give rise to a different final mRNA sequence and, as a result, alternate protein sequence (McManus and Graveley, 2011). Commonly, specific cell types give rise to alternate spliced forms and therefore distinct protein isoforms; as will be discussed later in the chapter, a different isoform of a protein may be found in osteoblasts in comparison with dermal fibroblasts. These different polypeptide sequences can have distinct functions, although the protein isoforms originally arose from the same gene. In essence, alternate splicing acts to increase the size of the proteome relative to the number of genes present in a given genome (McManus and Graveley, 2011). There are now microarrays available that allow assessment of alternate splicing, by monitoring each splicing event through exon–exon junction probes.

6.2.2.2 Posttranslational modifications

A further mechanism to increase the functional diversity of proteins is through the addition of functional groups to the —C or —N terminus of amino acids in the polypeptide chain of the protein (Lothrop et al., 2013). There are several different types of modifications that can be made to proteins, including phosphorylation, glycosylation, methylation, and acetylation. Each type of modification can confer changes in protein function through cellular recognition, as well as alter protein stability and degradation profiles.

6.3 Using gene expression for analysis of cell response to biomaterials

When first defined, biocompatibility referred to the properties of a material related to inflammation and foreign body response; initial materials were designed to be inert—to not elicit a response in a biological environment (Williams, 2003). While these materials did function to an extent in certain applications in certain tissues, their efficacy was limited by the fact that they could not be incorporated into the host tissues into which they were implanted.

Functional incorporation of any given biomaterial into a host tissue requires quantifying how cells respond to the basic chemical and topographical features of the material, ensuring that the material elicits an appropriate response from these cells (Lim and Donahue, 2007). Although certain materials, such as contact lenses, are designed to prevent cell attachment (Dutta et al., 2012), the vast majority of new generation biomaterials are bioactive, and they are functionalized to promote cell attachment and tissue integration (Sakiyama-Elbert and Hubbell, 2001). If we consider cell adhesion as the initial step toward alterations in gene expression, then what processes are altered and how can they be measured through mRNA analysis?

Gene functions can be assigned to different categories in all cell types. First are those that are active in all cell types related to adhesion, survival, and proliferation. The second classification reflects those genes specific to the differentiated function of each cell type, which are therefore much more restricted in expression. While mRNA analysis can be utilized to assess whether cells are dying or proliferating on a given material, this is a cumbersome and expensive way to analyze these types of processes. Complementary assays would need to be used to actually confirm that the mRNA activation could be linked to either cell death or cell division.

In the remainder of this chapter, we will illustrate how changes in gene expression can be accurately measured when cells are cultured on or in biomaterials, as well as the potential pitfalls that researchers can fall into. Specifically, we will discuss measuring gene expression in two tissue systems: in vitro analysis of bone formation/osteogenesis and in vivo quantification of skin healing.

6.3.1 Example 1: influence of biomaterials on osteogenic gene expression and mineralization in hPDL cells

In the first example, we will consider how to utilize gene expression to assess whether biomaterial "X" can induce bone formation or osteogenesis. There are multiple ways in which these experiments can be conducted, and proper quantification of bone formation must be assayed using different, but complementary, methods, of which mRNA analysis is only one.

6.3.1.1 Choosing an appropriate cell model

Before testing the osteogenic properties of a biomaterial, the first criterion that has to be established is what type of cells will be used in the study. The endogenous transcriptome of different cell populations is highly variable; the amount and types of mRNA transcripts they express can differ greatly. Such differences are particularly noticeable when mesenchymal progenitor cells, osteoblasts, or osteogenic cell lines are used as a starting point.

Cell culture experiments often include osteogenic cell lines (MC3T3-E1, MG-63), which have the advantage of well-characterized patterns of mineralization and predictable gene expression profiles. Yet, they have limited value as the cells are transformed and as their overall phenotype is not necessarily indicative of cells in the human body (Czekanska et al., 2012). Primary cell cultures are always preferable, particularly if human cells can be utilized, but these typically are more heterogeneous with respect to the phenotypes of the cells (Czekanska et al., 2012).

6.3.1.2 Experimental design

In the following example from our laboratory, we will describe our analysis of human periodontal ligament cell (hPDL) differentiation on biomaterial "X". The main variable to be investigated is whether the addition of osteogenic media (β-glycerophosphate and L-ascorbic acid) is required for the hPDL cells to mineralize on the material. As these are primary cells derived from human teeth, it is critical to use cells isolated from multiple donors and to have certain information related to the patients the cells were isolated from (age, gender, tooth location, periodontal disease status), which could be confounding variables in data analysis.

Two approaches could be taken to assess osteoblast differentiation and mineralization. First, time points could be selected at which gene expression is assessed to look for upregulation of mRNAs consistent with osteoblast differentiation. Alternatively, cultures could be established to assess when mineralization and nodule formation become evident on the material.

In our study, we opted to investigate temporal formation of mineral in the cultures using Alizarin red staining for calcium, which confirmed that the hPDL cells produced a mineralized matrix in response to osteogenic culture conditions only, with nodule formation evident at 14 days (Fig. 6.2(a)). Without osteogenic supplementation, hPDL cells did not significantly mineralize on biomaterial "X". Of potential significance is that the level of mineralization varied significantly in cells isolated from different patients, and regression analysis revealed that the amount of calcium deposited was inversely related to age of the donor at both 2 and 4 weeks postseeding (Fig. 6.2(b) and (c)). Therefore, by first performing simple mineralization assays, we immediately have quantified that not all hPDL cell cultures used in the experiment mineralize to the same level, even when cultured under the same conditions and osteogenic supplementation is a prerequisite for hPDL differentiation to osteoblasts. This data suggests that when considering mRNA analysis, these cultures will possibly show differences in transcript levels for genes required for mineralization, which is the next set of experiments we performed.

6.3.1.3 Gene expression analysis

In our study, we selected a panel of genes that can be classified depending on cellular function. Depending on what genes are analyzed, the information that can be derived requires additional assays of not only protein expression, but also localization of these proteins to certain compartments within the cells. If we want to quantify the differentiated phenotype and maturation of the cells, which genes are the most appropriate to investigate?

Transcriptional genes

One of the main transcription factors required for osteogenic differentiation is runt-related transcription factor 2 (RUNX2) (Camilleri and McDonald, 2006; Komori, 2006). RUNX2 can bind to the promoter region of proteins required for osteogenic differentiation, including bone sialoprotein (*BSP*), collagen type I (*COL1A1*), and osteocalcin (*BGLAP*). While other transcription factors are also involved in osteogenic

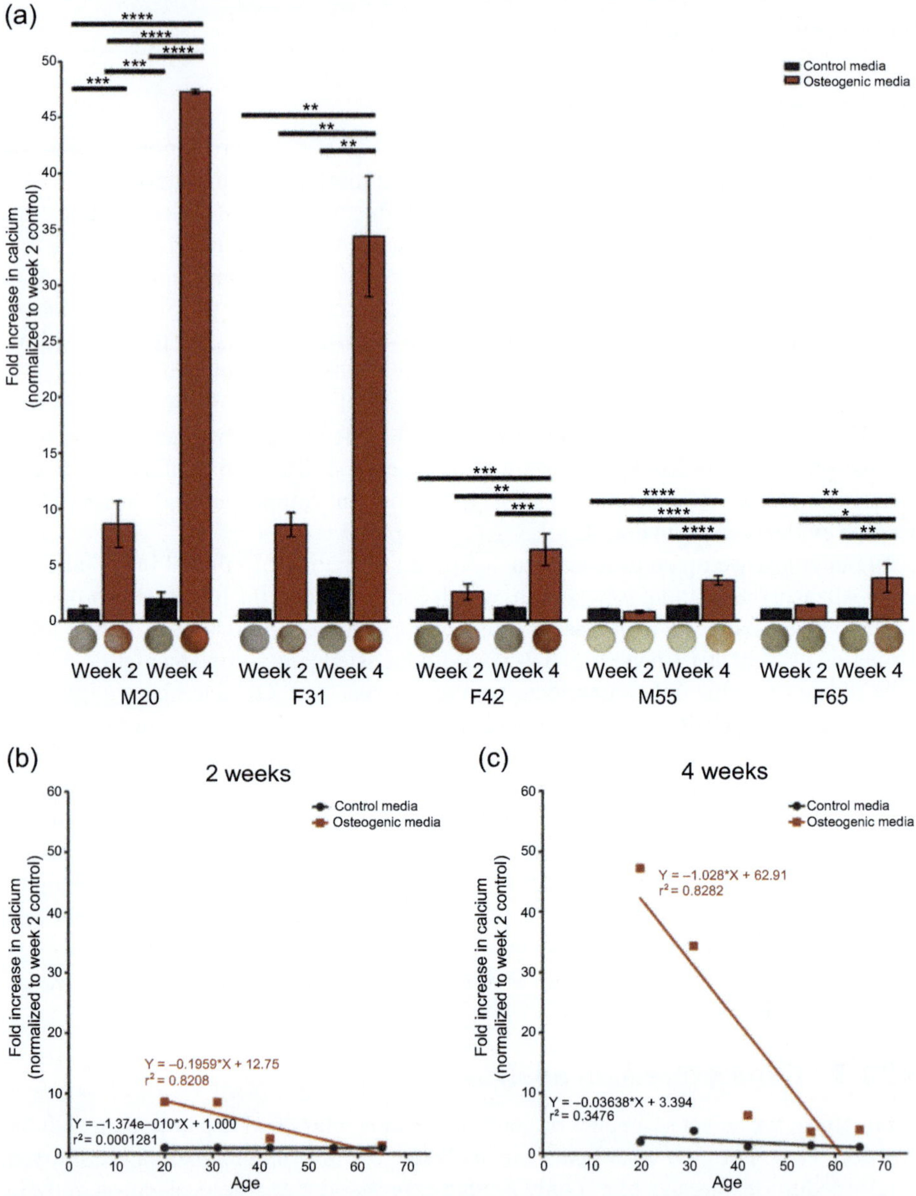

Figure 6.2 Alizarin Red S staining of calcium in hPDL cells during osteogenic differentiation. (a) Alizarin Red S staining was used to visualize calcium (stained red) deposited by cells at 2 and 4 weeks postseeding. Dye was subsequently eluted to quantify calcium content. Data for each patient is shown separately and presented as mean ± SD of three internal replicates from one experiment (except patient F31, two internal replicates); patient gender, age, and cell passage is designated under graphs. Two-way ANOVA with Tukey posttest for multiple comparisons was completed and multiplicity-adjusted p-values are reported. *$p<.05$, **$p<.01$, ***$p<.001$, ****$p<.0001$. Regression analysis at (b) 2 weeks and (c) 4 weeks indicated that calcium deposition was negatively correlated with age at 2 and 4 weeks in response to osteogenic media ($r^2 = 0.8208$, $r^2 = 0.8282$; $p<.05$), while deposition of calcium in control media was not significantly related to age.

differentiation, including β-catenin and the transcription factor Sp7 (also known as osterix), genetic deletion of *RUNX2* results in mice that contain no bone, with osteoblasts unable to express osteoblast markers (Komori, 2006). Although also essential for bone formation, Sp7 is downstream of *RUNX2* expression, and therefore many studies on osteogenesis look at *RUNX2* mRNA levels as a measure of osteogenic activity of the cells (Hamilton and Brunette, 2007; Miron et al., 2010).

If we consider differentiation of hPDL cultures on material "X", *RUNX2* mRNA levels showed little variation between cells cultured on material "X" between osteogenic and control conditions (Fig. 6.3(a) and (b)). While the role of Runx2 in osteogenic differentiation has been well characterized at the protein level (Komori, 2006), there are a number of studies that have indicated that its mRNA levels are a poor indicator of osteogenic activity (Miron et al., 2010; Prowse et al., 2013). As RUNX2 protein is endogenously expressed within the cytoplasm of most types of osteogenic cells, its translocation to the nucleus is more accurate of a switch to a differentiated phenotype, rather than alterations at the mRNA level. While variable, in the presence of osteogenic media, immunoreactivity of RUNX2 was localized to the nucleus of cells, but not in cells cultured in control media (Fig. 6.3(c)). Therefore on material "X", the presence of osteogenic media appears to be required for nuclear translocation of RUNX2, but very little variation in mRNA levels are evident.

Extracellular matrix and mineralization markers

Prior to initiating studies related to osteoblast mineralization markers, it is important to be aware of the temporal patterns of expression for each mRNA being investigated. In general, mineralized nodules become apparent in various osteogenic cell cultures (such as rat calvarial cells, bone marrow stromal cells, MC3T3-E1, and hPDL) around day 10–14 after plating. One of the first markers of osteoblast differentiation is an increase in alkaline phosphatase (*ALPL*), an enzyme that removes phosphate groups from molecules, likely providing a source of phosphate for mineralization, although this has yet to be demonstrated definitively (Golub and Boesze-Battaglia, 2007). mRNA transcripts for BSP also increase at early time points, but *BGLAP* is considered a late marker of mineralization and osteoblast maturation, with transcript levels increasing at days 14 onwards. In late-stage mineralizing cultures (2–4 weeks), *ALPL* (Jaiswal et al., 1997) and *BSP* (Chen et al., 1992, 1993) decrease, while *BGLAP* transcript levels remain high (Miron et al., 2010; Prowse et al., 2013). Analysis of these genes using RT-qPCR makes it possible to assess changes in mineralization patterns, and any perturbations away from this pattern of gene expression provides additional information on the maturation state of the cultures.

In our hPDL cell cultures, our data demonstrated that cultures established from younger patients showed increased mineralization in the presence of osteogenic supplementation on material "X". Cells isolated from M20 and F39 showed a gene expression pattern that was characteristic of osteogenic differentiation and osteoblast maturation as outlined in the previous paragraph (Fig. 6.4(a) and (b)). Specifically, expression of the early osteogenic marker *ALPL* was suppressed as early as 2 weeks after osteogenic induction, with simultaneous increase in *BGLAP*.

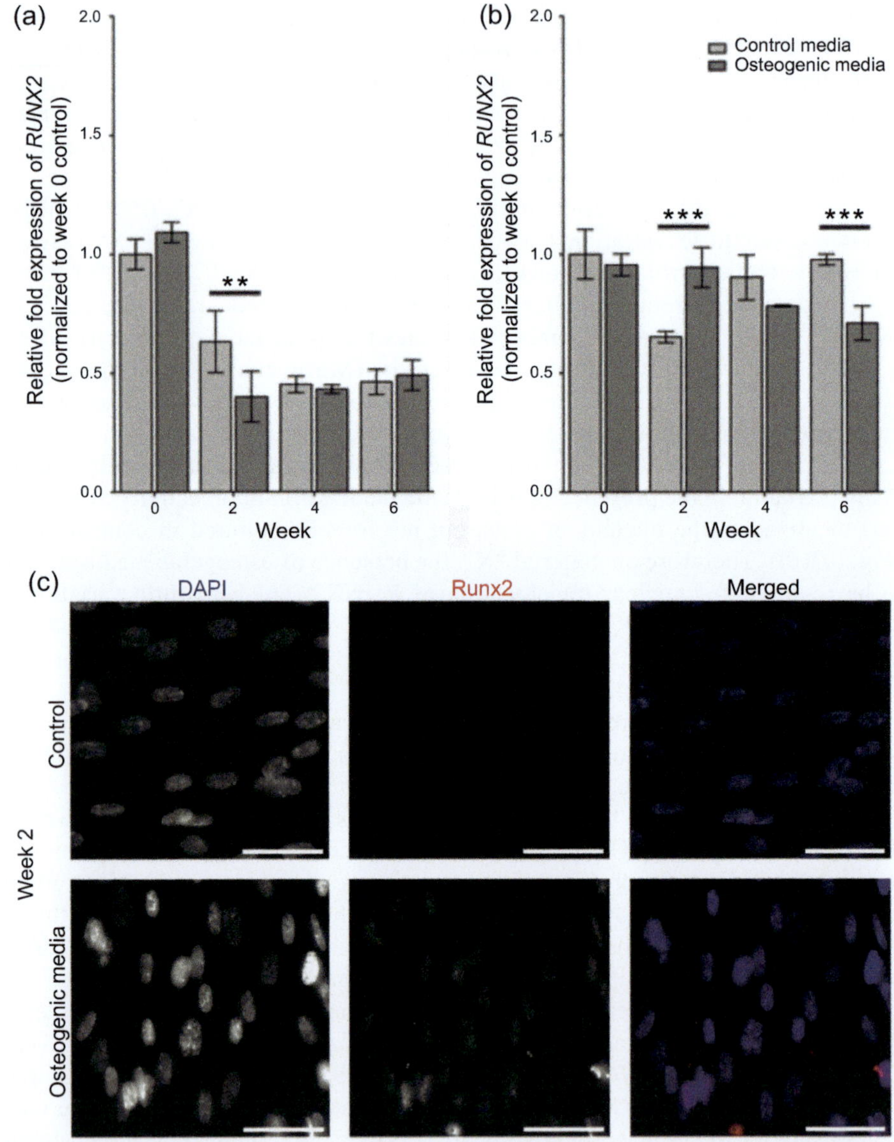

Figure 6.3 *RUNX2* mRNA levels in hPDL cells cultured in osteogenic media. (a) Cells isolated from a male, 20 years old, and (b) cells from a female, 39 years old. (c) RUNX2 localization in hPDL cells induced to undergo osteogenic differentiation, patient F29, at 2 weeks postseeding.

Genes not associated with osteogenesis

In these types of experiments, analysis of gene transcripts that should be downregulated or not expressed by cells that are committed to a specific cell lineage, in the case of osteoblast lineage, is often overlooked by investigators. hPDL cells often express markers associated with cementoblasts, including *CEMP1* (Cementum protein 1).

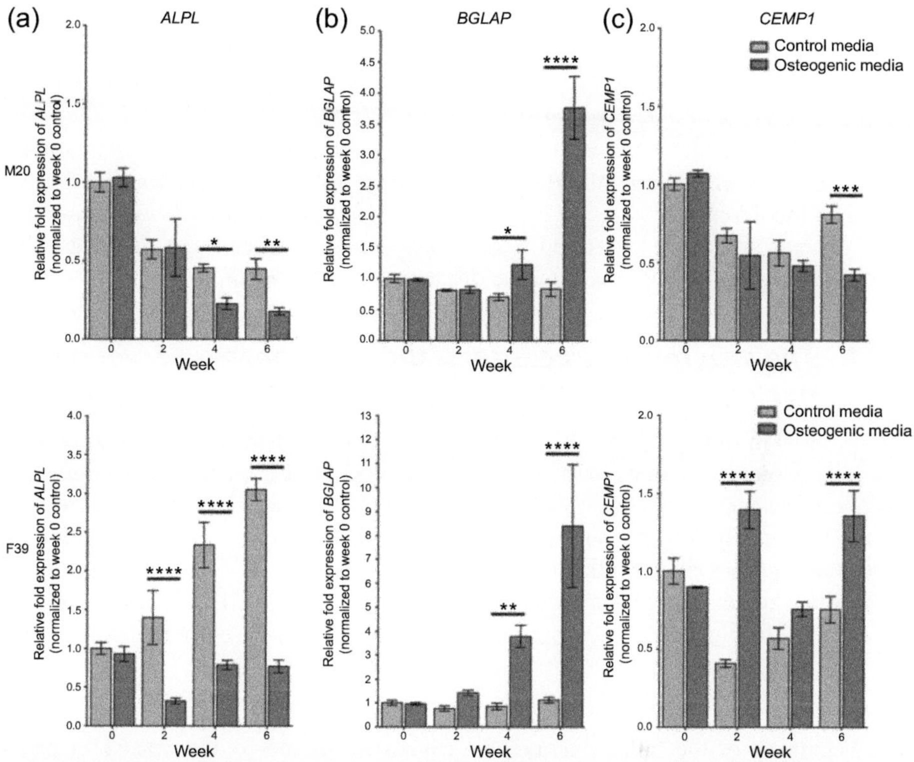

Figure 6.4 Gene expression of hPDL cells during osteogenic differentiation. Cells were isolated from a male, 20 years old and from a female, 39 years old. Expression of *ALPL* (alkaline phosphatase), *BGLAP* (osteocalcin), and *CEMP1* (cementum protein 1) was assessed in hPDL cells that were induced to undergo osteogenic differentiation (osteogenic media) compared to controls (control media) at 0, 2, 4, and 6 weeks. Cells from patient M20 showed gene expression typical of osteogenic differentiation, indicating mature osteoblast phenotype at 4 and 6 weeks as (a) *ALPL* expression decreased and (b) *BGLAP* increased relative to controls. Cells from patient F39 showed a decrease in expression of *ALPL* at 2, 4, and 6 weeks and expression of *BGLAP* at 4 and 6 weeks in response to osteogenic stimuli. For M20, expression of (c) *CEMP1* at 6 weeks was significantly lower in osteogenic condition, which was consistent with terminal differentiation of the cells. However, in F39, *CEMP1* levels remained significantly higher in osteogenic conditions, which correlates with a more immature phenotype. Data for each patient is presented as mean ± SD of three internal replicates from one experiment. Two-way ANOVA, Bonferroni posttest for multiple comparisons within time points, multiplicity-adjusted p-values reported. *$p<.05$, **$p<.01$, ***$p<.001$, ****$p<.0001$.

While expression of *CEMP1* is not specific to cementoblasts, it has been shown to be downregulated in hPDL cells induced to undergo osteogenic differentiation (Komaki et al., 2012). In M20, our results were consistent with the findings of Komaki and colleagues, although gene expression in cells from F39 contradicted the literature (Fig. 6.4(c)). As such, our results show that there is variability in the expression of *CEMP1* by hPDL cells during osteogenic induction. This emphasizes that it can be pertinent to consider genes that should be downregulated, rather than upregulated, in the design of experiments.

6.4 Gene expression in a context of skin healing

Promotion of skin repair through the use of bioactive material is an important and clinically relevant research field. In this section, we will present a hypothetical study assessing the efficacy of a biomaterial to promote wound healing in a diabetic murine model. In skin, the temporal expression of genes following wounding is strongly linked to the temporal phases of wound healing. However, before documenting how gene expression can be measured during skin healing, the cell and molecular processes leading to skin repair need to be discussed in more depth.

6.4.1 The skin repair process and the three phases of wound healing

Following skin injury, a cascade of complex cellular mechanisms occurs in order to repair the wounded tissues. In mice, the animal model to be used in this example, the temporal mechanisms are classically grouped into three major overlapping phases. In the case of full-thickness wounds where the dermis and the epidermis are both damaged, three phases of (1) inflammation, (2) proliferation, and (3) remodeling occur to facilitate repair (Singer and Clark, 1999; Walker et al., 2015). These phases are summarized in Fig. 6.5.

6.4.1.1 Inflammatory phase

The beginning of the inflammatory phase is characterized by the release of proinflammatory molecules by the platelets, forming the hemostasis clot and damaged host cells. These cytokines and growth factors initiate recruitment of immune cells to the wound site, initially large numbers of neutrophils (Walker et al., 2015). Neutrophils are a type of granular white blood cell that phagocytose foreign particles and bacteria. Their action is very aggressive; they will secrete proteases, reactive oxygen species, and cytokines such as MCP-1, TNF-α, and IL-1 to recruit monocytes at the wound site. Their presence is maximal at the wound site two days after injury.

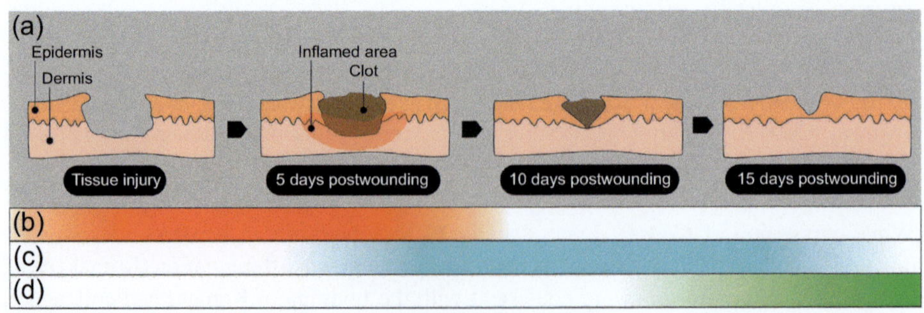

Figure 6.5 Schematic representation of the skin-healing process. (a) Representation of a wound cross section at key time points. Temporal representation of (b) inflammatory phase, (c) proliferative phase, and (d) the remodeling phase.

Temporally, monocytes are recruited to the wound bed in the inflammatory phase, differentiating into macrophages at the wound site (Lucas et al., 2010). Besides possessing phagocytic activity, macrophages also release proinflammatory molecules to potentiate the inflammatory response but also crucially release proproliferative molecules that will initiate the subsequent stages of healing (Mahdavian Delavary et al., 2011). Different subtypes of macrophages orchestrate those two processes (Martinez et al., 2008). Macrophages can be polarized toward the proinflammatory end of the spectrum (classic or M1 polarization) or the proregenerative end of the spectrum (alternative or M2 polarization) (Mahdavian Delavary et al., 2011), although a clear distinction of these phenotypes can be difficult to observe. The maintenance of the inflammatory response is mainly mediated through the release of proinflammatory cytokines such as TNF-α and IL-1 by M1 macrophages, while TGF-β, VEGF, PDGF, and IGF-1 are associated with M2 macrophages to initiate the proliferative phase. Finally, macrophages are also involved in humoral immunity by presenting antigens to lymphocytes when they arrive at the wound site around day 5 and peak at day 7 (Schaffer and Barbul, 1998).

6.4.1.2 Proliferative phase

The proliferative phase can be subdivided into three major processes: reepithelialization (regeneration of the epidermis), the granulation tissue formation (dermal repair), and angiogenesis (revascularization of the granulation tissue) (Gurtner et al., 2008). In a normal situation, these processes will typically lead to the formation of scar tissue, depending on the size and depth of the original injury. In order for appropriate completion of these cellular processes, communication must be coordinated between multiple different cell populations, including immune cells, myofibroblasts, endothelial cells, and keratinocytes (Eming et al., 2014). This can make assessing gene expression particularly challenging and difficult to interpret. These cells, as well as specific gene expression markers that allow identification of their presence in the wound, are shown in Fig. 6.6.

Neutrophils and macrophages produce trophic factors that will activate the resident cells of the wound during the inflammatory phase. Among those, the surrounding keratinocytes will facilitate reepithelialization by proliferating and migrating across the damaged area to reestablish barrier function. Two days after wounding, keratinocytes will upregulate the expression of keratin 10, 1, and 2 (K10, K1, and K2), as well as laminin 332 (Fuchs and Weber, 1994; Laplante et al., 2001). Concurrently, stromal cells are activated and upregulate secrete periostin, a protein that mediates stromal cell differentiation into myofibroblasts (Elliott et al., 2012). Myofibroblasts migrate into the wound bed to secrete a temporary granulation tissue made out of type I/III collagens and fibronectin in order to fill the space left empty by the injury. Other resident cell populations, including endothelial cells and pericytes, also invade the granulation tissue to revascularize the healing tissue (Morikawa and Ezaki, 2011).

6.4.1.3 Remodeling phase

Toward the end of the proliferative phase, there is a shift in the role of the myofibroblast as they start to turn over the extracellular matrix (ECM) through the secretion of

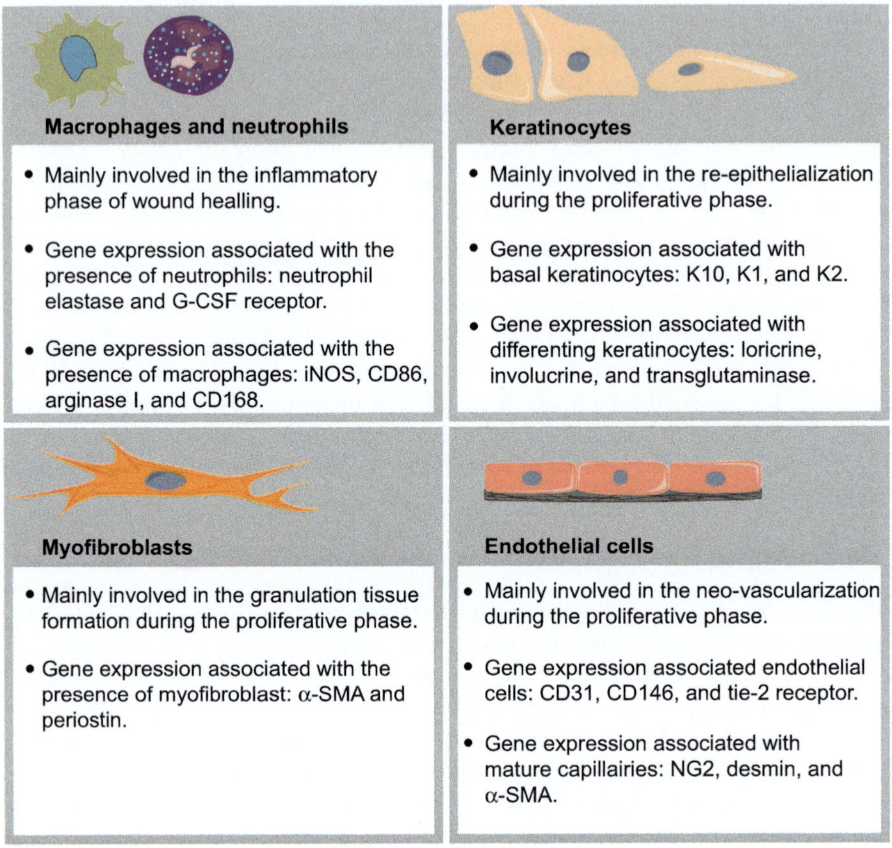

Figure 6.6 Main cell types contributing to the wound-healing response. *α-SMA*, α-smooth muscle actin; *G-CSF*, granulocyte-colony stimulating factor; *iNOS*, inducible nitric oxide synthases; *K10, K1, and K2*, keratin 10, 1, and 2; *NG2*, neural/glial antigen 2; *Tie-2*, tyrosine kinase with immunoglobulin and EGF homology domains 2.

matrix metalloproteinases (MMPs), combined with the synthesis of new ECM components, including collagen type I (Gurtner et al., 2008). The remodeling phase is also characterized by the regression of the overdeveloped capillary network that was formed during the proliferative phase, with endothelial cells undergoing apoptosis, reducing the number of capillaries.

6.4.2 Biomaterials and their effect on wound healing: a practical example

As explained thoroughly in Section 4.1, wound healing is a very complex process that requires spatial and temporal fine-tuning of multiple genes in several different cell populations. Any researchers studying biomaterial development for applications in cutaneous wound-healing context need to factor this knowledge into their experimental design.

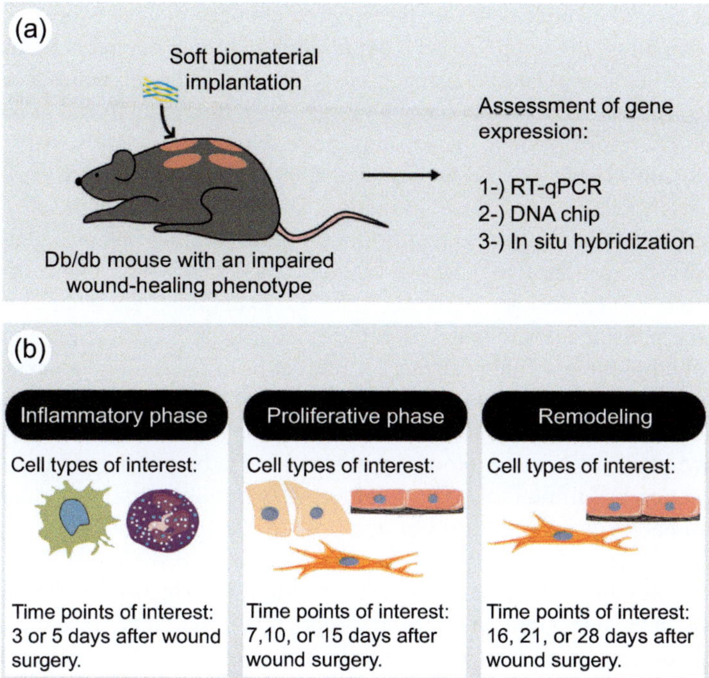

Figure 6.7 Experimental design of hypothetical experiment to investigate the effect of biomaterial "X" on gene expression in wound healing. (a) Animal model and downstream assays. (b) Cell types and time points of interest in the three phases of wound healing.

To probe how gene expression could be utilized in the assessment of a biomaterial on wound healing, we will use the dorsal full-thickness wound-healing model in C57BLKS-Leprdb (also named db/db) mice. db/db mice have a mutation in the leptin receptor (*LEPR*), which leads to the development of type II diabetes, and the mice harbor a well-described impairment in skin healing (Michaels et al., 2007). This model is commonly used in wound-healing experiments and is a useful tool to study wound healing in a manner representing impaired repair (Nambu et al., 2009; Tkalcevic et al., 2009; Van Slyke et al., 2009). The experimental design of our practical example illustrated in Fig. 6.7 will be the creation of four full-thickness 6-mm wounds on the back of each db/db mouse, with a soft biomaterial "X" implanted into half of the wounds (see Fig. 6.7(a)). In this impaired wound-healing model, the inflammatory phase is ongoing from day 0 to day 7, the proliferative phase begins around day 4 to day 15, and the remodeling phase starts at wound closure and is ongoing for several months (Tsuboi and Rifkin, 1990). Knowing how the impairment influences the timing of each stage of healing in the db/db mice is very important information, since the spatiotemporal expression of the target genes related to the phases of healing will vary, and how gene expression patterns are changed provides essential information on the efficacy of the biomaterial (Cooper et al., 2005; Deonarine et al., 2007; Lefebvre-Lavoie et al., 2005).

So what should be considered with respect to changes in gene expression? If scaffolds speed healing, the temporal gene expression pattern expected in db/db mice and the phases of healing would be accelerated. This would change which genes will be active based on cell recruitment and which genes should be analyzed at any selected time point. Therefore prior to performing gene expression studies, it is prudent to perform closure kinetic assays, as we have done, to assess where the effect of the scaffold starts to change the closure kinetics. This allows assessment of whether the repair speed is increasing and therefore the phase of healing has changed, i.e., from inflammatory to proliferative. Closure kinetics illustrates which phase of healing is being affected by the presence of the scaffold. For example, if the wounds are reduced in size in the presence of the material between days 1 and 3 compared to controls, it is very likely that the scaffold is altering a number of inflammatory processes. In contrast, if wound closure were faster in the presence of the biomaterial versus controls between days 4 and 7, the scaffold is very likely to influence processes part of the proliferative phase of healing. However, it should also be considered that measuring closure kinetics has limitations. For instance, it is possible that a biomaterial could alter inflammatory events that do not manifest in changes in closure rates until the proliferative phase.

Finally, although gene expression can give a lot of information on the effects of the scaffolds on the resident cell types of the wound, it is important to also include assessments at the protein level. This is particularly important since it is recognized that several posttranscriptional modifications affect the regulation of genes involved in wound healing. Besides, discoveries have also highlighted more than 21 microRNAs that can act as regulators of gene transcripts implicated in wound healing (Moura et al., 2014).

6.4.2.1 *Methods for in vivo gene expression analysis*

As indicated in Fig. 6.7, there are three main techniques for analyzing or quantifying gene expression that can be used effectively in assessment of the efficacy of a biomaterial on enhancing skin closure: RT-qPCR, microarray, and in situ hybridization. With these methods singularly or in combination, it is possible to quantify the effect of a given biomaterial on wound healing through gene expression, but it must also be combined with histological analysis, as will be illustrated, to get the most meaningful data. When assessing gene expression in vivo, temporally the cell populations change, and subsequently, so do the genes expressed. The advantages and the drawback of each method will be explained in the following section using the context of one of the three wound-healing phases.

In situ hybridization and inflammation

Extraction of mRNA and RT-qPCR could be used to get a screen of the types of genes expressed, but this information by itself will be of limited value, as it will not provide the abundance of each cell type. Neutrophils and macrophages are the main cell types that are present in the inflammatory phase of wound healing (Walker et al., 2016) (Fig. 6.6). The balance of neutrophils to macrophages, and further, presence of specific macrophage subpopulations is more pertinent information. The best method for assessing these genes would be in situ hybridization, which uses a labeled complementary RNA or DNA probe to localize a specific DNA or RNA sequence in a section of tissue (Zhou et al., 2010). Using this technique would demonstrate the influence of a biomaterial on the relative number and location of neutrophils and macrophages in the tissue at each specified time point. The advantage of this technique is that it localizes the signal to the specific cells expressing the mRNA, allowing identification and relative abundance of each cell type. Probes that could be used include neutrophil elastase (neutrophil marker, see Fig. 6.6), iNOS, and arginase I (macrophage markers). If sections were labeled for these markers at 1, 3, and 5 days postwounding, a direct measure could be made on the level and maturation of the inflammatory response. In situ hybridization results could be correlated with RT-qPCR for the same results and through immunohistochemistry to detect the active protein, giving a comprehensive analysis of the healing response.

Proliferative phase and microarrays

In the context of the proliferative phase of wound healing, measuring gene expression can be both complex and informative: the former because many different cell populations are still present. Inflammatory cells, mainly macrophages, persist during granulation tissue maturation and mesenchymal cell infiltration. While RT-qPCR can be used to quantify specific markers, as we have done in previous studies at this stage (Elliott et al., 2012; Walker et al., 2016), another method for analyzing gene expression that is relevant at this stage of healing is using a microarray-based approach. Advantages of this method are that it assesses global gene expression and can be used to assess up- and downregulation of gene clusters associated with reepithelialization, granulation tissue formation, and angiogenesis (Cole et al., 2001). Time points that should be used to study gene expression temporally in the proliferative phase are shown in Fig. 6.5.

As briefly mentioned earlier, one of the advantages of microarrays is that it allows analysis of gene clusters. By assigning genes into specific clusters, the transcriptome data generated can show which specific cellular functions have been altered, such as cell survival, cell migration, cell proliferation, etc. This analysis can reduce the number of genes of interest to a few candidates. Afterward, those genes can also be probed using different techniques, such as in situ hybridization, which allows confirmation of which cell populations are expressing the gene of interest, that is, are genes associated with reepithelialization, for example, actually localized to keratinocytes.

Microarrays can be used to measure the gene expression levels of all the known genes of a species genome at one time in one tissue sample. Not surprisingly, this generates a substantial amount of information, with analysis of microarray results requiring substantial bioinformatics knowledge (Zhang et al., 2009). Furthermore, the sensitivity of microarrays is much lower than RT-qPCR: the genes of interest will ultimately have to be confirmed using specific primers and RT-qPCR.

Remodeling phase of healing and RT-qPCR

Upon transition of the proliferative to the remodeling phase, in general, many of the gene clusters evident during proliferation will be downregulated, and the tissue will return to a quiescent state (Walker et al., 2015). As the granulation tissue ECM matures into a connective tissue resembling dermis, the gene expression of profibrotic clusters (including the cell proliferation and ECM secretion genes) should decrease following wound closure, while the gene expression of apoptotic and matrix-remodeling genes (including MMPs and TIMPs (tissue inhibitors of metalloproteinases)) should increase. One of the major areas to investigate with respect to a biomaterial for skin healing in the remodeling phase is whether or not it induces scar formation. Due to decades of research, many of the genes associated with scar healing are very well defined and thus, RT-qPCR is a more suitable method for use at this stage of healing. For instance, RT-qPCR directed against α-smooth muscle actin (Hinz, 2007), type I collagen (Gauglitz et al., 2011), and periostin (Crawford et al., 2014) could be correlated to an increase a profibrotic state within the wound.

For a biomaterial to be considered as having a positive impact on scarring, it should suppress cellular proliferation and matrix deposition during the remodeling phase of healing. In contrast, prolonged activation of myofibroblasts and matrix deposition during that phase would infer that the material is having a pro-scarring effect, which could limit its clinical applicability. Gene expression analysis can provide a useful insight of the effect of biomaterials on these processes.

6.5 Future trends/conclusions

The rapid development of techniques for assessing gene expression has exponentially expanded our knowledge of cell response at the molecular level, allowing identification of how cells regulate specific processes and behaviors. With the increasing use of biomaterials in medicine, understanding how cells respond to foreign materials from a molecular standpoint will be instrumental in development of more appropriate materials. As highlighted within this chapter, utilizing gene expression properly can be a challenging task, particularly in vivo, and the relevance of the data by itself must always be questioned. However, it is clear that gene expression technology will play a pivotal role in future years in the development of rational biomaterials for specific medical applications.

References

Bellows, C.G., Aubin, J.E., Heersche, J.N., Antosz, M.E., 1986. Mineralized bone nodules formed in vitro from enzymatically released rat calvaria cell populations. Calcif. Tissue Int. 38, 143–154.

Camilleri, S., McDonald, F., 2006. Runx2 and dental development. Eur. J. Oral Sci. 114, 361–373.

Chen, J., Shapiro, H.S., Sodek, J., 1992. Development expression of bone sialoprotein mRNA in rat mineralized connective tissues. J. Bone Miner. Res. 7, 987–997.

Chen, J., Singh, K., Mukherjee, B.B., Sodek, J., 1993. Developmental expression of osteopontin (OPN) mRNA in rat tissues: evidence for a role for OPN in bone formation and resorption. Matrix 13, 113–123.

Cole, J., Tsou, R., Wallace, K., Gibran, N., Isik, F., 2001. Early gene expression profile of human skin to injury using high-density cDNA microarrays. Wound Repair Regen. 9, 360–370.
Cooper, L., Johnson, C., Burslem, F., Martin, P., 2005. Wound healing and inflammation genes revealed by array analysis of 'macrophageless' *PU.1* null mice. Genome Biol. 6, R5.
Crawford, J., Nygard, K., Gan, B.S., O'Gorman, D.B., 2014. Periostin induces fibroblast proliferation and myofibroblast persistence in hypertrophic scarring. Exp. Dermatol.
Czekanska, E.M., Stoddart, M.J., Richards, R.G., Hayes, J.S., 2012. In search of an osteoblast cell model for in vitro research. Eur. Cell Mater. 24, 1–17.
Deonarine, K., Panelli, M.C., Stashower, M.E., Jin, P., Smith, K., Slade, H.B., Norwood, C., Wang, E., Marincola, F.M., Stroncek, D.F., 2007. Gene expression profiling of cutaneous wound healing. J. Transl. Med. 5, 11.
Dutta, D., Cole, N., Willcox, M., 2012. Factors influencing bacterial adhesion to contact lenses. Mol. Vis. 18, 14–21.
Elliott, C.G., Wang, J., Guo, X., Xu, S.W., Eastwood, M., Guan, J., Leask, A., Conway, S.J., Hamilton, D.W., 2012. Periostin modulates myofibroblast differentiation during full-thickness cutaneous wound repair. J. Cell Sci. 125, 121–132.
Eming, S.A., Martin, P., Tomic-Canic, M., 2014. Wound repair and regeneration: mechanisms, signaling, and translation. Sci. Transl. Med. 6, 265sr266.
Fuchs, E., Weber, K., 1994. Intermediate filaments: structure, dynamics, function, and disease. Annu. Rev. Biochem. 63, 345–382.
Gauglitz, G.G., Korting, H.C., Pavicic, T., Ruzicka, T., Jeschke, M.G., 2011. Hypertrophic scarring and keloids: pathomechanisms and current and emerging treatment strategies. Mol. Med. 17, 113–125.
Gilbert, S.F., 2000. Control of gene expression at the level of translation. In: Developmental Biology. Sinauer Associates, Inc., Sunderland, Massachusetts.
Golub, E.E., Boesze-Battaglia, K., 2007. The role of alkaline phosphatase in mineralization. Curr. Opin. Orthop. 18, 444–448.
Goodkind, J.R., Edwards, J.S., 2005. Gene expression measurement technologies: innovations and ethical considerations. Comput. Chem. Eng. 29, 589–596.
Groen, N., Guvendiren, M., Rabitz, H., Welsh, W.J., Kohn, J., de Boer, J., 2016. Stepping into the omics era: opportunities and challenges for biomaterials science and engineering. Acta Biomater. 34, 133–142.
Gurtner, G.C., Werner, S., Barrandon, Y., Longaker, M.T., 2008. Wound repair and regeneration. Nature 453, 314–321.
Hamilton, D.W., Brunette, D.M., 2007. The effect of substratum topography on osteoblast adhesion mediated signal transduction and phosphorylation. Biomaterials 28, 1806–1819.
Hanagata, N., 2015. Global gene expression analysis for the assessment of nanobiomaterials. Front. Oral Biol. 17, 78–89.
Heid, C.A., Stevens, J., Livak, K.J., Williams, P.M., 1996. Real time quantitative PCR. Genome Res. 6, 986–994.
Hinz, B., 2007. Formation and function of the myofibroblast during tissue repair. J. Invest. Dermatol.
Jaiswal, N., Haynesworth, S.E., Caplan, A.I., Bruder, S.P., 1997. Osteogenic differentiation of purified, culture-expanded human mesenchymal stem cells in vitro. J. Cell. Biochem. 64, 295–312.
Kim, S.S., Wen, W., Prowse, P., Hamilton, D.W., 2015. Regulation of matrix remodelling phenotype in gingival fibroblasts by substratum topography. J. Cell Mol. Med. 19, 1183–1196.
Komaki, M., Iwasaki, K., Arzate, H., Narayanan, A.S., Izumi, Y., Morita, I., 2012. Cementum protein 1 (CEMP1) induces a cementoblastic phenotype and reduces osteoblastic differentiation in periodontal ligament cells. J. Cell. Physiol. 227, 649–657.

Komori, T., 2006. Regulation of osteoblast differentiation by transcription factors. J. Cell. Biochem. 99, 1233–1239.

Laplante, A.F., Germain, L., Auger, F.A., Moulin, V., 2001. Mechanisms of wound reepithelialization: hints from a tissue-engineered reconstructed skin to long-standing questions. FASEB J. 15, 2377–2389.

Lefebvre-Lavoie, J., Lussier, J.G., Theoret, C.L., 2005. Profiling of differentially expressed genes in wound margin biopsies of horses using suppression subtractive hybridization. Physiol. Genomics 22, 157–170.

Li, C., Wong, W.H., 2001. Model-based analysis of oligonucleotide arrays: expression index computation and outlier detection. Proc. Natl. Acad. Sci. U.S.A. 98, 31–36.

Lim, J.Y., Donahue, H.J., 2007. Cell sensing and response to micro- and nanostructured surfaces produced by chemical and topographic patterning. Tissue Eng. 13, 1879–1891.

Liu, W.,F., Chen, C.S., 2005. Engineering biomaterials to control cell function. Mater.Today 8, 28–35.

Lothrop, A.P., Torres, M.P., Fuchs, S.M., 2013. Deciphering post-translational modification codes. FEBS Lett. 587, 1247–1257.

Lucas, T., Waisman, A., Ranjan, R., Roes, J., Krieg, T., Muller, W., Roers, A., Eming, S.A., 2010. Differential roles of macrophages in diverse phases of skin repair. J. Immunol. 184, 3964–3977.

Mahdavian Delavary, B., van der Veer, W.M., van Egmond, M., Niessen, F.B., Beelen, R.H., 2011. Macrophages in skin injury and repair. Immunobiology 216, 753–762.

Martinez, F.O., Sica, A., Mantovani, A., Locati, M., 2008. Macrophage activation and polarization. Front. Biosci. 13, 453–461.

McManus, C.J., Graveley, B.R., 2011. RNA structure and the mechanisms of alternative splicing. Curr. Opin. Genet. Dev. 21, 373–379.

Michaels, J., Churgin, S.S., Blechman, K.M., Greives, M.R., Aarabi, S., Galiano, R.D., Gurtner, G.C., 2007. db/db mice exhibit severe wound-healing impairments compared with other murine diabetic strains in a silicone-splinted excisional wound model. Wound Repair Regen. 15, 665–670.

Miron, R.J., Oates, C.J., Molenberg, A., Dard, M., Hamilton, D.W., 2010. The effect of enamel matrix proteins on the spreading, proliferation and differentiation of osteoblasts cultured on titanium surfaces. Biomaterials 31, 449–460.

Morikawa, S., Ezaki, T., 2011. Phenotypic changes and possible angiogenic roles of pericytes during wound healing in the mouse skin. Histol. Histopathol. 26, 979–995.

Moura, J., Borsheim, E., Carvalho, E., 2014. The role of microRNAs in diabetic complications – special emphasis on wound healing. Genes 5, 926–956.

Nambu, M., Kishimoto, S., Nakamura, S., Mizuno, H., Yanagibayashi, S., Yamamoto, N., Azuma, R., Kiyosawa, T., Ishihara, M., Kanatani, Y., 2009. Accelerated wound healing in healing-impaired db/db mice by autologous adipose tissue-derived stromal cells combined with atelocollagen matrix. Ann. Plast. Surg. 62, 317–321.

Prowse, P.D., Elliott, C.G., Hutter, J., Hamilton, D.W., 2013. Inhibition of Rac and ROCK signalling influence osteoblast adhesion, differentiation and mineralization on titanium topographies. PLoS One 8, e58898.

Roth, C.M., 2002. Quantifying gene expression. Curr. Issue. Mol. Biol. 4, 93–100.

Sakiyama-Elbert, S.E., Hubbell, J.A., 2001. Functional biomaterials: design of novel biomaterials. Annu. Rev. Mater. Res. 31, 183–201.

Schaffer, M., Barbul, A., 1998. Lymphocyte function in wound healing and following injury. Br. J. Surg. 85, 444–460.

Singer, A.J., Clark, R.A., 1999. Cutaneous wound healing. N. Engl. J. Med. 341, 738–746.

Tkalcevic, V.I., Cuzic, S., Parnham, M.J., Pasalic, I., Brajsa, K., 2009. Differential evaluation of excisional non-occluded wound healing in db/db mice. Toxicol. Pathol. 37, 183–192.

Tsuboi, R., Rifkin, D.B., 1990. Recombinant basic fibroblast growth factor stimulates wound healing in healing-impaired db/db mice. J. Exp. Med. 172, 245–251.

Van Slyke, P., Alami, J., Martin, D., Kuliszewski, M., Leong-Poi, H., Sefton, M.V., Dumont, D., 2009. Acceleration of diabetic wound healing by an angiopoietin peptide mimetic. Tissue Eng. Part A 15, 1269–1280.

Walker, J.T., Elliott, C.G., Forbes, T.L., Hamilton, D.W., 2016. Genetic deletion of galectin-3 does not impair full-thickness excisional skin healing. J. Invest. Dermatol. 136, 1042–1050.

Walker, J.T., Kim, S.S., Michelsons, S., Creber, K., Elliott, C.G., Leask, A., Hamilton, D.W., 2015. Cell–matrix interactions governing skin repair: matricellular proteins as diverse modulators of cell function. Res. Rep. Biochem. 5, 73–88.

Williams, D., 2003. Revisiting the definition of biocompatibility. Med. Device Technol. 14, 10–13.

Wong, M.L., Medrano, J.F., 2005. Real-time PCR for mRNA quantitation. BioTechniques 39, 75–85.

Zhang, Y., Szustakowski, J., Schinke, M., 2009. Bioinformatics analysis of microarray data. Methods Mol. Biol. 573, 259–284.

Zhou, H.M., Wang, J., Elliott, C., Wen, W., Hamilton, D.W., Conway, S.J., 2010. Spatiotemporal expression of periostin during skin development and incisional wound healing: lessons for human fibrotic scar formation. J. Cell Commun. Signal. 4, 99–107.

Part Three

Monitoring and evaluation of functional biomaterial performance in vivo

Monitoring and tracking metallic nanobiomaterials in vivo

7

D. Pissuwan
Mahidol University, Bangkok, Thailand

7.1 Metallic nanobiomaterials

Many metal nanomaterials have shown excellent properties that are suitable for in vivo biomedical applications. Gold nanoparticles and iron oxide magnetic nanoparticles have especially shown a high potential as diagnostic markers and therapeutic tools in various diseases (Hudoklin et al., 2013; Liu et al., 2008, 2015; Lara-González et al., 2013). These metallic nanobiomaterials are easy to synthesize. Furthermore, their surfaces can be modified and functionalized with various types of chemical and biological molecules (Neouze and Schubert, 2008). Their unique optical properties also make these metallic nanobiomaterials attractive candidates in biomedical fields (Huang and El-Sayed, 2010; Coronado et al., 2011). A brief introduction of gold and magnetic iron oxide nanobiomaterials are in the following lists.

7.1.1 Gold nanoparticles

Gold nanoparticles (GNPs) can be easily synthesized using various techniques, depending on the required shape and size (Pérez-Juste et al., 2005). Their surfaces can also be simply modified and attached with several molecules, such as antibody, protein, carbohydrate, and lipid (Di Pasqua et al., 2009; Pissuwan et al., 2007). According to the review by Dykman and Khlebtsov (2011), many shapes of GNPs have been applied in biomedical applications, such as spherical and rod shapes (Fig. 7.1). However, it seems that spherical and rod-shaped GNPs are the most common shapes used in biomedical applications. Spherical GNPs can be synthesized by chemical reduction, and rod-shaped GNPs are generally synthesized by the seed-mediated synthesis method. The difference in shape and size of GNPs leads to different optical properties and cellular uptakes that can increase the wide use of GNPs in modern biomedical applications both in vitro and in vivo (Kim et al., 2015). For example, they can be applied as a potential tool for the diagnosis of various diseases (Mieszawska et al., 2013; Pissuwan et al., 2008). Due to their surface plasmon property, the light absorbed by GNPs can be converted into heat, which makes gold nanoparticles suitable for photothermal therapy (Huang and El-Sayed, 2011; Pissuwan et al., 2006). Rod-shaped GNPs or gold nanorods (GNRs) are especially well-known for having high photothermal efficiency. Their optical absorption can also be tuned to the near-infrared region, which can reduce the risk of healthy tissue damage from light exposure because of the low light absorption of biological tissues at near-infrared wavelengths. Besides this decent property, GNRs also have strong surface

Monitoring and Evaluation of Biomaterials and their Performance in vivo. http://dx.doi.org/10.1016/B978-0-08-100603-0.00007-9

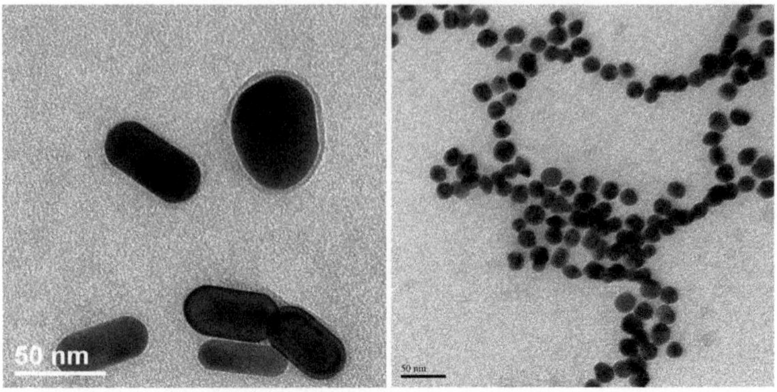

Figure 7.1 SRod and spherical shapes of gold nanoparticles.

plasmon absorption and a high light-scattering ability that make them useful in therapeutic, diagnostic, and imaging applications (Pissuwan et al., 2008).

7.1.2 Magnetic iron oxide nanoparticles

Magnetic iron oxide nanoparticles (MINPs) are also attractive nanoparticles with an excellent magnetic property that is suitable for application in biomedical approaches. Although MINPs are easily oxidized with air, similar to GNPs, their surface can be modified to provide better stability than the naked form. Various types of inorganic coatings, such as metal substance, silica, sulfide, metal oxide, and nonmetal material, can be used for coating the surface of MINPs. Besides these inorganic materials, MINPs can also be indirectly or directly coated with organic materials. The common organic materials that have been used to coat the surface of MINPs are dextran, starch, poly(ethylene glycol) (PEG), poly(D, L-lactide), and polyethylenimine. In general, after coating MINPs with these materials, they can be further modified with designed molecules (Wu et al., 2008, 2015). It is commonly known that there are three popular forms of MINPs: hematite (α-Fe_2O_3), magnetite (Fe_2O_4), and maghemite (γ-Fe_2O_3) (Fig. 7.2) (Wu et al., 2015). Their morphology relies on an iron oxide precursor with other processes such as nucleation, growth, and adsorption, which cause more difficulty in controlling the shape and size of MINPs than gold nanoparticle synthesis. Nevertheless, different shapes and sizes of MINPs can be prepared through various techniques, such as hydrothermal synthesis, thermal decomposition, coprecipitation, and sonochemical synthesis (Roca et al., 2009; Wu et al., 2008). The aggregation is an important factor on synthesis of MINPs (Mohapatra and Anand, 2010). Different techniques for MINP synthesis were reviewed by Laurent et al. (2008). As mentioned previously, it is important to make MINPS stable against aggregation stimulated by the magnetic field and biological fluid. To overcome this aggregation problem, controlling electrostatic and steric repulsions is a key factor. Therefore many approaches of surface coatings have been applied to increase the stability of MINPs. However, the coating effect on magnetic property and biocompatibility of MINPs needs to be taken into consideration.

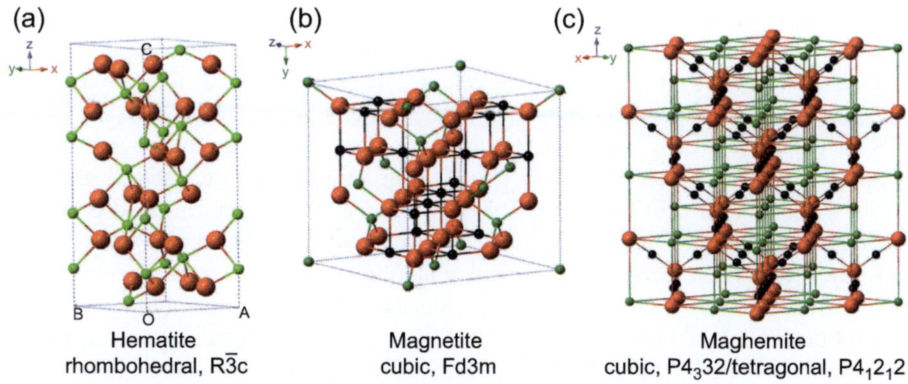

Figure 7.2 Different crystal structure of different MINPs. The black, green, and red *balls* represent Fe^{2+}, Fe^{3+}, and O^{2-} respectively. *MINPs*, magnetic iron oxide nanoparticles. Waiting for permission from Wu, W., Wu, Z., Yu, T., Jiang, C., Kim, W.S., 2015. Recent progress on magnetic iron oxide nanoparticles: synthesis, surface functional strategies and biomedical applications. Science and Technology of Advanced Materials 16, 023501.

7.2 Metallic nanobiomaterials for monitoring and tracking in vivo

Many imaging techniques and instrumentation have been developed to increase the efficiency of diagnostics and the treatment of diseases in vivo. To achieve this, many contrast agents and molecular imaging probes have been used in imaging systems to potentially visualize interesting biological features or biological signals in an in vivo system. For example, to monitor the reaction or mechanism of drugs or other therapeutic materials in vivo, fluorescent dyes have been used as probes and signal transducers for many years (Yamaoka et al., 2010; Carlson et al., 2013; Mérian et al., 2012; Ghoroghchian et al., 2009; Lisy et al., 2008). However, the loss of fluorescent signal always occurs because of bleaching fluorescent dyes. The adverse effect from fluorescent dyes to cells and tissues is another concerning issue (Jensen, 2021). Due to the fast growth of nanotechnology, the use of metallic nanobiomaterials in biomedical/biological applications is also quite attractive. It is well-known that metallic nanoparticles provide an interesting optical property that makes them useful for imaging modalities as a contrast agent or probe (Trequesser et al., 2013; Nune et al., 2009; Mody et al., 2010). The applications of using metallic nanobiomaterials (gold and magnetic iron oxide nanoparticles) are discussed here.

7.2.1 Tracking cellular regeneration

In recent years, stem cells have shown a great potential in regenerative medicine. However, a greater understanding in mechanism, function, and distribution of stem cells used for cellular regeneration in vivo is strongly needed. To investigate stem cell activities in vivo, labeling and tracking stem cells with metallic nanoparticles are quite attractive techniques. As mentioned previously, metallic nanoparticles have excellent physical and chemical properties, especially their optical property that supports metallic nanoparticles for use in various imaging systems. For example, rod-shaped gold nanoparticles (gold nanorods, GNRs) were coated with silica and used as a photoacoustic contrast agent to track stem cells in the musculature of living mice. After an injection of mesenchymal stem cells labeled with silica-coated GNRs, the labeled mesenchymal stem cells were detected in mice after photoacoustic imaging (Jokerst et al., 2012). The monitoring of skin tissue construction of adipose-derived stem cells (ASCs) labeled with PEGylated GNRs that coated a silica layer was also performed by Nam et al. (2015). With this technique, they could detect ASCs in the burn tissue of rats. The former work carried out by Nam et al. (2012) also labeled mesenchymal stem cells with 20 nm GNPs (citrate reduction gold nanospheres). The signal from the optical absorption of GNP labeling on mesenchymal stem cells could be monitored and tracked in Lewis rats using ultrasound-guided spectroscopic imaging and photoacoustic imaging. After GNPs were intramuscularly injected to rats, mesenchymal stem cell monitoring was detected through the spatial distribution of labeled cells for 3, 7, and 10 days (Fig. 7.3). It is worth noting here that GNPs used in their study were contained in a PEGylated fibrin gel system.

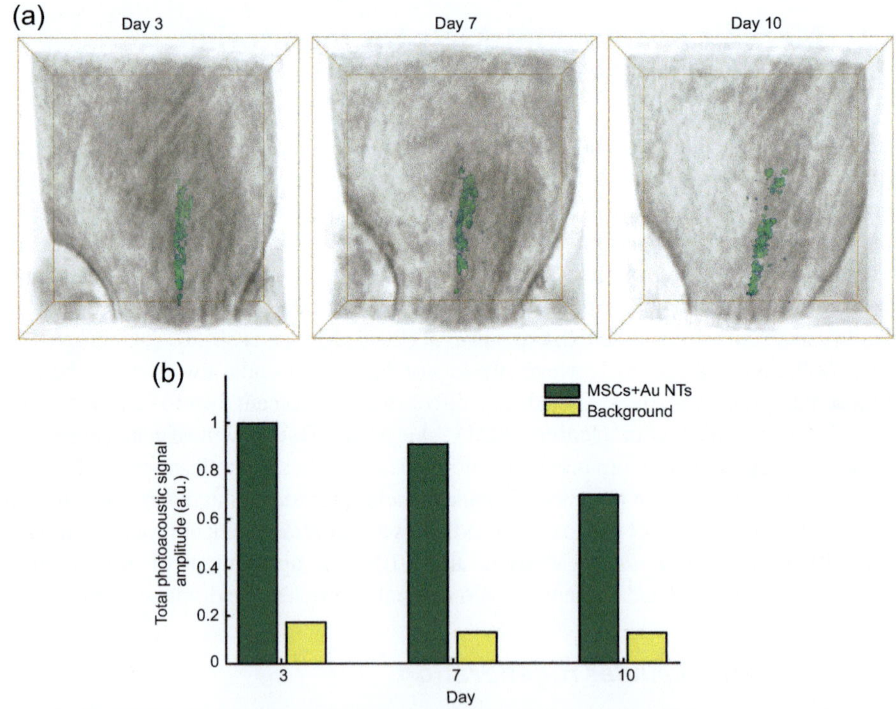

Figure 7.3 Monitoring of mesenchymal stem cells labeled with GNPs (a, shown in green) using ultrasound-guided spectroscopic imaging at 3, 7, and 10 days. The photoacoustic signals of mesenchymal stem cells labeled with GNPs (b). *GNPs*, gold nanoparticles.
Reproduced with permission from Nam, S.Y., Ricles, L.M., Suggs, L.J., Emelianov, S.Y., 2012. In vivo ultrasound and photoacoustic monitoring of mesenchymal stem cells labeled with gold nanotracers. PLoS One 7, e37267.

Magnetic resonance imaging (MRI) is another technique that can be used to monitor and assess cell activities and cell conditions. Cho et al. (2014) prepared iron oxide nanocrystals combined with bacterial genes, referred to as MagA, to monitor stem cell grafts in mice induced by doxycycline through diet (Tet-On; tetracycline inducible gene expression). This MagA acted as a genetic MRI reporter that could control the level of MRI contrast and also assess the cell grafts used for regenerative medicine. The tracking of mesenchymal stem cells labeled with chitosan-superparamagnetic iron oxide nanoparticles in rabbit brains under MRI was also performed by Reddy et al. (2010). Superparamagnetic iron oxide nanoparticles labeled with mesenchymal stem cells were also used to track how mesenchymal stem cells could be involved in the treatment of rheumatoid arthritis in vivo. With MRI, this technique can help gain information on mesenchymal stem cell mechanisms such as cell migration, cell localization, and rate of tissue repair by tracking stem cells (Markides et al., 2013).

7.2.2 Biodistribution monitoring of metallic nanobiomaterials to target tissue

Metallic nanobiomaterials can play a vital role in tissue targeting. Many techniques can be used to monitor how these materials interact with target tissues or how they are located in target tissues. A recent promising technique that can be used is surface-enhanced Raman spectroscopy (SERS). It was reported that the in vivo SERS spectra were detected in nude mice after injecting GNPs conjugated with the single chain variable fragment (ScFv) antibody into mice. The ScFV-GNP conjugates could target tumors in vivo and produce the SERS signals after exposure to a 785-nm laser beam at the tumor site (Fig. 7.4) (Qian et al., 2008).

A similar example using SERS nanomaterials to detect target tissue in vivo was reported by Samanta et al. (2014). They prepared a combination of Raman reporter (Cy7LA) with GNPs (60 nm citrate capped GNPs) encapsulated with polymers named as Cy7LA@GNPs@PEG-anti-CD184 nanotag. This nanotag could target teratoma after 4 h postinjection. The strong SERS signals were detected from the germ layer of teratoma. In the case of nanotag without anti-CD184, no SERS signal was detected from teratoma. Due to the excellent plasmonic properties of GNRs, they can be applied with optical coherence tomography (OCT) for in vivo imaging. It is commonly known that long GNRs have a stronger light scattering than short ones. To have high quality in vivo OCT imaging, it is important to have a strong signal from exogenous agents that can overcome the intrinsic signal of living tissues. SoRelle et al. (2015) used long GNRs (~100 nm in length and 30 nm in width) as OCT contrast agents for in vivo imaging. GNRs were coated with PSS (polystyrene sulfonate) and PEG (Polyethylene glycol) referred to GNR-PSS-mPEG. Then they were injected into a nude mouse-bearing tumor (a U87MG tumor xenograft in the right pinna of a mouse) through a tail vein. The enhancement of the OCT signal in blood vessels at tumor tissues was detected.

MINPs can be also used to target tissues in vivo. The recent work contributed by NDong et al. (2015) has shown that 30 nm MINPs conjugated with Trastuzufab (Tfab) protein sequence could be well-concentrated at the target tumor tissue of NSG (NOD *scid* gamma) mice bearing human HER2 positive BT-474 tumors after intravenous

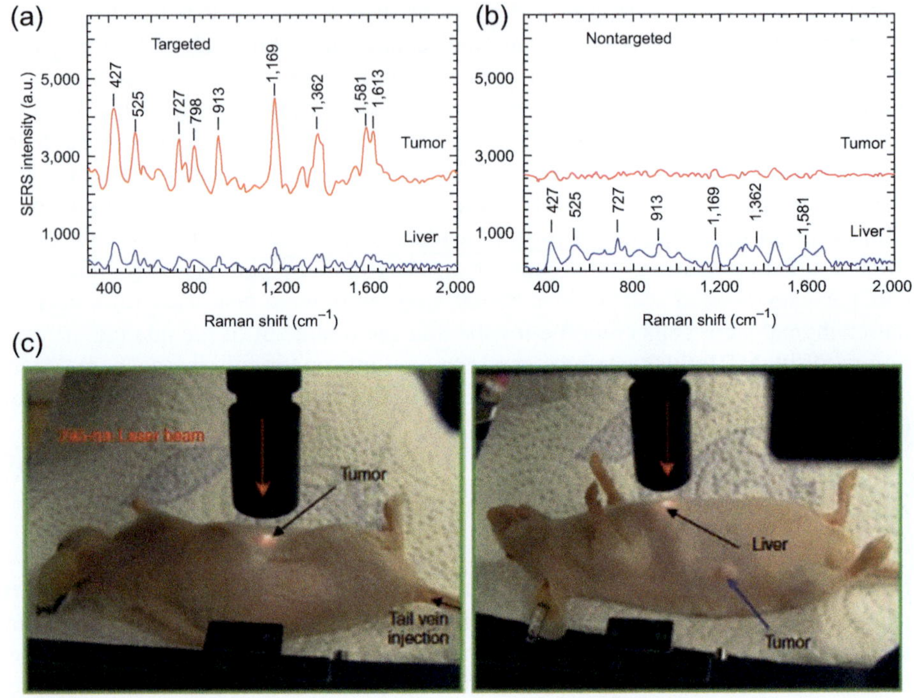

Figure 7.4 In vivo detection of SERS spectra in nude mice after injecting with ScFV-GNP conjugates. SERS spectra detected at tumor and liver after injecting ScFV-GNP conjugates respectively (a, b). When nude mice were injected with nonconjugated GNPs, the SERS signal detected at the tumor tissue of mice was totally different from the one that was injected with ScFV-GNP conjugates. Malachite green was used as a Raman reporter in the structure of nanoparticles, and mice were exposed to a laser beam, as shown in (c). *ScFV-GNP*, single chain variable fragment-gold nanoparticle; *SERS*, surface-enhanced Raman spectroscopy. Reproduced with permission from Qian, X., Peng, X.H., Ansari, D.O., Yin-Goen, Q., Chen, G.Z., Shin, D.M., Yang, L., Young, A.N., Wang, M.D., Nie, S., 2008. In vivo tumor targeting and spectroscopic detection with surface-enhanced Raman nanoparticle tags. Nature Biotechnology 26, 83–90.

injection. The accumulation of MINPs at tumor tissues in vivo was also reported by Melanie et al. (2011). They found that superpara-MINPs were mostly located at tumor tissues. But in the meantime, only the low amounts of particles were detected in the liver and spleen.

7.2.3 Metallic nanobiomaterials for monitoring inflamed tissue

Inflammation can be used as an indicator of many diseases, such as cancer, as well as cardiovascular and autoimmune diseases (Tlaskalova-Hogenova et al., 1998; Lu et al., 2006; Balta et al., 2015). Therefore the detection of inflamed tissue or inflammatory responses can help in the diagnosis of these diseases. Similar to earlier sections, imaging techniques can be used to observe the inflammation of tissues in vivo.

However, the improvement of imaging diagnostics is needed to increase the efficiency of this technique. CT imaging has been used for visualization of inflammation of hard tissues through X-ray transmission (Abel et al., 2013). Iodine-based molecules have been injected intra-articularly as a contrast agent to enhance the signal of soft tissues by CT imaging. However, there are some negative points, such as toxic induction and increasing risk of infection and allergy (Berquist, 1997). Because of these reasons, GNPs have been used as a contrast agent for CT imaging due to their high X-ray attenuation that can provide a high vasculature contrast. The use of GNPs to detect an early stage of edema, which is a swelling caused by inflammation, has been reported (Domey et al., 2015). The contrast agent, which was a 15 nm spherical GNP, could enhance the signal of micro-CT at the edema area of edema-bearing mice after 2 h postinjection. The outcome of this study confirmed that GNPs could be used to increase micro-CT signaling for an early detection of soft tissue inflammation in vivo (Domey et al., 2015).

The use of MINPs for inflammation detection was also reported. Radermacher et al. (2009) prepared PEGylation of iron oxide particles at a very small size and combined them with a natural ligand of selectin produced by endothelial cells (E-selectin): the tetrasaccharide, sialyl Lewis X. The whole particle was called "USPIO-PEG-sLeX". Generally, selectins are surface adhesion molecules that can be enhanced by inflammatory cytokines. The overexpression of E-selectin can be used as an early marker of inflammation (Macías et al., 2003). USPIO-PEG-sLeX particles were injected into the tail vein of mice. The electron paramagnetic resonance (EPR) signal was detected in stimulated mice that were enhanced for E-selectin expression. Furthermore, the strong accumulation of USPIO-PEG-sLeX at the inflamed area could be detected in vivo under MRI (Radermacher et al., 2009). Their results show that MINPs can be used as a contrast agent for inflammation detection.

7.3 Biodistribution and elimination of metallic nanobiomaterials

7.3.1 *Biodistribution and elimination of gold nanoparticles in vivo*

Many investigations on the toxic effects of GNPs have been performed. Generally, the nanoparticles (NPs) can induce oxidative stress, cell apoptosis, and damage of DNA, mitochondria, and cell membranes, leading to adverse effects on cells (Elsaesser and Howard, 2012). In comparing various types of metal NPs, many reports have shown that GNPs have less toxicity than others. The concentration and the surface of GNPs are likely to be the key factor on toxic induction. The recent review by Alkilany and Murphy (2010) has shown that the surface of GNPs plays a major role on the toxic effect. However, the effect of size, shape, zeta potential value, and even exposure time of GNPs on toxic induction cannot be avoided. Mironava et al. (2010) reported that different sizes of spherical GNPs lead to different penetration pathways and cellular uptakes. This can result in different impacts on biological responses of cells and tissues. The recent review by Shang et al. (2014) has demonstrated that the smaller the size of the NPs, the higher the toxic effects. In the case of zeta potential values, it was reported that the cellular uptakes of different values of zeta potential of GNRs were dissimilar, and the inflammatory cytokine inductions of cells treated with these GNRs were also different (Pissuwan et al., 2013).

Nevertheless, due to the higher complexity and variation of in vivo systems, it is important to evaluate the toxic effect of GNPs in vivo. Likewise, in vitro, the impact of GNPs on in vivo toxicity also depends on size, shape, concentration, exposure time, and surface property of GNPs. The other factor that is very important on toxic induction by GNPs in vivo is the administration route of GNPs. It was reported that the injection of 13.5 nm spherical GNPs in mice through oral and intraperitoneal routes caused a higher toxicity than that of the tail-vein route. However, it seems that size and surface properties of GNPs play a major role in the in vivo biological activities. It is commonly known that GNPs without good surface stabilizers could lead to aggregation in biological fluid (Zhang et al., 2012) and then cause aggregation in organs (Jong et al., 2010). It was reported that the major organs where the accumulation of different surface coatings of GNPs were detected were the liver and spleen (De Jong et al., 2008; Morais et al., 2012).

The injection of cetyltrimethylammonium bromide (CTAB)-GNRs through an intravenous route showed that they were mainly accumulated in the liver and spleen after administration for one day and 6 days. However, GNRs coated with polyethylene glycol (PEG-GNRs) still circulated in the blood and were mostly accumulated in the spleen and then the liver at day 6 after administration. These results showed evidence that the surface coating of GNRs also impacts the distribution of particles in vivo (Lankveld et al., 2011). It was reported that the possibility of different distributions of CTAB-GNRs and PEG-GNRs should be affected from the binding degree of opsonin proteins to GNRs. These proteins can enhance cellular uptake by cells in the reticuloendothelial system, resulting in the rapid clearance of CTAB-GNRs from blood (Zhang et al., 2012). Different shapes of GNPs also affected biodistribution. Wang et al. (2015) demonstrated that the levels of accumulation between star- and rod-shaped GNPs were different. They found that there was a rapid accumulation in the spleen after intravenous injection of star-shaped GNPs coated with chitosan. In the case of rod-shaped GNPs coated with chitosan, there was a slower rate of accumulation detected than that of star-shaped GNPs. The higher accumulations of rod-shaped GNPs in the kidney and lung were higher than star-shaped GNPs. Their results confirm that the shape of GNPs also has an impact on biodistribution.

Besides biodistribution, the knowledge of the elimination process of NPs applied in vivo is essential. Renal clearance is one of the pathways to remove NPs from the body. With this pathway, NPs can be eliminated through glomerular filtration, tubular secretion, and finally urinary excretion (Longmire et al., 2008). It was reported that size, surface property, concentration, and stability of injected NPs are important factors of the clearance process of NPs. Choi et al. (2007) reported that NPs at the hydrodynamic size less than 5.5 nm could be eliminated by the renal clearance. Nevertheless, it is important to not ignore the fact that the initial size of NPs, especially naked NPs, injected into the body can interact with proteins in blood. This interaction can lead to a change in the size of NPs, resulting in the change of a clearance mechanism. In this case, sizes larger than 5.5 nm are faced with the difficulty of overcoming the renal clearance barrier and therefore cannot be removed from the body through urine excretion (Fig. 7.5).

Zhang et al. (2012) investigated the interaction of gold nanoclusters (Au_{25}-NCs) with human blood plasma. They prepared two different surface coatings of Au_{25}-NCs called as GSH-Au_{25}-NCs (glutathione coating gold nanoclusters; size ~2.1 nm) and BSA-Au_{25}-NCs (bovine serum albumin coating gold nanoclusters; size ~8.2 nm) and found that BSA-Au_{25}-NCs formed a larger size (40–80 nm) than GSH-Au_{25}-NCs (5–30 nm) after interacting with human blood plasma for 24 h. They also found that the amount of GSH-Au_{25}-NCs eliminated through renal clearance was higher than that of BSA-Au_{25}-NCs. Their results suggest that the size of NPs was a key factor to removing particles via the renal pathway. However, it seems that not only size has a major impact on renal clearance. The charge of NPs also is involved in the elimination process, as proposed by Hirn et al. (2011). They reported that a higher number of negative GNPs (carboxylate GNPs) was detected in urine after 24 h intravenous injection rather than positive GNPs (Aminated GNPs).

Hepatic clearance is another important pathway to eliminate NPs from the body. This type of clearance is more complicated than that of the renal clearance. Basically, catabolism and biliary excretion are major mechanisms of hepatic clearance. Phagocytic Kupffer cells play a key role in this clearance, and these cells are reticuloendothelial (liver and spleen). These Kupffer cells can eliminate foreign materials/particles through phagocytosis. Besides Kupffer cells, hepatocytes are also the cells in the liver that are involved in the elimination of particles by endocytosis and enzymatic digestion. NPs taken up by hepatocytes are processed in biliary excretion and are further excreted into the bile at the end (Longmire et al., 2008). It was reported that different surface coatings of GNPs were entrapped by both hepatocytes and Kupffer cells (Morais et al., 2012). However, it seems that Kuppfer cells (cells located in the liver) play a major role in the elimination of GNPs injected through an intravenous route (Sadauskas et al., 2007, 2009). As far as we are aware, more information of hepatic clearance of GNPs by hepatocytes and Kupffer cells is required

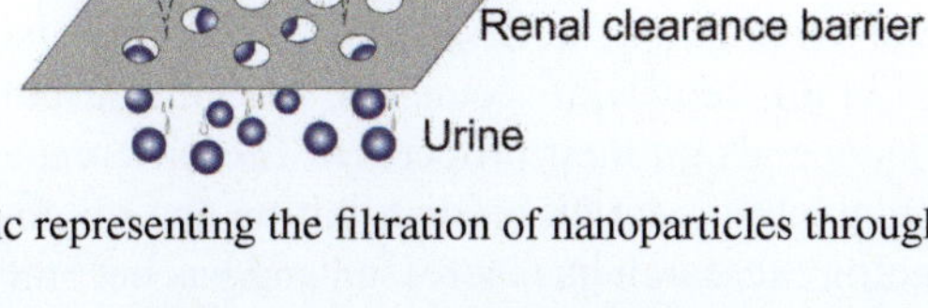

Figure 7.5 Schematic representing the filtration of nanoparticles through the renal clearance barrier.

and should be further investigated, because the knowledge on elimination GNPs through this clearance system is still scarce.

7.3.2 Biodistribution and elimination of magnetic iron oxide nanoparticles in vivo

Similar to GNPs, the biodistribution of MINPs relies on size, shape, and surface property. Yang et al. (2015) have recently investigated the impact of size of MINPs on biodistribution. This group evaluated the biodistribution of MINPs coated with a carboxyl group. The sizes of MINPs in their evaluation were 10, 20, 30, and 40 nm. After tail–vein injection in mice for 1 day, they found that 10 nm MINPs coated with a carboxyl group were highly taken up in the liver. In contrast, larger sizes of MINPS coated with a carboxyl group were highly accumulated in the spleen. Compared to GNPs, it was also reported that there was a high accumulation of 10 nm GNPs coated with PEG in the liver (Zhang et al., 2011). These results implied that although these particles were made from different metals and had different zeta potentials, the size of these metal nanoparticles seems to have a vital role on biodistribution. The amount of 10 nm MINPs in the liver was decreased after 7 days postinjection (Zhang et al., 2011). This decrease could occur from the elimination of the biological system that will be discussed in the next section.

As discussed previously for GNPs, MINPs could also be distributed to other organs and tissues such as the brain, heart, lungs, and kidneys, depending on the property of MINPs. The interaction between MINPs and plasma proteins in biological fluid is also another important factor that affects biodistribution of MINPs. Unlike GNPs, it is worth noting that the use of an external magnetic field could enhance the distribution of MINPs into target tissues or organs (Jimeno et al., 2012). However, it is necessary to investigate what will happen in the term of biodistribution after removal of an external magnetic field. Similar to GNPs, MINPs can be taken up by the liver and spleen, whereby both organs act as a key player in clearance pathways of particles in blood circulation. Generally, the mechanism of clearance of MINPS is the same with that of GNPs (Arami et al., 2015).

7.4 Conclusion

Both GNPs and MINPs are potential nanobiomaterials that can be promisingly used in biomedical applications for in vivo monitoring and tracking. Both nanobiomaterials can be prepared in different sizes, shapes, concentrations, and surface functionalization to be fit for the specific application. These properties can have an impact on biodistribution and elimination of GNPs and MINPs in vivo. According to the information provided in this review, it seems that the biodistribution and elimination of GNPs and MINPs depends on their properties. The difference in the type of metals seems not to have much impact on biodistribution and elimination. However, the amount of nanotoxicology research has increased and has become attractive to people in the field. Therefore the toxic effects of applying both types of nanobiomaterials for in vivo monitoring and tracking need to be considered.

Acknowledgments

The author acknowledges the support of the Talent Management Project and the Faculty of Science, Mahidol University, Thailand. The author also thanks Ms. Sunisa Chaicherd and the Center of Nanoimaging, Mahidol University for the technical support of TEM images.

Nanobiomaterials can be defined as the use of materials in a level of nanoscale for biomedical applications. In this chapter an overview of gold and magnetic iron oxide nanoparticles that have been recently applied in biological systems in vivo for diagnostic imaging and treatment of diseases is provided.

References

Abel, R., Prime, M., Jin, A., Cobb, J., Bhattacharya, R., 2013. 3D imaging bone quality: bench to bedside. Hard Tissue 2, 42.

Alkilany, A.M., Murphy, C.J., 2010. Toxicity and cellular uptake of gold nanoparticles: what we have learned so far? Journal of Nanoparticle Research 12, 2313–2333.

Arami, H., Khandhar, A., Liggitt, D., Krishnan, K.M., 2015. In vivo delivery, pharmacokinetics, biodistribution and toxicity of iron oxide nanoparticles. Chemical Society Reviews 44, 8576–8607.

Balta, S., Mikhailidis, D.P., Demirkol, S., Ozturk, C., Celik, T., Iyisoy, A., 2015. Endocan: a novel inflammatory indicator in cardiovascular disease? Atherosclerosis 243, 339–343.

Berquist, T., 1997. Imaging of articular pathology: MRI, CT, arthrography. Clinical Anatomy 10, 1–13.

Carlson, A.L., Fujisaki, J., Wu, J., Runnels, J.M., Turcotte, R., Celso, C.L., Scadden, D.T., Strom, T.B., Lin, C.P., 2013. Tracking single cells in live animals using a photoconvertible near-infrared cell membrane label. PLoS One 8, e69257.

Cho, I.K., Moran, S.P., Paudyal, R., Nitsche, K.P., Cheng, P.H., Zhang, X., Mao, H., Chan, A.W.S., 2014. Longitudinal monitoring of stem cell grafts in vivo using magnetic resonance imaging with inducible maga as a genetic reporter. Theranostics 4, 972–989.

Choi, H.S., Liu, W., Misra, P., Tanaka, E., Zimmer, J.P., Ipe, B.I., Bawendi, M.G., Frangioni, J.V., 2007. Renal clearance of nanoparticles. Nature Biotechnology 25, 1165–1170.

Coronado, E.A., Encina, E.R., Stefani, F.D., 2011. Optical properties of metallic nanoparticles: manipulating light, heat and forces at the nanoscale. Nanoscale 3, 4042–4059.

Domey, J., Teichgräber, U., Hilger, I., 2015. Gold nanoparticles allow detection of early-stage edema in mice via computed tomography imaging. International Journal of Nanomedicine 10, 3803–3814.

Dykman, L.A., Khlebtsov, N.G., 2011. Gold nanoparticles in biology and medicine: recent advances and prospects. Acta Naturae 3, 34–55.

Elsaesser, A., Howard, C.V., 2012. Toxicology of nanoparticles. Advanced Drug Delivery Reviews 64, 129–137.

Ghoroghchian, P.P., Therien, M.J., Hammer, D.A., 2009. In vivo fluorescence imaging: a personal perspective. Wiley Interdisciplinary Reviews: Nanomedicine and Nanobiotechnology 1, 156–167.

Hirn, S., Semmler-Behnke, M., Schleh, C., Wenk, A., Lipka, J., Schäffler, M., Takenaka, S., Möller, W., Schmid, G., Simon, U., Kreyling, W.G., 2011. Particle size-dependent and surface charge-dependent biodistribution of gold nanoparticles after intravenous administration. European Journal of Pharmaceutics and Biopharmaceutics 77, 407–416.

Huang, X., El-Sayed, M.A., 2010. Gold nanoparticles: optical properties and implementations in cancer diagnosis and photothermal therapy. Journal of Advanced Research 1, 13–28.

Huang, X., El-Sayed, M.A., 2011. Plasmonic photo-thermal therapy (PPTT). Alexandria Journal of Medicine 47, 1–9.

Hudoklin, S., Zupančič, D., Makovec, D., Kreft, M.E., Romih, R., 2013. Gold nanoparticles as physiological markers of urine internalization into urothelial cells in vivo. International Journal of Nanomedicine 8, 3945–3953.

De Jong, W.H., Hagens, W.I., Krystek, P., Burger, M.C., Sips, A.J., Geertsma, R.E., 2008. Particle size-dependent organ distribution of gold nanoparticles after intravenous administration. Biomaterials 29.

Jensen, E.C., 2012. Use of fluorescent probes: their effect on cell biology and limitations. Anaomical Record (Hoboken) 295, 2031–2036.

Jimeno, S.G., Escribano, E., Queralt, J., Estelrich, J., 2012. External magnetic field-induced selective biodistribution of magnetoliposomes in mice. Nanoscale Research Letter 7, 452.

Jokerst, J.V., Thangaraj, M., Kempen, P.J., Sinclair, R., Gambhir, S.S., 2012. Photoacoustic imaging of mesenchymal stem cells in living mice via silica-coated gold nanorods. ACS Nano 6, 5920–5930.

Jong, W.H.D., Burger, M.C., Verheijen, M.A., Geertsma, R.E., 2010. Detection of the presence of gold nanoparticles in organs by transmission electron microscope. Materials 3, 4681–4694.

Kim, E.Y., Kumar, D., Khang, G., Lim, D.-K., 2015. Recent advances in gold nanoparticle-based bioengineering applications. Journal of Materials Chemistry B 3, 8433–8444.

Lara-González, J.H., Gomez-Flores, R., Tamez-Guerra, P., Monreal-Cuevas, E., Tamez-Guerra, R., Rodríguez-Padilla, C., 2013. In vivo antitumor activity of metal silver and silver nanoparticles in the L5178Y-R murine lymphoma model. British Journal of Medicine and Medical Research 3, 1308–1316.

Lankveld, D.P., Rayavarapu, R.G., Krystek, P., Oomen, A.G., Verharen, H.W., Leeuwen, T.G.v, Jong, W.H.D., Manohar, S., 2011. Blood clearance and tissue distribution of PEGylated and non-PEGylated gold nanorods after intravenous administration in rats. Nanomedicine 6, 339–349.

Laurent, S., Forge, D., Port, M., Roch, A., Robic, C., Vander Elst, L., Muller, R.N., 2008. Magnetic iron oxide nanoparticles: synthesis, stabilization, vectorization, physicochemical characterizations, and biological applications. Chemical Reviews 108, 2064–2110.

Lisy, M.-R., Goermar, A., Thomas, C., Pauli, J., Genger, U.R., Kaiser, W.A., Hilger, I., 2008. In vivo near-infrared fluorescence imaging of carcinoembryonic antigen–expressing tumor cells in mice. Radiology 247, 779–787.

Liu, W., Dahnke, H., Jordan, E.K., Schaeffter, T., Frank, J.A., 2008. In vivo MRI using positive-contrast techniques in detection of cells labeled with superparamagnetic iron oxide nanoparticles. NMR in Biomedicine 21, 242–250.

Liu, Y., Ashton, J.R., Moding, E.J., Yuan, H., Register, J.K., Fales, A.M., Choi, J., Whitley, M.J., Zhao, X., Qi, Y., Ma, Y., Vaidyanathan, G., 2015. A plasmonic gold nanostar theranostic probe for in vivo tumor imaging and photothermal therapy. Theranostics 5, 946–960.

Longmire, M., Choyke, P.L., Kobayashi, H., 2008. Clearance properties of nano-sized particles and molecules as imaging agents: considerations and caveats. Nanomedicine 3, 703–717.

Lu, H., Ouyang, W., Huang, C., 2006. Inflammation, a key event in cancer development. Molecular Cancer Research 4, 221–233.

Macías, C., Villaescusa, R., del Valle, L., Boffil, V., Cordero, G., Hernández, A., Hernández, P., Ballester, J.M., 2003. Endothelial adhesion molecules ICAM-1, VCAM-1 and E-Selectin in patients with acute coronary syndrome. Revista Española de Cardiología 56, 137–144.

Markides, H., Kehoe, O., Morris, R.H., Haj, A.J.E., 2013. Whole body tracking of superparamagnetic iron oxide nanoparticle-labelled cells – a rheumatoid arthritis mouse model. Stem Cell Research and Therapy 4, 126.

Melanie, K., Heike, R., Frank, W., Sibylle, B.-S., Lutz, T., Werner Alois, K., Ingrid, H., 2011. Minimal-invasive magnetic heating of tumors does not alter intra-tumoral nanoparticle accumulation, allowing for repeated therapy sessions: an in vivo study in mice. Nanotechnology 22, 505102.

Mérian, J., Gravier, J., Navarro, F., Texier, I., 2012. Fluorescent nanoprobes dedicated to in vivo imaging: from preclinical validations to clinical translation. Molecules 17, 5564–5591.

Mieszawska, A.J., Mulder, W.J.M., Fayad, Z.A., Cormode, D.P., 2013. Multifunctional gold nanoparticles for diagnosis and therapy of disease. Molecular Pharmacology 10, 831–847.

Mironava, T., Hadjiargyroub, M., Simonc, M., Jurukovskic, V., Rafailovicha, M.H., 2010. Gold nanoparticles cellular toxicity and recovery: effect of size, concentration and exposure time. Nanotoxicology 4 (1), 120–137.

Mody, V.V., Siwale, R., Singh, A., Mody, H.R., 2010. Introduction to metallic nanoparticles. Journal of Pharmacy and Bioallied Sciences 2, 282–289.

Mohapatra, M., Anand, S., 2010. Synthesis and applications of nano-structured iron oxides/hydroxides – a review. International Journal of Engineering Science and Technology 2, 127–146.

Morais, T., Soares, M.E., Duarte, J.A., Soares, L., Maia, S., Gomes, P., Pereira, E., Fraga, S., Carmo, H., Bastos, M.d L., 2012. Effect of surface coating on the biodistribution profile of gold nanoparticles in the rat. European Journal of Pharmaceutics and Biopharmaceutics 80, 185–193.

Nam, S.Y., Chung, E., Suggs, L.J., Emelianov, S.Y., 2015. Combined ultrasound and photoacoustic imaging to noninvasively assess burn injury and selectively monitor a regenerative tissue-engineered construct. Tissue Engineering Part C 21, 557–566.

Nam, S.Y., Ricles, L.M., Suggs, L.J., Emelianov, S.Y., 2012. In vivo ultrasound and photoacoustic monitoring of mesenchymal stem cells labeled with gold nanotracers. PLoS One 7, e37267.

NDong, C., Tate, J.A., Kett, W.C., Batra, J., Demidenko, E., Lewis, L.D., Hoopes, P.J., Gerngross, T.U., Griswold, K.E., 2015. Tumor cell targeting by iron oxide nanoparticles is dominated by different factors in vitro versus in vivo. PLoS One 10, e0115636.

Neouze, M.-A., Schubert, U., 2008. Surface modification and functionalization of metal and metal oxide nanoparticles by organic ligands. Monatshefte für Chemie – Chemical Monthly 139, 183–195.

Nune, S.K., Gunda, P., Thallapally, P.K., Lin, Y.-Y., Forrest, M.L., Berkland, C.J., 2009. Nanoparticles for biomedical imaging. Expert Opinion on Drug Delivery 6, 1175–1194.

Di Pasqua, A.J., Mishler Ii, R.E., Ship, Y.-L., Dabrowiak, J.C., Asefa, T., 2009. Preparation of antibody-conjugated gold nanoparticles. Materials Letters 63, 1876–1879.

Pérez-Juste, J., Pastoriza-Santos, I., Liz-Marzán, L.M., Mulvaney, P., 2005. Gold nanorods: synthesis, characterization and applications. Coordination Chemistry Reviews 249, 1870–1901.

Pissuwan, D., Valenzuela, S., MB, C., 2008. Prospects for gold nanorod particles in diagnostic and therapeutic applications. Biotechnology & Genetic Engineering Reviews 25, 93–112.

Pissuwan, D., Cortie, C.H., Valenzuela, S.M., Cortie, M.B., 2007. Gold nanosphere-antibody conjugates for hyperthermal therapeutic applications. Gold Bulletin 40, 121–129.

Pissuwan, D., Kumagai, Y., Smith, N.I., 2013. Effect of surface-modified gold nanorods on the inflammatory cytokine response in macrophage cells. Particle & Particle Systems Characterization 30, 427–433.

Pissuwan, D., Valenzuela, S.M., Cortie, M.B., 2006. Therapeutic possibilities of plasmonically heated gold nanoparticles. Trends in Biotechnology 24, 62–67.

Qian, X., Peng, X.H., Ansari, D.O., Yin-Goen, Q., Chen, G.Z., Shin, D.M., Yang, L., Young, A.N., Wang, M.D., Nie, S., 2008. In vivo tumor targeting and spectroscopic detection with surface-enhanced Raman nanoparticle tags. Nature Biotechnology 26, 83–90.

Radermacher, K.A., Beghein, N., Boutry, S., Laurent, S., Elst, L.V., Muller, R.N., Jordan, B.F., Gallez, B., 2009. In vivo detection of inflammation using pegylated iron oxide particles targeted at E-selectin: a multimodal approach using MR imaging and EPR spectroscopy. Investigative Radiology 77, 398–404.

Reddy, A.M., Kwak, B.K., Shim, H.J., Ahn, C., Lee, H.S., Suh, Y.J., Park, E.S., 2010. In vivo tracking of mesenchymal stem cells labeled with a novel chitosan-coated superparamagnetic iron oxide nanoparticles using 3.0T MRI. Journal of Korean Medical Science 25, 211–219.

Roca, A.G., Costo, R., Rebolledo, A.F., Veintemillas-Verdaguer, S., Tartaj, P., González-Carreño, T., Morales, M.P., Serna, C.J., 2009. Progress in the preparation of magnetic nanoparticles for applications in biomedicine. Journal of Physics D: Applied Physics 42, 224002.

SoRelle, E.D., Liba, O., Hussain, Z., Gambhir, M., de la Zerda, A., 2015. Biofunctionalization of large gold nanorods realizes ultrahigh-sensitivity optical imaging agent. Langmuir 31, 12339–12347.

Sadauskas, E., Danscher, G., Stoltenberg, M., Vogel, U., Larsen, A., Wallin, H., 2009. Protracted elimination of gold nanoparticles from mouse liver. Nanomedicine: Nanotechnology, Biology and Medicine 5, 162–169.

Sadauskas, E., Wallin, H., Stoltenberg, M., Vogel, U., Doering, P., Larsen, A., Danscher, G., 2007. Kupffer cells are central in the removal of nanoparticles from the organism. Particle and Fibre Toxicology 4, 10.

Samanta, A., Das, R.K., Park, S.J., Maiti, K.K., Chang, Y.T., 2014. Multiplexing SERS nanotags for the imaging of differentiated mouse embryonic stem cells (mESC) and detection of teratoma in vivo. American Journal of Nuclear Medicine and Molecular Imaging 4, 114–124.

Shang, L., Nienhaus, K., Nienhaus, G.U., 2014. Engineered nanoparticles interacting with cells: size matters. Journal of Nanobiotechnology 12.

Tlaskalova-Hogenova, H., Stěpánková, R., Tucková, L., Farré, M., Funda, D., Verdú, E., Sinkora, J., Hudcovic, T., Reháková, Z., Cukrowska, B., Kozáková, H., Prokesová, L., 1998. Autoimmunity, immunodeficiency and mucosal infections: chronic intestinal inflammation as a sensitive indicator of immunoregulatory defects in response to normal luminal microflora. Folia Microbiology (Praha) 43, 545–550.

Trequesser, Q.L., Seznec, H., Delville, M.-H., 2013. Functionalized nanomaterials: their use as contrast agents in bioimaging: mono- and multimodal approaches. Nanotechnology Reviews 2, 125–169.

Wang, J., Xie, Y., Wang, L., Tang, J., Li, J., Kocaefe, D., Kocaefe, Y., Zhang, Z., Li, Y., Chen, C., 2015. In vivo pharmacokinetic features and biodistribution of star and rod shaped gold nanoparticles by multispectral optoacoustic tomography. RSC Advances 5, 7529–7538.

Wu, W., He, Q., Jiang, C., 2008. Magnetic iron oxide nanoparticles: synthesis and surface functionalization strategies. Nanoscale Research Letters 3, 397–415.

Wu, W., Wu, Z., Yu, T., Jiang, C., Kim, W.S., 2015. Recent progress on magnetic iron oxide nanoparticles: synthesis, surface functional strategies and biomedical applications. Science and Technology of Advanced Materials 16, 023501.

Yamaoka, N., Kawasaki, Y., Xu, Y., Yamamoto, H., Terada, N., Okamura, H., Kubo, S., 2010. Establishment of in vivo fluorescence imaging in mouse models of malignant mesothelioma. International Journal of Oncology 37, 273–279.

Yang, L., Kuang, H., Zhang, W., Aguilar, Z.P., Xiong, Y., Lai, W., Xu, H., Wei, H., 2015. Size dependent biodistribution and toxicokinetics of iron oxide magnetic nanoparticles in mice. Nanoscale 7, 625–636.

Zhang, X.-D., Di Wu, X.S., Liu, P.-X., Yang, N., Zhao, B., Zhang, H., Sun, Y.-M., Zhang, L.-A., Fan, F.-Y., 2011. Size-dependent in vivo toxicity of PEG-coated gold nanoparticles. International Journal of Nanomedicine 6, 2071–2081.

Zhang, X.D., Yang, J., Song, S.S., Long, W., Chen, J., Shen, X., Wang, H., Sun, Y.M., Liu, P.X., Fan, S., 2014. Passing through the renal clearance barrier: toward ultrasmall sizes with stable ligands for potential clinical applications. International Journal of Nanomedicine 9, 2069–2072.

Zhang, X.-D., Wu, D., Shen, X., Liu, P.-X., Fan, F.-Y., Fan, S.-J., 2012. In vivo renal clearance, biodistribution, toxicity of gold nanoclusters. Biomaterials 33, 4628–4638.

High-resolution imaging techniques in tissue engineering

8

S. Wang, I.V. Larina
Baylor College of Medicine, Houston, TX, United States

8.1 Introduction

The rapid development of the tissue engineering field is producing attractive techniques to replace and regenerate damaged or lost tissues for restoration of proper tissue functions. In order to evaluate tissue engineering techniques, visualization and monitoring of cellular behavior, extracellular matrix composition, and scaffold structure and biocompatibility are essential. Traditionally, histology and scanning electron microscopy are the gold standards for high-resolution imaging and characterization in tissue engineering. However, the invasive nature of these two approaches requires destruction of the sample, which consequentially prevents live analysis and functional assessment as well as three-dimensional (3-D) quantifications. The application of live, 3-D, and nondestructive imaging techniques in tissue engineering is growing rapidly due to the increased capability to achieve a better understanding of the critical biological processes during the formation and growth of tissues and organs. Such ability plays a critical role in developing new and powerful biomaterials as well as advancing tissue engineering techniques to improve human health.

A number of noninvasive live imaging techniques have been utilized in tissue engineering (Nam et al., 2015; Vielreicher et al., 2013; Appel et al., 2013), including X-ray computed tomography (Izadifar et al., 2014), magnetic resonance imaging (Xu et al., 2008), nuclear imaging (positron emission tomography and single photon emission computed tomography) (Ventura et al., 2014), ultrasonic imaging (Kreitz et al., 2011), optical imaging (Smith et al., 2010), and photoacoustic imaging (Cai et al., 2013b). These techniques have been widely used for the characterization of biomaterials, visualization of important structures, and monitoring of major processes in tissue engineering, as reviewed by several studies (Nam et al., 2015; Vielreicher et al., 2013; Appel et al., 2013). Fig. 8.1 summarizes the spatial imaging scales (resolution and field of view) of these techniques. It can be seen that due to employing a short wavelength of radiation, optical imaging and photoacoustic imaging are able to provide micro and submicroscale spatial resolution, capable of resolving cellular and microstructural information in tissue engineering. This high-resolution information can provide great insights into the developmental processes of functional tissue constructs such as cell viability and growth, extracellular matrix orientation, and scaffold degradation.

In this chapter, we review high-resolution imaging techniques in tissue engineering, focusing on the optical and photoacoustic imaging techniques that have

Monitoring and Evaluation of Biomaterials and their Performance in vivo. http://dx.doi.org/10.1016/B978-0-08-100603-0.00008-0

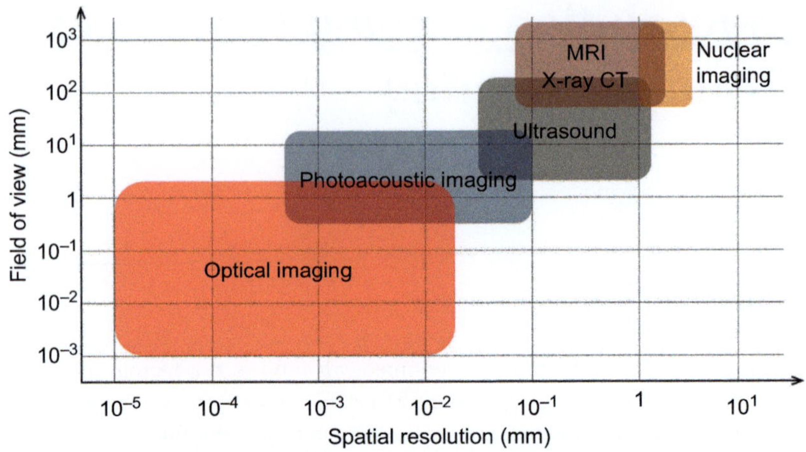

Figure 8.1 Spatial imaging scales of commonly used imaging techniques in tissue engineering. Each imaging technique is assigned a space with respect to the spatial resolution and the field of view. *CT*, computed tomography; *MRI*, magnetic resonance imaging.

micron level and submicron level spatial resolving capability. Specifically, we include phase contrast microscopy (PCM), confocal microscopy (CM), multiphoton microscopy (MPM), optical coherence tomography (OCT), photoacoustic microscopy (PAM), Raman spectroscopy (RS), and multimodality imaging based on these techniques. For each technique, we first describe its basic principle, with emphasis on the spatial imaging scales and contrast mechanisms, and then review in detail the specific imaging approaches and applications of each technique in tissue engineering. Lastly, we discuss emerging high-resolution techniques that have an attractive potential in the tissue engineering field. Throughout the review, we will emphasize the applications in three aspects: (1) morphological imaging with structural visualization and dynamic monitoring, (2) functional imaging with biomechanical characterization and perfusion analysis, and (3) molecular imaging with subcellular component identification and molecule distribution. We aim for this review to provide useful references for the researchers working in the tissue engineering field.

8.2 Phase contrast microscopy

8.2.1 General

Phase contrast microscopy (PCM) is generally composed of a bright-field microscope with the addition of a condenser annulus and a phase plate. Traditional bright-field imaging with transmitted light illumination solely relies on the intensity of light to form contrast based on the visible light absorption from the sample. However, due to the requirement of relative transparency of the imaging subject (cell culture in most cases), the contrast formed by the absorption is typically very limited within the cell, thus resulting in cellular structures that are hardly visible and therefore significantly restricting its usefulness for cell observation. Although exogenous staining can be introduced for bright-field microscopy to increase the imaging contrast, staining methods are often toxic to cells and reduce experimental efficiency due to the extra procedures (Smith et al., 2010).

Utilizing the phase of light, PCM employs coherent light interference to transform the phase difference of light into an amplitude difference that can be directly picked up by the eye or detected by the camera. Here, the interference is formed between the light diffracted from the sample and the light passed through or around the sample. Since the optical phase retardation is related to the optical path length from the sample, differences of both the refractive index and the thickness of the structure contribute to the imaging contrast of PCM. Because of the ultra-high sensitivity of the optical phase to the change of path length of light, as well as the great transforming efficiency and amplifying effect from phase to amplitude by using light interference, PCM possesses a significant improvement of contrast for live cell imaging without a large sacrifice of the resolution compared with bright-field microscopy (Zernike, 1955). This has positioned PCM as an efficient and convenient imaging tool for screening a thin, transparent layer of cultured cells without staining or labeling (Yang et al., 2005; Schmedlen et al., 2002; Fukuda, 2001).

The lateral resolution of PCM is mainly determined by the objective lens and condenser as well as the reduction of aperture introduced by the condenser annulus and phase plate. Under optimal conditions, PCM can reach a spatial resolution of ~0.3 μm (Snyder et al., 1987). Due to the lack of depthwise sectioning capability, PCM is primarily used for two-dimensional (2-D) visualizations. PCM has been widely utilized for the morphological imaging of cells in culture, and various image processing and analyzing methods have been developed for PCM to achieve cell detection (Pan et al., 2009) and segmentation (Su et al., 2013; Ambuhl et al., 2012). With time-lapse PCM imaging, these methods have successfully enabled the large-scale tracking of cell migration and proliferation (Kang et al., 2006), the automatic mitosis identification of stem cell populations (Huh et al., 2011), and the dynamic monitoring of cell apoptosis (Huh and Kanade, 2013).

8.2.2 Quantitative phase imaging

Traditional PCM only provides inherently qualitative phase shift information because the interference amplitude of light is mixed with the absorption-induced optical amplitude variations. This leads to poor subcellular specificity and makes the longitudinal quantitative study of cellular dynamics challenging, as the pixel intensity alteration is not linearly related with the morphological change of the cell (Zernike, 1955). By mapping the absolute phase of light, quantitative phase imaging (QPI) has been developed as an emerging technique (Popescu, 2011) that addresses this limitation and extends the application range of phase contrast imaging in tissue engineering. Based on coherent interferometry, unwrapped optical phase shifts introduced by the sample are extracted from the whole field of view to form a phase image that is independent of the amplitude image (Mir et al., 2012), thus providing quantification of the optical path length change with nanometer scale sensitivity. With QPI, time-lapse nanoscale measurement of the fluctuations from the membrane of cells can be obtained (Popescu et al., 2008).

Recently, high-resolution (hundreds of nanometers) 3-D tomography of unlabeled live cells has been achieved based on QPI (Kim et al., 2014), opening great opportunities for subcellular structural examination of cultured cells. Specifically, light interferometry is utilized to achieve depthwise optical gating (i.e., short coherence length) and significantly reduced speckle noise level, which is hard to obtain with coherent light illumination. Full-field sectioning in depth by moving the objective lens allows depth-resolved cellular imaging, resulting in 3-D quantitative phase tomography. For applications, Mir et al. utilized QPI to measure the fundamental properties of neural networks in culture from a subcellular to cell population level scale and discovered the correlations between the growing, transporting, and spatially organizing trends of a human stem cell-derived neural system (Mir et al., 2014). Also, combined QPI quantitative assessment of single cell motility with dry mass measurements was demonstrated with Drosophila S2 cells on poly-L-lysine substrate (Sridharan et al., 2011). The capability of QPI to quantify the thermal fluctuations of cell membranes with nanometer accuracy has enabled the mechanical assessment of cells (Park et al., 2010), which, in addition to morphological characterization provided by QPI, serves as a novel application that pushes the optical phase-based microscopic techniques toward the functional analysis of cell cultures.

8.3 Confocal microscopy

8.3.1 General

Confocal microscopy (CM) is one of the most widely used high-resolution imaging techniques in tissue engineering (Smith et al., 2010). By introducing a spatial pinhole at the confocal plane in front of the detector, the out-of-focus light from the sample is eliminated, leading to a major improvement in axial resolution compared with a conventional wide field microscope (Gu, 1996). The spatial resolution of CM is mainly controlled by the diameter of the pinhole and is diffraction limited. Generally, with optimized conditions, the highest spatial resolution can reach ~0.8 μm in the axial direction and ~0.3 μm in the lateral direction. In comparison with traditional phase contrast microscopy, the confocal configuration of CM produces superior depthwise sectioning capability and is therefore able to provide high-resolution 3-D reconstruction. The imaging depth of CM is limited to the superficial layer of the sample (approximately 100–200 μm), which is dependent on the sample transparency and the wavelength of illumination. Current CM techniques largely rely on the scanning of the laser beam and have been extensively used for live imaging of cells and tissues, as well as structural characterization of scaffolds in tissue engineering (Hanke et al., 2003; Aigner et al., 1998; Engelmayr et al., 2008).

8.3.2 Confocal reflectance microscopy

Confocal reflectance microscopy (CRM) directly probes the reflected light from the sample, allowing for minimum specimen preparation and instrument reconfiguration. Because no labeling is required, CRM is well-suited for in vivo imaging of cells and tissue structures such as the skin (Calzavara-Pinton et al., 2008) and the cornea (Jalbert et al., 2003). For applications in tissue engineering, CRM has been mainly utilized to characterize extracellular matrix structure, such as collagen fibers, and their interactions with cells through time-lapse imaging (Barnes et al., 2014; Gillette et al., 2011; Brightman et al., 2000). As an example, the formation of ducts and acini from single human breast cells and the reorganization of the collagen fiber network were observed and quantitatively assessed using time-lapse CRM (Barnes et al., 2014). Although the whole imaging preparation process is very facile, the reflectance contrast of CRM lacks good imaging quality and might lead to artifacts in many cases, such as suffering from the dependence of signal amplitude on fiber orientation when imaging biopolymer networks (Jawerth et al., 2010), which results in a limited application range of CRM for tissue engineering.

8.3.3 Confocal florescence microscopy

By fluorescent labeling of cellular components with either vital reporters or exogenous staining, confocal florescence microscopy (CFM) is a powerful imaging technique that has highly specific molecular contrast to resolve the targeted subcellular structures (Muller, 2006). Based on the absorption and emission spectra of the florescent proteins or dyes, CFM utilizes a set of optical filters to selectively excite and detect the wavelengths of light, which contrasts out the florescence-labeled components of cells. Through combining different settings of illumination/detection, a multichannel registered image can be produced to have simultaneous visualization of multiple subcellular structures. The high degree of molecular information as well as the superior sensitivity and specificity enabled by CFM are of significant value for 3-D monitoring and evaluation of cells and scaffold structures during the engineering and regeneration of tissue (Mierke et al., 2010; Pampaloni et al., 2007; Chwalek et al., 2014). The design of florescent labeling usually requires careful selections of the florescent proteins or dyes to separate out the emission spectra for efficient detection.

The application of CFM covers many aspects of tissue engineering, including the time-resolved monitoring of 3-D cell migration and neurite outgrowth in a novel photo-labile hydrogel (Luo and Shoichet, 2004), the high-resolution visualization of collagen fiber formation in live cell culture (Krahn et al., 2006), the detailed characterization of knitted biodegradable polyester-based hybrid scaffolds for improvement of cell attachment and proliferation (Sambit et al., 2007), and the longitudinal assessment of the growth of human dermal microvascular endothelial cells on the fibronectin-coated nano/microfiber-combined scaffolds (Santos et al., 2008), as shown in Fig. 8.2(a). In addition to the imaging of cells and scaffolds, CFM has also been utilized to evaluate the engineered vasculature networks. Moon et al. have applied CFM for longitudinal dynamic 3-D analysis of hydrogel-induced angiogenesis (Moon et al., 2010), as shown

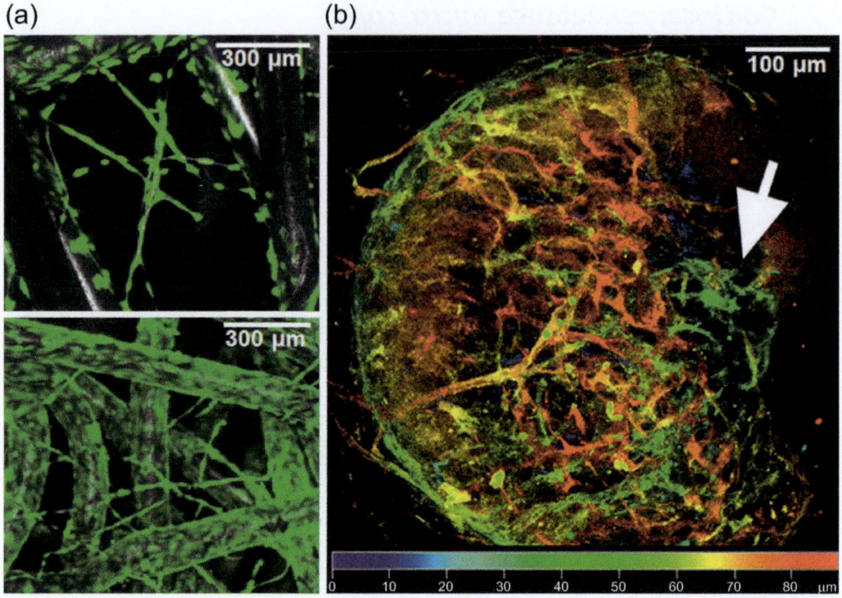

Figure 8.2 High-resolution cellular imaging in tissue engineering with confocal florescence microscopy. (a) Projection of 3-D imaging of human dermal microvascular endothelial cell growth on the fibronectin-coated nano/microfiber-combined scaffolds after three (top) and seven (bottom) days. *Reprinted from Biomaterials, 29, Santos, M.I., Tuzlakoglu, K., Fuchs, S., Gomes, M.E., Peters, K., Unger, R.E., Piskin, E., Reis, R.L., Kirkpatrick, C.J., Endothelial cell colonization and angiogenic potential of combined nano- and micro-fibrous scaffolds for bone tissue engineering, 4306-4313, Copyright (2008), with permission from Elsevier.* (b) Depth-encoded 3-D visualization of robust neovascularization adjacent to the hydrogels and extensive infiltration of host vasculature into the hydrogels in the mouse cornea. The *arrow* shows a portion hydrogel undergoing active degradation. *Reprinted from Biomaterials, 31, Moon, J.J., Saik, J.E., Poche, R.A., Leslie-Barbick, J.E., Lee, S.H., Smith, A.A., Dickinson, M.E., West, J.L., Biomimetic hydrogels with pro-angiogenic properties, 3840–3847, Copyright (2010), with permission from Elsevier.*

in Fig. 8.2(b), demonstrating the feasibility to promote neovascularization both in vitro and in vivo in completely synthetic biomaterials. Recently, Hsu et al. have taken a further step and employed CFM to show that incorporating macrophage-recruiting factors into the biomaterial scaffolds is able to improve angiogenesis (Hsu et al., 2015).

Based on the high spatial resolvability, both CRM and CFM have been used for microbiomechanical analysis of biomaterials and tissue constructs (Voytik-Harbin et al., 2003). Specifically, a miniature mechanical loading unit is combined with CM, and the load-induced changes of the sample (such as the strain) is noninvasively monitored with high accuracy by CRM and CFM to analyze the sample biomechanics (Voytik-Harbin et al., 2003). This CM-based biomechanical characterization technique has been successfully utilized to assess the structural–mechanical properties of 3-D tissue-derived biomaterials and cell–scaffold interactions (Voytik-Harbin et al., 2003), which is promising for functional imaging of tissue engineering.

8.4 Multiphoton microscopy

8.4.1 General

Multiphoton microscopy (MPM) encompasses a group of microscopy modalities that are characterized by a nonlinear optical process where two or three photons are utilized for quasi-simultaneous absorption with emission of a single photon (Ustione and Piston, 2011). In contrast to single photon excitation, such as CFM, where the relationship between the emission and excitation amplitude is linear, MPM relies on nonlinear interaction (second or third order relation from excitation to emission) between photons and the molecule (Masters, 2006), resulting in several advantages and important features for cellular imaging. The longer wavelength of infrared light employed by MPM for excitation leads to higher penetration depth into the tissue sample as compared to CM because of the reduced diffraction of light. Generally, the imaging depth of MPM is ~400 μm, though it can reach up to ~1 mm and even higher depending on the transparency of the sample. The multiphoton excitation requires a high photon density from the illumination beam, which is only achieved at the focal volume, thus producing a natural pinhole effect that eliminates the out-of-focus light. Since a spatial pinhole aperture in CM rejects part of the light from the focal region inside the sample due to scattering, in comparison, MPM collects all emission light from the multiphoton excitation, minimizing the signal loss. Also, compared with CFM, where molecules along the whole illumination path are excited, MPM possesses significantly less photo-bleaching effect due to excitation only in the focal zone (Niesner and Hauser, 2011).

Because the wavelength of illumination is longer than the one used for CFM, the focal size that can be achieved in MPM is relatively larger, resulting in lower spatial resolution, but still featuring at the micron and submicron level (Scientist and Technology, 2008). Specifically, for two-photon excitation, the spatial resolution is about twice of CFM. As the pinhole effect in MPM is intrinsically achieved by focusing the light, the spatial resolution of MPM is mainly determined by the numerical aperture of the objective lens. Similar to CM, the depthwise sectioning of MPM is obtained with axial movement of the imaging lens, and laser scanning is generally employed for a 3-D reconstruction of the sample. Multiphoton excitation is a powerful approach that has served as the basis for a number of imaging modalities (Masters, 2006). Here, we focus our discussions on two-photon fluorescence and second harmonic generation microscopy, which have both been used largely in tissue engineering.

8.4.2 Two-photon fluorescence microscopy

As the most commonly used form of MPM, two-photon fluorescence microscopy (2-PFM) utilizes near-infrared light with a wavelength of about twice as long as the one required for excitation of the fluorescent molecule (Palikaras and Tavernarakis, 2001). As an intrinsic property, cells can produce fluorescence emission from endogenous fluorophores, such as NADH, NADPH, flavins, collagen and elastin, which are excitable with the visible spectrum (Monici, 2005). By probing this auto-fluorescence signal, 2-PFM does not require fluorescence labeling of the sample, providing convenient imaging and characterization of cellular and tissue structures. In tissue engineering, cell viability assessment has been achieved by imaging the auto-fluorescence using 2-PFM, where the viable and dead cells can be easily distinguished with spectral analysis of the auto-fluorescence emissions (Dittmar et al., 2012), representing a simple and efficient approach. Also, depth-resolved 2-PFM imaging of the mitochondrial NADH auto-fluorescence has been demonstrated to be able to differentiate between normal and precancerous engineered tissues (Levitt et al., 2007). Additionally, time-lapse 2-PFM dynamic monitoring of the fluorescence contribution from the intrinsic cellular fluorophores, such as flavoproteins and lipofuscin, were reported with human mesenchymal stem cells (Rice et al., 2010). In addition to cells, extracellular matrix components, including collagen and elastin, have also been probed and assessed based on auto-fluorescence via 2-PFM (Schenke-Layland, 2008; Schenke-Layland et al., 2009; Schade et al., 2010). As an example, 3-D auto-fluorescence imaging of the elastic fibers in tissue-engineered heart valves has been demonstrated with 2-PFM in the diagnosis of tissue conditions prior to implantation (König et al., 2005).

With fluorescence labeling, 2-PFM has more extended applications in tissue engineering. With various types of proteins and dyes, different structures of the cell can be well resolved, such as the nuclei (Filova et al., 2010), membrane (Diaspro et al., 2005), and cytoplasm (Rubbens et al., 2009). Boerboom et al. achieved improved structural imaging of collagen using 2-PFM and a novel collagen fluorescence probe, leading to high-resolution visualization of the collagen in engineered cardiovascular constructs (Boerboom et al., 2007). Also, Liu et al. (2007) employed 2-PFM for 3-D deep imaging and quantitative characterization of the microstructures (such as porosity and pore size) and cell–substrate interactions (such as cellular morphological patterns) in microporous scaffold substrates fabricated from synthetic biodegradable polymers. In addition, similar to CFM, 2-PFM can also be used for vasculature imaging in tissue engineering, but with relatively higher penetration depth. Hegen et al. (2011) have successfully characterized intrascaffold microvessel self-assembly efficiency in a physiological in vivo tissue engineering implant context. Yanez et al. (2013) demonstrated 3-D reconstruction of vascular plexus formation at an imaging depth of up to 1.6 mm within the regenerating wound tissue, using 2-PFM and an integrin fluorescent probe.

8.4.3 Second harmonic generation microscopy

While 2-PFM provides specificity to the type of molecules, second harmonic generation microscopy (SHGM) is highly specific to the molecular structure, i.e., the orientation and organization, in tissues and cells (Chen et al., 2012). Although also relying on two-photon illumination, SHGM imaging contrast arises from the induced polarization instead of the excitation-emission mechanism in fluorescence imaging (Campagnola, 2011). Upon strong coherent photon illumination, noncentrosymmetric molecular structure can generate second-harmonic light with the wavelength exactly half the illumination light, which is probed by SHGM. As the imaging contrast of SHMG is from an endogenous molecular structure, no labeling process is required in this technique and efficient in vivo imaging is possible. The imaging scale of SHGM is very similar to the one from 2-PFM (Campagnola et al., 2001). Since not based on photon absorption, SHGM is energy-conserving and has substantially reduced photo-bleaching and heating effect compared with CFM and 2-PFM. These features make SGHM a powerful high-resolution 3-D live imaging approach for collagen, microtubules, and muscle myosin (Campagnola and Loew, 2003; Nucciotti et al., 2010; Campagnola et al., 2002), which is exceedingly useful in tissue engineering.

Structural imaging of type I fibrillar collagen has been one of the major applications of SHGM in tissue engineering (Williams et al., 2005). SHGM has been applied to probe the depth-resolved collagen organization in the calvarial structure microenvironment during osteogenesis (Villa et al., 2013), to quantitatively characterize the collagen organization and structure subcutaneously generated in mice upon polystyrene particle injection (Akilbekova and Bratlie, 2015), and to dynamically assess the spatial organization of collagen fibers in a sparsely distributed collagen scaffold sample (Kabir et al., 2013). Because SHGM and 2-PFM imaging can be achieved with one single microscope setup, these two imaging techniques are usually combined to provide high-resolution visualization (Chen et al., 2010). The integration of SHGM and auto-fluorescence imaging with 2-PFM was reported by Sun et al. to study the 3-D microstructure and nonlinear optical properties of different types of scaffolds used in tissue engineering (Sun et al., 2008). By combining SHGM with fluorescence imaging using 2-PFM, Villa et al. have shown longitudinal visualization of the bone formation in a tissue-engineered construct both in vivo with single cell resolution and in situ with 3-D information (Villa et al., 2013). This combined imaging has enabled in vivo assessment of the host cells, donor cells, scaffold, and collagen matrix during a repair process.

The combination of 2-PFM and SHGM has also been used to probe the mechanics of collagen gel through microstructural analysis (Raub et al., 2007). Specifically, Raub et al. have demonstrated that the differential microscopic features of collagen hydrogel characterized by 2-PFM and SHGM correlate well with its bulk mechanical properties (Raub et al., 2007). This indirect MPM functional analysis approach is an interesting direction for a more robust assessment in tissue engineering.

8.5 Optical coherence tomography

8.5.1 General

Optical coherence tomography (OCT) is a 3-D imaging technique based on low-coherence interferometry (Huang et al., 1991; Schmitt, 1999). OCT has a typical spatial resolution of 1–15 μm in the axial direction, which is decoupled from lateral resolution and solely determined by the bandwidth of the imaging light source. Generally, the laser source of OCT is in the infrared spectral range, providing a depth of penetration of up to several millimeters in scattering tissues. To ensure the imaging depth and avoid the axial scanning, a scan lens with low numerical aperture is usually utilized in OCT, which leads to a typical microscale lateral resolution. Fourier domain OCT (FDOCT) is currently the most widely used OCT technique, as it features greater sensitivity and higher imaging speed as compared to time domain OCT (TDOCT) (Leitgeb et al., 2003). In FDOCT, the depth-resolved scan (A-scan) is obtained through a simple Fourier transform of the interference fringes with respect to the wavenumber, where the amplitude information is utilized to form the structural OCT image, and the phase of light is extracted to achieve high sensitivity of tissue and cell displacement for functional imaging, such as Doppler OCT (Fercher et al., 2003). Three-dimensional OCT reconstruction is achieved by lateral scanning of the imaging beam with a field of view generally at the millimeter level. By employing a swept laser source (Choma et al., 2003), current FDOCT imaging provides a typical A-scan rate of up to hundreds of kHz (Drexler et al., 2014), and with an ultrafast swept laser source (such as Fourier domain mode-locked laser), OCT A-scan rate at MHz level has been demonstrated (Klein et al., 2013). With the unique imaging scale and only relying on the endogenous contrast, both structural and functional OCT imaging has been applied as useful tools for tissue engineering (Liang et al., 2009; Boppart et al., 2008).

8.5.2 Structural imaging

Structural OCT imaging, based on the scattering contrast from refractive index mismatch inside the tissue, can be utilized to monitor structural development and cell dynamics in tissue-engineered constructs with a relatively large field of view (Mason et al., 2004b). Tan et al. have demonstrated longitudinal OCT 3-D imaging of the microarchitecture during the developmental process of engineered tissues (Tan et al., 2004), where interior details deep inside the tissue can be well visualized with arbitrary sectioning planes. Additionally, cell activities with the tissue growth, including the interactions between cells and extracellular matrix, have been probed in 3-D over time with OCT (Tan et al., 2004). In another study, OCT has been used to characterize the structural morphology of the engineered bone tissue under development (Yang et al., 2006). Furthermore, scaffold assessment has been performed by OCT (Yang et al., 2008; Bagnaninchi et al., 2007; Chen et al., 2011). As an example, Chen et al. have shown that the key morphological design parameters for macroporous hydrogel scaffolds can be quantitatively measured, including the volume porosity, pore interconnectivity, and pore size, which was utilized to discriminate scaffolds made from different formulations (Chen et al., 2011). In addition, cell dynamic behaviors, including chemotaxis migration, proliferation, deadhesion, and cell–material interactions, in three-dimensional thick-tissue models have been successfully imaged in four dimensions (3-D with time) in a quantitative fashion (Tan et al., 2006). For skin repair analysis in wound-healing experiments, OCT demonstrated the ability to resolve and distinguish between different layers of skin equivalents, providing a convenient way for evaluation of the quality of skin equivalents prior to transplantation (Spoler et al., 2006). Recently, Haraguchi et al. achieved noninvasive 3-D analysis of cell sheet tissue fabrication using OCT, which enabled detailed observations of adhesions between layered cell sheets, as well as the beating of a rat cardiac cell sheet (Haraguchi et al., 2015).

Optical coherence microscopy (OCM) is the high-resolution form of OCT that utilizes a lens with higher numerical aperture to achieve greater lateral resolving capability (submicron level) for cellular imaging (Aguirre et al., 2015). Full-field OCM, based on TDOCT configuration and a 2-D camera, provides *en face* imaging with further improved lateral resolution (Beaurepaire et al., 1998). Reported by Yang et al. (2006) OCM was used to delineate the morphology of cells and constructs in tissue engineering. Orwin et al. (2004) utilized OCM to evaluate the structure of tissue-engineered artificial cornea over time and its optical properties. Recently, living cells and 3-D tissue from cell sheet fabrication has been imaged with OCM with clearly distinguished cell nuclei and cytoplasm; 3-D migration of the cells was also successfully detected (Hasegawa et al., 2015). Endoscopic OCT with a miniature imaging probe is a promising technique for both intravascular assessment (Yabushita et al., 2002) as well as characterization of gastrointestinal and respiratory tracts (Tearney et al., 1997). The ability of endoscopic OCT for visualization of the cellular lining of a tissue-engineered blood vessel mimic and the response of this lining to a bare metal stent has been evaluated (Bonnema et al., 2007).

8.5.3 Polarization sensitive OCT

Polarization sensitive OCT (PSOCT) generates tissue-specific contrast by probing the polarization state of light that can be altered by tissue–light interaction (Park and Boer, 2008). A number of tissue types, such as tendon and muscle, exhibit form birefringence, where the optical phase difference between orthogonal polarization components is nonzero. This optical property of tissue is one of the widely used parameters characterized by PSOCT (Everett et al., 1998). Based on OCT, PSOCT provides additional contrast and enhanced specificity for identifying the tissue structures. Major applications of PSOCT are emerging in dentistry, ophthalmology, and dermatology (de Boer and Milner, 2002). For tissue engineering, PSOCT has been employed for the nondestructive online monitoring of the growth of engineered tendon constructs (Yang et al., 2008). Recently, PSOCT was demonstrated with the capability to map the "brushing direction" of collagen fibers in articular cartilage, which is useful to optimize the design of scaffolds for cartilage repair (Lu et al., 2014). In regards to articular cartilage, PSOCT is considered to be well suited for in situ assessment of the development and integration of the 3-D tissue-engineered cartilage constructs (Matcher, 2009).

8.5.4 Optical coherence elastography

Using OCT to probe tissue biomechanics, optical coherence elastography (OCE) is a rapidly developing technique that provides both qualitative and quantitative measures of tissue elasticity (Schmitt, 1998; Kennedy et al., 2014). Combining a tissue-loading approach with OCT, the mechanical response of tissue to the stimulus is assessed with high sensitivity to produce mechanical parameters, such as strain, shear wave velocity, and natural frequency. These parameters serve as the imaging contrast of OCE and can be further used to reconstruct quantitative tissue elasticity (Kennedy et al., 2014;

Wang and Larin, 2014). The spatial imaging scale of OCE features a relatively wide range, with the resolution from microscale to hundreds of microns and the field of view at the millimeter level, depending on the specific OCE method and the employed mechanical contrast (Kennedy et al., 2014). At this imaging scale, OCE fills in the gap from traditional mechanical imaging techniques and has enabled a broad range of applications, revealing the tissue biomechanical information that was previously unavailable (Wang and Larin, 2014). Several studies of OCE have focused on the tissue engineering applications and are promising to establish OCE as an essential functional imaging and characterization tool in the engineering and regeneration of tissues. Specifically, Ko et al. (2006) have demonstrated that OCE can be used to monitor the mechanical property of the developing, engineered tissue over time and is able to obtain the relative elasticity differences during cell proliferation. Additionally, a study on OCE of myocardium has shown the capability of OCE for noncontact quantitative elasticity measurement of mouse cardiac muscle tissue, which led to the observation that the genetically altered adult cardiomyocytes with regenerative capability appear to be more elastic than normal ones (Wang et al., 2014). Since regaining cardiomyocyte regeneration ability through genetic manipulation is an emerging approach for repairing the heart after heart failure (Heallen et al., 2011), this application of OCE to assess the cardiac mechanical function has significant value for evaluating the regeneration of myocardium.

8.5.5 Doppler optical coherence tomography

Based on the OCT phase signal, Doppler OCT (DOCT) employs the Doppler frequency shift induced by moving scatters to obtain the velocity information and is extensively utilized for functional blood flow imaging and measurement (Yang et al., 2003). With the known angle between flow direction and imaging beam, the absolute flow velocity can be quantified. Usually relying on inter-A-scan signal analysis, DOCT possesses the same spatial and temporal imaging scales with OCT, thus providing a powerful 3-D flow imaging technique with high spatiotemporal resolution (Chen and Zhang, 2008). Fluid flow is a critical aspect of successful tissue engineering in certain cases (Hillsley and Frangos, 1994; Gemmiti and Guldberg, 2006), and quantitative assessment of the flow dynamics can provide great insight into understanding tissue development. The application of DOCT on tissue engineering was first reported by Mason et al., who demonstrated the imaging of a fully developed laminar flow in a tissue-engineered construct in situ within a bioreactor (Mason et al., 2004a). In another study, Veksler et al. used DOCT to monitor the complex microflow in the porous scaffolds and estimated the shear stress acting on the cells (Veksler et al., 2008). Furthermore, by measuring the flow profile and estimating the shear stress within low- and high-porosity chitosan scaffolds using DOCT, Jia et al. found that the fluid flow and the flow-induced shear stress in micropores are largely affected by the size of pores, porosity, and micropore interconnectivity (Jia et al., 2009), as shown in Fig. 8.3(a). These studies indicate that the high resolution and quantitative assessment characteristics of DOCT are highly useful in analyzing fluid flow in tissue engineering.

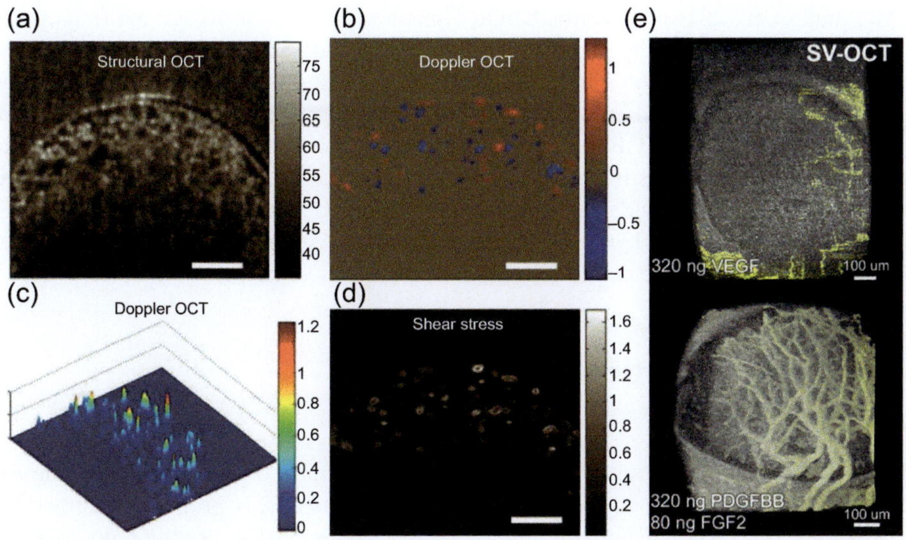

Figure 8.3 Structural and functional optical coherence tomography imaging in application to tissue engineering. (a) Depth-resolved optical coherence tomography imaging of the low-porosity chitosan scaffolds shows the microstructures. Color bar: dB. (b) Depth-resolved Doppler optical coherence tomography imaging of the fluid flow inside the scaffolds shows the map of bidirectional flow velocity. Color bar: mm/s. (c) 3-D magnitude plot of the flow velocities measured in scaffolds shows the laminar flow profile. Color bar: mm/s. (d) Depth-resolved mapping of the quantified shear stress induced by the fluid flow inside the scaffolds. Color bar: dyn/cm^2. Scale bars for (a–d) correspond to 200 μm. (e) In vivo 3-D speckle variance optical coherence tomography imaging of the perfusion of vasculature network induced by growth factors in the mouse cornea. Results show that PDGFBB/FGF2-releasing hydrogels introduce better-perfused blood vessels than VEGF-releasing hydrogels. (a–d) are *reproduced with permission from Jia, Y., Bagnaninchi, P.O., Yang, Y., Haj, A.E., Hinds, M.T., Kirkpatrick, S.J., Wang, R.K., 2009. Doppler optical coherence tomography imaging of local fluid flow and shear stress within microporous scaffolds. Journal of Biomedical Optics 14, 034014.* (e) is *reproduced with permission from Hsu, C.W., Poché, R.A., Saik, J.E., Ali, S., Wang, S., Yosef, N., Calderon, G.A., Scott, L., Vadakkan Jr., T.J., Larina, I.V., West, J.L., Dickinson, M.E., 2015. Improved angiogenesis in response to localized delivery of macrophage-recruiting molecules. PLoS One 10, e0131643.*

8.5.6 Speckle variance optical coherence tomography

The vascularization of tissue scaffolds with proper function is required for successful engineering of complex organs (Bramfeldt et al., 2010). Speckle variance OCT (SVOCT), based on the OCT speckle fluctuations introduced by moving scatters, is able to provide 3-D mapping of the vasculature network inside the tissue (Mariampillai et al., 2008). As SVOCT relies on endogenous blood perfusion to form the contrast, SVOCT imaging of blood vessels directly reveals the function of the vasculature and is thus useful in assessing engineered blood vessels. Based on the imaging scale of OCT, SVOCT can resolve single capillaries with a millimeter-range field of view

(Mahmud et al., 2013). Recently, SVOCT has been utilized to image the function of vascularization induced by proangiogenic growth factors in vivo in the mouse cornea (Hsu et al., 2015), as shown in Fig. 8.3(b). In this study, 3-D SVOCT reconstruction shows better perfusion of the blood vessels from PDGFBB/FGF2-releasing hydrogels compared with VEGF-releasing hydrogels in the cornea tissue, which help to define improved engineering strategies for vascularization. Further data analysis has enabled SVOCT to provide measurements of flux and velocity of red blood cells in capillaries (Lee et al., 2013), which may facilitate more robust functional blood vessel characterization in tissue engineering.

8.6 Photoacoustic microscopy

8.6.1 General

Photoacoustic microscopy (PAM) is the microscopic form of photoacoustic imaging, where the laser-induced tissue photoacoustic phenomenon is probed by ultrasound transducer for image reconstruction (Yao and Wang, 2013). Relying on acoustic detection of tissue optical absorption contrast, PAM can reach an imaging depth of up to several millimeters in tissue over the optical diffusion limit (Wang, 2008). In PAM, the excitation light and the ultrasonic detection are cofocused on the sample to achieve one-dimensional depth-resolved A-scan, which is used for 3-D imaging based on mechanical scanning of the excitation and detection beams (Wang and Gao, 2014). The lateral resolution and imaging depth of PAM are adjustable based on the selective tightening between the optical and acoustic foci, while the axial resolution of PAM is dependent on the bandwidth of the photoacoustic signal that is detected by the ultrasonic detector (Yao and Wang, 2013). With a high-frequency transducer (e.g., 50 MHz), PAM can achieve an axial resolution of ~15 μm (Yao and Wang, 2013). The scalability and unique optical absorption contrast of PAM provides a useful tool to characterize 3-D tissue-engineered samples, specifically, scaffolds, cells, and blood vessels (Cai et al., 2013b).

8.6.2 Acoustic resolution photoacoustic microscopy

Acoustic resolution PAM (AR-PAM) has a relatively tighter acoustic focusing than optical focusing, featuring dark-field illumination with a ring-shape light excitation (Zhang et al., 2006). In AR-PAM, the spatial imaging scale is mainly determined by the ultrasound part of the system, which provides a lateral resolution of tens of microns and an imaging depth over several millimeters with a high-frequency ultrasonic transducer (Yao and Wang, 2013). Although this scale of imaging is similar to the high-frequency ultrasonic imaging, the contrast of imaging formed by optical absorption enables applications that are not achievable with solely acoustic imaging. AR-PAM has been utilized for 3-D imaging of the porous scaffolds with quantification of the porosity and pore size (Cai et al., 2012). Also, Zhang et al. (2010a) have employed AR-PAM for label-free 3-D evaluation of how seeding and culturing methods influence the spatial distribution of melanoma cells inside porous scaffolds. The quantification of the number of melanoma cells and the monitoring of the cell proliferation profile are demonstrated with AR-PAM (Zhang et al., 2010a). In addition to imaging cells with intrinsic absorption contrast, contrast agents, such as 3-(4,5-Dimethylthiazol-2-yl)-2,5-diphenyltetrazolium bromide (MTT) formazan (Mosmann, 1983), have been used with AR-PAM for cell imaging in the case of low optical absorption from the targets. Following a three-hour MTT staining, AR-PAM can be utilized to longitudinally assess fibroblast growth in the inverse opal scaffolds with visualization of cell invasion (Zhang et al., 2011). Additionally, based on the high optical absorption from blood, AR-PAM has also been used to probe the vasculature network deep inside porous scaffolds, providing visualization and characterization of neovascularization (Cai et al., 2013a).

8.6.3 Optical resolution photoacoustic microscopy

With highly focused light excitation within the optical diffusion limit, optical resolution PAM (OR-PAM) provides improved spatial resolution to resolve more detailed tissue structures (Maslov et al., 2008). Since the optical focal spot can be achieved much more tightly than the acoustic focus, the lateral resolution of OR-PAM can reach microscale and even submicron level, with the depth of penetration typically around 1 mm (Hu and Wang, 2013). While sharing a similar imaging scale with OCT that employs optical scattering as the imaging contrast, the optical absorption contrast from OR-PAM makes it a powerful technique for direct high-resolution imaging and characterization of vasculature networks without extra image processing efforts (Hu and Wang, 2010). For example, Cai et al. (2013a) utilized OR-PAM to image the development of vasculature in the inverse opal scaffolds, revealing the effect of pore size of the scaffold on neovascularization. In addition, OR-PAM has been employed for quantitative measures of 3 D porous scaffolds incorporating single-walled carbon nanotube (Cai et al., 2012). Recent development of OR-PAM enabled an oxygen-metabolic assessment (Yao et al., 2011), providing advanced noninvasive label-free functional analysis of blood vessels in tissue engineering.

8.7 Raman spectroscopy

8.7.1 General

Raman spectroscopy (RS) is a noninvasive label-free spectroscopic technique that probes molecular information of a sample with light (Ferraro and Nakamoto, 2012). The contrast of RS comes from the inelastic scattering (Raman scattering) of photons by the molecules, where a gain or loss of energy occurs, leading to a frequency shift of the scattered light. In RS, the Raman scattering is usually analyzed with respect to wavenumber, where the peaks of the spectrum serve as fingerprint identifications of different molecules (Ferraro and Nakamoto, 2012). The time required to produce the Raman spectrum is generally within seconds to minutes, allowing for a rapid biochemical analysis. Near-infrared light ranging from ~700 nm to ~1064 nm has been most commonly used to illuminate the biological samples in RS due to the auto-fluorescence in the visible light range and the photo-degradation of tissue by the light in the ultra-violet spectral range (Movasaghi et al., 2007).

Imaging with RS can provide high-resolution 3-D distribution of the specific molecules in a heterogeneous biological sample by spatially mapping the Raman spectrum information (Zhang et al., 2010b). The spatial scale of RS imaging of cells and tissues is similar to the traditional optical microscopy but with reduced resolution and higher penetration depth due to the larger wavelength of light that is employed. Specifically, the spatial resolution can reach the submicron level and is limited by optical diffraction (Zhang et al., 2010b). Utilizing a confocal configuration, confocal RS imaging has an improved spatial resolving capability and is able to provide depthwise sectioning with a penetration depth of up to the millimeter level (Dieing et al., 2011). Hyperspectral RS imaging data can be achieved with both point scanning and line scanning schemes for 3-D molecular imaging with high specificity (Zoubir, 2012).

Since Raman scattering is significantly weaker compared with Rayleigh scattering and fluorescence, traditional RS might suffer from low signal-to-noise ratio, thus requiring a longer time of data collection. The development of Raman scattering-based spectroscopic methods has led to a number of advanced RS techniques, such as surface-enhanced resonance RS (McNay et al., 2011) and coherent anti-Stokes RS (Evans and Xie, 2008), which provide increased Raman scattering and improved resolution and sensitivity. Although molecular specific imaging can be achieved with fluorescence labeling in CM and MPM, the unique features of RS that include utilizing endogenous contrast, requiring minimum sample preparation, and simultaneously obtaining a large amount of molecular composition data are very attractive and make RS a useful molecular imaging tool for both cells and tissue constructs in tissue engineering (Jell et al., 2010; Perlaki et al., 2014).

8.7.2 Cell analysis with Raman spectroscopy

Raman spectroscopy can provide characterization of cellular process and response in tissue engineering by analyzing cell biomolecular composition (Weeks and Huser, 2010). Swain et al. (2008a) have demonstrated the use of RS to assess the biochemical changes related to cell cycle dynamics through the analysis of Raman spectra from human osteosarcoma cells as a function of the cell cycle phase. Also, cell differentiation in culture has been noninvasively monitored based on RS and statistical analysis. Specifically, Jell et al. (2008) reported the application of RS combined with multivariate statistical analysis for rapid and noninvasive identification of the biomaterial-accelerated differentiation of fetal osteoblasts. A similar approach has been utilized by the same group for successful detection of the spontaneous differentiation of the live human alveolar epithelial type II cells in culture (Swain et al., 2008b). Biochemical markers have also been investigated and determined based on RS to identify the differentiation status of mouse embryonic stem cells cultured on biomaterials, including undifferentiated, spontaneously differentiated, and differentiated cell status (Notingher et al., 2004). In addition to monitoring the cell cycle and differentiation, cell proliferation can be characterized using RS based on the measurement of Raman spectra of cells and nuclei in culture during the nonproliferating and proliferating

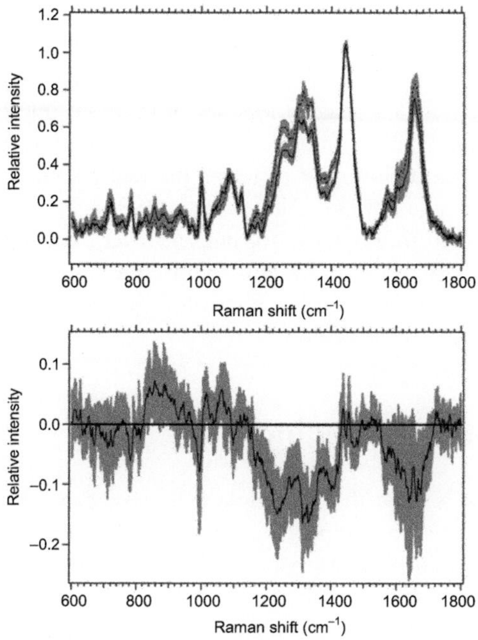

Figure 8.4 Raman spectroscopy characterization of cell proliferation Raman spectra of nonproliferating (*solid line*) and proliferating (*dotted line*) MR1 cells with the mean value as the lines and standard deviations as the shaded areas (top); Difference spectrum for the average of nonproliferating cells minus proliferating cells with the standard deviation shown as the shaded area (bottom). *Reprinted from Biophysical Journal, 88, Short, K.W., Carpenter, S., Freyer, J.P., Mourant, J.R., Raman spectroscopy detects biochemical changes due to proliferation in mammalian cell cultures, 4274–4288, Copyright (2005), with permission from Elsevier.*

phases, as shown in Fig. 8.4 (Short et al., 2005). RS imaging of human cells at various mitotic stages has also been reported to reveal a complete cell division cycle using spectroscopic techniques (Matthaus et al., 2006). These monitoring and assessments of cell behavior enabled by RS are critically important for understanding the molecular changes in primary cellular processes and developing functional tissue constructs.

8.7.3 Biomaterial analysis with Raman spectroscopy

Molecular modification of the biomaterial surface is an important way to make biomimetic materials, which is of great significance for obtaining desired cell behavior and manipulating tissue formation (Shin et al., 2003). As a nondestructive approach, biochemical characterization of the biomaterial surface can be efficiently conducted with RS (Perlaki et al., 2014). Rice et al. (2008) has demonstrated that RS can be a useful tool to assist and confirm the optical structural analysis of silk fibroin biomaterials. RS imaging was also reported as a way to differentiate between polymer species and to quantify the volume fractions of degradable polymer, promising to provide advanced analysis of degradation rates of polymer scaffolds (Nandagawali et al., 2007). Additionally, confocal RS imaging has been employed to study the intracellular degradation of poly(lactic-co-glycolic acid) microspheres inside individual macrophages, showing a heterogeneous degradation manner of ingested microspheres that is more rapid in the center (van Apeldoorn et al., 2004). In bone implants, RS has been used to investigate the biocompatibility of different implant coatings and their integrations with bone (Bertoluzza et al., 1994; Dippel et al., 1998). In addition, longitudinal RS analysis was reported to monitor the formation of an extracellular matrix in a 3-D medium-throughput pellet culture system (Kunstar et al., 2011). Recently, Kunstar et al. (2013) have shown the use of a fiber-optic RS setup to monitor extracellular matrix formation inside 3-D scaffolds.

8.8 Multimodality imaging

As reviewed above, it is clear that no single technique can fulfill all the high-resolution imaging needs in tissue engineering. The spatial imaging scale and the contrast mechanism of the technique determine, but also limit, the information it can provide and thus inform the range of its applicability. To overcome this limitation, multimodality imaging, the combination of generally two or three imaging techniques, has been employed to achieve a more robust assessment of a sample with multidimensional information.

An integrated OCM and 2-PFM system was built by Tan et al. to simultaneously provide optical scattering and fluorescence imaging from the same sample region (Tan et al., 2007; Graf and Boppart, 2010). Specifically, the 2-PFM can image individual cells, and the OCM allows structural visualization of the substrates. This multimodal approach has been applied to investigate cellular responses to mechanical stimuli in 3-D tissue constructs through the imaging of fibroblasts cultured in 3-D PDMS substrates and polymer scaffolds, (Tan et al., 2007). The combination of OCT and CFM has been used for longitudinal visualization of the cell dynamics in chitosan scaffold culture (Graf and Boppart, 2010). Dunkers et al. have reported a collinear OCM and CFM instrument for simultaneous scattering and fluorescence imaging deep inside a PCL scaffold with fetal chick osteoblasts (Dunkers et al., 2003). Complementary information provided by OCT and SHGM has been applied for time-dependent monitoring of the wound-healing process in a skin-equivalent raft tissue (Yeh et al., 2004). In this approach, OCT imaging was used to delineate the injured region and collagen microstructure organization, while fibroblast cell migration in response to injury was visualized by SHGM (Yeh et al., 2004). In addition, since both rely on two-photon excitation, 2-PFM and SHGM are often combined to image collagen-related tissue constructs and cell behavior in tissue engineering (Villa et al., 2013; Filova et al., 2010; Schenke-Layland et al., 2003; Cortiella et al., 2010). As an example, the extracellularly distributed collagen in a PCL scaffold was visualized, and the volume of collagen was quantified using combined 2-PFM and SHGM imaging (Filova et al., 2010).

8.9 Perspectives

We want to end this chapter by briefly introducing three high-resolution imaging techniques from the aspects of super-resolution visualization, dirцct biomechanical characterization, and deep molecular imaging. We expect increased application of these techniques in the exciting field of tissue engineering due to their unique and powerful individual properties.

Spatial resolution is one of the most critical parameters of microscopy, and improvement in spatial resolution has always expanded the limit of what people can see and therefore understand at new spatial levels. Resolutions of traditional optical microscopy techniques, as discussed above, are all limited by diffraction, which is on the order of a half-wavelength of the light (Born et al., 1999). Relying on fluorescence imaging, super-resolution microscopy techniques, such as stimulated emission depletion microscopy (Hell and Wichmann, 1994), stochastic optical reconstruction microscopy (Huang et al., 2008), and photo-activated localization microscopy (Hess et al., 2006), have been developed to break the diffraction limit and can feature spatial resolutions as good as ~20 nm (Huang et al., 2009). This spatial imaging scale allows time-resolved localization of individual molecules in live cells (Godin et al., 2014). This technology can prove useful in providing detailed molecular analysis of the cellular response to scaffolds and external stimuli.

Brillouin scattering is the inelastic light scattering between photons and acoustic phonons, which allows viscoelastic characterization of the material (Dil, 1982). Scarcelli et al. have developed confocal Brillouin microscopy that employs Brillouin scattering in tissue to probe biomechanics (Scarcelli and Yun, 2007). With a highly sensitive spectrometer, the Brillouin shift from tissue can be measured noninvasively with a 3-D spatial resolution as high as that seen in confocal microscopy. The Brillouin shift can be utilized as a quantitative measure of tissue elasticity and is well correlated with the traditionally used elastic modulus (Scarcelli et al., 2011). Confocal Brillouin microscopy has been extensively employed to study ocular tissue biomechanics (Scarcelli et al., 2011, 2014, 2015a), including the acrylic intraocular lens (Scarcelli and Yun, 2007). Noncontact 3-D mapping of intracellular hydromechanical properties using Brillouin microscopy has been demonstrated (Scarcelli et al., 2015b), which can be utilized as a new and efficient approach to assess the cellular biomechanical changes in tissue engineering.

For a long time, molecular imaging has suffered from a limited depth of view in highly scattering tissues. Photothermal OCT, which employs the OCT phase signal to probe the externally induced photothermal expansion inside tissue (Tucker-Schwartz et al., 2012; 2015), can achieve 3-D molecular contrast with millimeter-level imaging depth in scattering samples (Zhou et al., 2010). With photon-absorption nanostructures targeting specific molecules, upon modulated light excitation, molecular specificity can be obtained, which has been used for cell identification (Skala et al., 2008). Since the unique imaging scale of OCT is highly useful in a number of applications in tissue engineering, the addition of molecular contrast holds the promise for robust structural, functional, and molecular characterization of tissue constructs within a single system.

8.10 Conclusions

It is clear that each of the high-resolution imaging techniques has unique features for specific applications in tissue engineering. In deciding the best imaging strategy, the detailed properties of the imaging techniques should be taken into careful consideration to drive the selection of particular techniques to fulfill the imaging requirements. This review has described the imaging properties of the widely used high-resolution techniques and discussed their representative applications in tissue engineering, which provides a helpful reference to determine the most appropriate imaging tools for tissue engineering studies.

Acknowledgments

We would like to thank the funding support from the National Institute of Health with the grants R01HL120140 and U54HG006348. S. W. was supported by the American Heart Association with the grant 16POST30990070. We also want to thank Mr. David S. Lakomy (Baylor College of Medicine) for a careful reading and editing of the text.

References

Aguirre, A.D., Zhou, C., Lee, H.-C., Ahsen, O.O., Fujimoto, J.G., 2015. Optical coherence microscopy. In: Drexler, W., Fujimoto, G.J. (Eds.), Optical Coherence Tomography: Technology and Applications. Springer International Publishing, Cham.

Aigner, J., Tegeler, J., Hutzler, P., Campoccia, D., Pavesio, A., Hammer, C., Kastenbauer, E., Naumann, A., 1998. Cartilage tissue engineering with novel nonwoven structured biomaterial based on hyaluronic acid benzyl ester. Journal of Biomedical Materials Research 42, 172–181.

Akilbekova, D., Bratlie, K.M., 2015. Quantitative characterization of collagen in the fibrotic capsule surrounding implanted polymeric microparticles through second harmonic generation imaging. PLoS One 10, e0130386.

Ambuhl, M.E., Brepsant, C., Meister, J.J., Verkhovsky, A.B., Sbalzarini, I.F., 2012. High-resolution cell outline segmentation and tracking from phase-contrast microscopy images. Journal of Microscopy 245, 161–170.

Appel, A.A., Anastasio, M.A., Larson, J.C., Brey, E.M., 2013. Imaging challenges in biomaterials and tissue engineering. Biomaterials 34, 6615–6630.

Bagnaninchi, P.O., Yang, Y., Zghoul, N., Maffulli, N., Wang, R.K., Haj, A.J., 2007. Chitosan microchannel scaffolds for tendon tissue engineering characterized using optical coherence tomography. Tissue Engineering 13, 323–331.

Barnes, C., Speroni, L., Quinn, K.P., Montevil, M., Saetzler, K., Bode-Animashaun, G., Mckerr, G., Georgakoudi, I., Downes, C.S., Sonnenschein, C., Howard, C.V., Soto, A.M., 2014. From single cells to tissues: interactions between the matrix and human breast cells in real time. PLoS One 9, e93325.

Beaurepaire, E., Boccara, A.C., Lebec, M., Blanchot, L., Saint-Jalmes, H., 1998. Full-field optical coherence microscopy. Optics Letters 23, 244–246.

Bertoluzza, A., Fagnano, C., Tinti, A., Morelli, M.A., Tosi, M.R., Maggi, G., Marchetti, P.G., 1994. Raman and infrared spectroscopic study of the molecular characterization of the biocompatibility of prosthetic biomaterials. Journal of Raman Spectroscopy 25, 109–114.

Boerboom, R.A., Krahn, K.N., Megens, R.T.A., Van Zandvoort, M.A.M.J., Merkx, M., Bouten, C.V.C., 2007. High resolution imaging of collagen organisation and synthesis using a versatile collagen specific probe. Journal of Structural Biology 159, 392–399.

Bonnema, G.T., Cardinal, K.O., Mcnally, J.B., Williams, S.K., Barton, J.K., 2007. Assessment of blood vessel mimics with optical coherence tomography. Journal of Biomedical Optics 12, 024018–024018-6.

Boppart, S.A., Yang, Y., Wang, R.K., 2008. Optical coherence tomography in tissue engineering. In: Drexler, W., Fujimoto, J.G. (Eds.), Optical Coherence Tomography: Technology and Applications. Springer Berlin Heidelberg, Berlin, Heidelberg.

Born, M., Wolf, E., Bhatia, A.B., 1999. Principles of Optics: Electromagnetic Theory of Propagation, Interference and Diffraction of Light. Cambridge University Press.

Bramfeldt, H., Sabra, G., Centis, V., Vermette, P., 2010. Scaffold vascularization: a challenge for three-dimensional tissue engineering. Current Medicinal Chemistry 17, 3944–3967.

Brightman, A.O., Rajwa, B.P., Sturgis, J.E., Mccallister, M.E., Robinson, J.P., Voytik-Harbin, S.L., 2000. Time-lapse confocal reflection microscopy of collagen fibrillogenesis and extracellular matrix assembly in vitro. Biopolymers 54, 222–234.

Cai, X., Paratala, B.S., Hu, S., Sitharaman, B., Wang, L.V., 2012. Multiscale photoacoustic microscopy of single-walled carbon nanotube-incorporated tissue engineering scaffolds. Tissue Engineering, Part C Methods 18, 310–317.

Cai, X., Zhang, Y., Li, L., Choi, S.W., Macewan, M.R., Yao, J., Kim, C., Xia, Y., Wang, L.V., 2013a. Investigation of neovascularization in three-dimensional porous scaffolds in vivo by a combination of multiscale photoacoustic microscopy and optical coherence tomography. Tissue Engineering, Part C Methods 19, 196–204.

Cai, X., Zhang, Y.S., Xia, Y., Wang, L.V., 2013b. Photoacoustic microscopy in tissue engineering. Materials Today 16, 67–77.

Calzavara-Pinton, P., Longo, C., Venturini, M., Sala, R., Pellacani, G., 2008. Reflectance confocal microscopy for in vivo skin imaging. Photochemistry and Photobiology 84, 1421–1430.

Campagnola, P., 2011. Second harmonic generation imaging microscopy: applications to diseases diagnostics. Analytical Chemistry 83, 3224–3231.

Campagnola, P.J., Clark, H.A., Mohler, W.A., Lewis, A., Loew, L.M., 2001. Second-harmonic imaging microscopy of living cells. Journal of Biomedical Optics 6, 277–286.

Campagnola, P.J., Loew, L.M., 2003. Second-harmonic imaging microscopy for visualizing biomolecular arrays in cells, tissues and organisms. Nature Biotechnology 21, 1356–1360.

Campagnola, P.J., Millard, A.C., Terasaki, M., Hoppe, P.E., Malone, C.J., Mohler, W.A., 2002. Three-dimensional high-resolution second-harmonic generation imaging of endogenous structural proteins in biological tissues. Biophysical Journal 82, 493–508.

Chen, C.-W., Betz, M.W., Fisher, J.P., Paek, A., Chen, Y., 2011. Macroporous hydrogel scaffolds and their characterization by optical coherence tomography. Tissue Engineering, Part C: Methods 17, 101.

Chen, W.L., Huang, C.H., Chiou, L.L., Chen, T.H., Huang, Y.Y., Jiang, C.C., Lee, H.S., Dong, C.Y., 2010. Multiphoton imaging and quantitative analysis of collagen production by chondrogenic human mesenchymal stem cells cultured in chitosan scaffold. Tissue Engineering, Part C: Methods 16, 913–920.

Chen, X., Nadiarynkh, O., Plotnikov, S., Campagnola, P.J., 2012. Second harmonic generation microscopy for quantitative analysis of collagen fibrillar structure. Nature Protocols 7, 654–669.

Chen, Z., Zhang, J., 2008. Doppler optical coherence tomography. In: Drexler, W., Fujimoto, G.J. (Eds.), Optical Coherence Tomography: Technology and Applications. Springer Berlin Heidelberg, Berlin, Heidelberg.

Choma, M.A., Sarunic, M.V., Yang, C., Izatt, J.A., 2003. Sensitivity advantage of swept source and Fourier domain optical coherence tomography. Optics Express 11, 2183–2189.

Chwalek, K., Tsurkan, M.V., Freudenberg, U., Werner, C., 2014. Glycosaminoglycan-based hydrogels to modulate heterocellular communication in in vitro angiogenesis models. Scientific Reports 4, 4414.

Cortiella, J., Niles, J., Cantu, A., Brettler, A., Pham, A., Vargas, G., Winston, S., Wang, J., Walls, S., Nichols, J.E., 2010. Influence of acellular natural lung matrix on murine embryonic stem cell differentiation and tissue formation. Tissue Engineering, Part A 16, 2565–2580.

de Boer, J.F., Milner, T.E., 2002. Review of polarization sensitive optical coherence tomography and stokes vector determination. Journal of Biomedical Optics 7, 359–371.

Diaspro, A., Chirico, G., Collini, M., 2005. Two-photon fluorescence excitation and related techniques in biological microscopy. Quarterly Reviews of Biophysics 38, 97–166.

Dieing, T., Hollricher, O., Toporski, J., 2011. Confocal Raman Microscopy. Springer Berlin Heidelberg.

Dil, J.G., 1982. Brillouin scattering in condensed matter. Reports on Progress in Physics 45, 285.

Dippel, B., Mueller, R.T., Pingsmann, A., Schrader, B., 1998. Composition, constitution, and interaction of bone with hydroxyapatite coatings determined by FT Raman microscopy. Biospectroscopy 4, 403–412.

Dittmar, R., Potier, E., Van Zandvoort, M., Ito, K., 2012. Assessment of cell viability in three-dimensional scaffolds using cellular auto-fluorescence. Tissue Engineering, Part C: Methods 18, 198–204.

Drexler, W., Liu, M., Kumar, A., Kamali, T., Unterhuber, A., Leitgeb, R.A., 2014. Optical coherence tomography today: speed, contrast, and multimodality. Journal of Biomedical Optics 19, 071412.

Dunkers, J., Cicerone, M., Washburn, N., 2003. Collinear optical coherence and confocal fluorescence microscopies for tissue engineering. Optics Express 11, 3074–3079.

Engelmayr, G.C., Cheng, M., Bettinger, C.J., Borenstein, J.T., Langer, R., Freed, L.E., 2008. Accordion-like honeycombs for tissue engineering of cardiac anisotropy. Nature Materials 7, 1003–1010.

Evans, C.L., Xie, X.S., 2008. Coherent anti-stokes Raman scattering microscopy: chemical imaging for biology and medicine. Annual Review of Analytical Chemistry 1, 883–909.

Everett, M.J., Schoenenberger, K., Colston, B.W., Da Silva, L.B., 1998. Birefringence characterization of biological tissue by use of optical coherence tomography. Optics Letters 23, 228–230.

Fercher, A.F., Drexler, W., Hitzenberger, C.K., Lasser, T., 2003. Optical coherence tomography – principles and applications. Reports on Progress in Physics 66, 239.

Ferraro, J.R., Nakamoto, K., 2012. Introductory Raman Spectroscopy. Elsevier Science.

Filova, E., Burdíková, Z., Rampichová, M., Bianchini, P., Čapek, M., Košt'áková, E., Amler, E., Kubínová, L., 2010. Analysis and three-dimensional visualization of collagen in artificial scaffolds using nonlinear microscopy techniques. Journal of Biomedical Optics 15, 066011–066011-7.

Fukuda, K., 2001. Development of regenerative cardiomyocytes from mesenchymal stem cells for cardiovascular tissue engineering. Artificial Organs 25, 187–193.

Gemmiti, C.V., Guldberg, R.E., 2006. Fluid flow increases type II collagen deposition and tensile mechanical properties in bioreactor-grown tissue-engineered cartilage. Tissue Engineering 12, 469–479.

Gillette, B.M., Rossen, N.S., Das, N., Leong, D., Wang, M., Dugar, A., Sia, S.K., 2011. Engineering extracellular matrix structure in 3D multiphase tissues. Biomaterials 32, 8067–8076.

Godin, A.G., Lounis, B., Cognet, L., 2014. Super-resolution microscopy approaches for live cell imaging. Biophysical Journal 107, 1777–1784.

Graf, B.W., Boppart, S.A., 2010. Imaging and analysis of three-dimensional cell culture models. Methods in Molecular Biology (Clifton, N.J.) 591, 211–227.

Gu, M., 1996. Principles of Three Dimensional Imaging in Confocal Microscopes. World Scientific.

Hanke, T., Wollenweber, M., Burmeister, B., Kruse De Pacheco, M., Gelinsky, M., Scharnweber, D., Worch, H., 2003. Confocal laser scanning microscopy examination of cell cultures in three-dimensional scaffolds for tissue engineering. Microscopy and Microanalysis 9, 452–453.

Haraguchi, Y., Shimizu, T., Mizuuchi, K., Kawata, H., Kobayashi, M., Hirai, Y., Iwana, S.-I., 2015. Noninvasive cross-sectional observation of three-dimensional cell sheet-tissue-fabrication by optical coherence tomography. Biochemistry and Biophysics Reports 2, 57–62.

Hasegawa, A., Haraguchi, Y., Oikaze, H., Kabetani, Y., Sakaguchi, K., Shimizu, T., 2015. Optical coherence microscopy of living cells and bioengineered tissue dynamics in high-resolution cross-section. Journal of Biomedical Materials Research Part B: Applied Biomaterials.

Heallen, T., Zhang, M., Wang, J., Bonilla-Claudio, M., Klysik, E., Johnson, R.L., Martin, J.F., 2011. Hippo pathway inhibits Wnt signaling to restrain cardiomyocyte proliferation and heart size. Science 332, 458–461.

Hegen, A., Blois, A., Tiron, C.E., Hellesøy, M., Micklem, D.R., Nör, J.E., Akslen, L.A., Lorens, J.B., 2011. Efficient in vivo vascularization of tissue engineering scaffolds. Journal of Tissue Engineering and Regenerative Medicine 5, e52–e62.

Hell, S.W., Wichmann, J., 1994. Breaking the diffraction resolution limit by stimulated emission: stimulated-emission-depletion fluorescence microscopy. Optics Letters 19, 780–782.

Hess, S.T., Girirajan, T.P.K., Mason, M.D., 2006. Ultra-high resolution imaging by fluorescence photoactivation localization microscopy. Biophysical Journal 91, 4258–4272.

Hillsley, M.V., Frangos, J.A., 1994. Bone tissue engineering: the role of interstitial fluid flow. Biotechnology and Bioengineering 43, 573–581.

Hsu, C.W., Poché, R.A., Saik, J.E., Ali, S., Wang, S., Yosef, N., Calderon, G.A., Scott, L., Vadakkan Jr., T.J., Larina, I.V., West, J.L., Dickinson, M.E., 2015. Improved angiogenesis in response to localized delivery of macrophage-recruiting molecules. PLoS One 10, e0131643.

Hu, S., Wang, L.V., 2010. Photoacoustic imaging and characterization of the microvasculature. Journal of Biomedical Optics 15, 011101–011101-15.

Hu, S., Wang, L.V., 2013. Optical-resolution photoacoustic microscopy: auscultation of biological systems at the cellular level. Biophysical Journal 105, 841–847.

Huang, B., Bates, M., Zhuang, X., 2009. Super resolution fluorescence microscopy. Annual Review of Biochemistry 78, 993–1016.

Huang, B., Wang, W., Bates, M., Zhuang, X., 2008. Three-dimensional super-resolution imaging by stochastic optical reconstruction microscopy. Science 319, 810–813.

Huang, D., Swanson, E.A., Lin, C.P., Schuman, J.S., Stinson, W.G., Chang, W., Hee, M.R., Flotte, T., Gregory, K., Puliafito, C.A., et al., 1991. Optical coherence tomography. Science 254, 1178–1181.

Huh, S., Kanade, T., 2013. Apoptosis detection for non-adherent cells in time-lapse phase contrast microscopy. Medical Image Computing and Computer-Assisted Intervention 16, 59–66.

Huh, S., Ker, D.F., Bise, R., Chen, M., Kanade, T., 2011. Automated mitosis detection of stem cell populations in phase-contrast microscopy images. IEEE Transactions on Medical Imaging 30, 586–596.

Izadifar, Z., Chapman, L.D., Chen, X., 2014. Computed tomography diffraction-enhanced imaging for in situ visualization of tissue scaffolds implanted in cartilage. Tissue Engineering, Part C: Methods 20, 140–148.

Jalbert, I., Stapleton, F., Papas, E., Sweeney, D.F., Coroneo, M., 2003. In vivo confocal microscopy of the human cornea. The British Journal of Ophthalmology 87, 225–236.

Jawerth, L.M., Münster, S., Vader, D.A., Fabry, B., Weitz, D.A., 2010. A blind spot in confocal reflection microscopy: the dependence of fiber brightness on fiber orientation in imaging biopolymer networks. Biophysical Journal 98, L1–L3.

Jell, G., Notingher, I., Tsigkou, O., Notingher, P., Polak, J.M., Hench, L.L., Stevens, M.M., 2008. Bioactive glass-induced osteoblast differentiation: a noninvasive spectroscopic study. Journal of Biomedical Materials Research Part A 86, 31–40.

Jell, G., Swain, R., Stevens, M., 2010. Raman spectroscopy: a tool for tissue engineering. In: Matousek, P., Morris, D.M. (Eds.), Emerging Raman Applications and Techniques in Biomedical and Pharmaceutical Fields. Springer Berlin Heidelberg, Berlin, Heidelberg.

Jia, Y., Bagnaninchi, P.O., Yang, Y., Haj, A.E., Hinds, M.T., Kirkpatrick, S.J., Wang, R.K., 2009. Doppler optical coherence tomography imaging of local fluid flow and shear stress within microporous scaffolds. Journal of Biomedical Optics 14, 034014.

Kabir, M.M., Inavalli, V.V.G.K., Lau, T.-Y., Toussaint, K.C., 2013. Application of quantitative second-harmonic generation microscopy to dynamic conditions. Biomedical Optics Express 4, 2546–2554.

Kang, L., Miller, E.D., Weiss, L.E., Campbell, P.G., Kanade, T., 2006. Online tracking of migrating and proliferating cells imaged with phase-contrast microscopy. In: Computer Vision and Pattern Recognition Workshop, 2006 (CVPRW '06). Conference on, June 17–22, 2006, p. 65.

Kennedy, B.F., Kennedy, K.M., Sampson, D.D., 2014. A review of optical coherence elastography: fundamentals, techniques and prospects. IEEE Journal of Selected Topics in Quantum Electronics 20, 1–17.

Kim, T., Zhou, R., Mir, M., Babacan, S.D., Carney, P.S., Goddard, L.L., Popescu, G., 2014. White-light diffraction tomography of unlabelled live cells. Nature Photonics 8, 256–263.

Klein, T., Wieser, W., Reznicek, L., Neubauer, A., Kampik, A., Huber, R., 2013. Multi-MHz retinal OCT. Biomedical Optics Express 4, 1890–1908.

Ko, H.-J., Tan, W., Stack, R., Boppart, S.A, 2006. Optical coherence elastography of engineered and developing tissue. Tissue Engineering 12, 63–73.

König, K., Schenke-Layland, K., Riemann, I., Stock, U.A., 2005. Multiphoton autofluorescence imaging of intratissue elastic fibers. Biomaterials 26, 495–500.

Krahn, K.N., Bouten, C.V.C., Van Tuijl, S., Van Zandvoort, M.A.M.J., Merkx, M., 2006. Fluorescently labeled collagen binding proteins allow specific visualization of collagen in tissues and live cell culture. Analytical Biochemistry 350, 177–185.

Kreitz, S., Dohmen, G., Hasken, S., Schmitz-Rode, T., Mela, P., Jockenhoevel, S., 2011. Nondestructive method to evaluate the collagen content of fibrin-based tissue engineered structures via ultrasound. Tissue Engineering, Part C: Methods 17, 1021–1026.

Kunstar, A., Leferink, A.M., Okagbare, P.I., Morris, M.D., Roessler, B.J., Otto, C., Karperien, M., Van Blitterswijk, C.A., Moroni, L., Van Apeldoorn, A.A., 2013. Label-free Raman monitoring of extracellular matrix formation in three-dimensional polymeric scaffolds. Journal of the Royal Society Interface 10.

Kunstar, A., Otto, C., Karperien, M., Van Blitterswijk, C., Van Apeldoorn, A., 2011. Raman microspectroscopy: a noninvasive analysis tool for monitoring of collagen-containing extracellular matrix formation in a medium-throughput culture system. Tissue Engineering, Part C: Methods 17, 737–744.

Lee, J., Wu, W., Lesage, F., Boas, D.A., 2013. Multiple-capillary measurement of RBC speed, flux, and density with optical coherence tomography. Journal of Cerebral Blood Flow & Metabolism 33, 1707–1710.

Leitgeb, R., Hitzenberger, C.K., Fercher, A.F., 2003. Performance of fourier domain vs. time domain optical coherence tomography. Optics Express 11, 889–894.

Levitt, J.M., Hunter, M., Mujat, C., Mclaughlin-Drubin, M., Münger, K., Georgakoudi, I., 2007. Diagnostic cellular organization features extracted from autofluorescence images. Optics Letters 32, 3305–3307.

Liang, X., Graf, B.W., Boppart, S.A., 2009. Imaging engineered tissues using structural and functional optical coherence tomography. Journal of Biophotonics 2, 643–655.

Liu, E., Treiser, M.D., Johnson, P.A., Patel, P., Rege, A., Kohn, J., Moghe, P.V., 2007. Quantitative biorelevant profiling of material microstructure within 3D porous scaffolds via multiphoton fluorescence microscopy. Journal of Biomedical Materials Research Part B: Applied Biomaterials 82B, 284–297.

Lu, Z., Kasaragod, D., Matcher, S.J., 2014. Conical scan polarization-sensitive optical coherence tomography. Biomedical Optics Express 5, 752–762.

Luo, Y., Shoichet, M.S., 2004. A photolabile hydrogel for guided three-dimensional cell growth and migration. Nature Materials 3, 249–253.

Mahmud, M.S., Cadotte, D.W., Vuong, B., Sun, C., Luk, T.W., Mariampillai, A., Yang, V.X., 2013. Review of speckle and phase variance optical coherence tomography to visualize microvascular networks. Journal of Biomedical Optics 18, 50901.

Mariampillai, A., Standish, B.A., Moriyama, E.H., Khurana, M., Munce, N.R., Leung, M.K.K., Jiang, J., Cable, A., Wilson, B.C., Vitkin, I.A., Yang, V.X.D., 2008. Speckle variance detection of microvasculature using swept-source optical coherence tomography. Optics Letters 33, 1530–1532.

Maslov, K., Zhang, H.F., Hu, S., Wang, L.V., 2008. Optical-resolution photoacoustic microscopy for in vivo imaging of single capillaries. Optics Letters 33, 929–931.

Mason, C., Markusen, J.F., Town, M.A., Dunnill, P., Wang, R.K., 2004a. Doppler optical coherence tomography for measuring flow in engineered tissue. Biosensors and Bioelectronics 20, 414–423.

Mason, C., Markusen, J.F., Town, M.A., Dunnill, P., Wang, R.K., 2004b. The potential of optical coherence tomography in the engineering of living tissue. Physics in Medicine and Biology 49, 1097.

Masters, B.R., 2006. Confocal Microscopy and Multiphoton Excitation Microscopy: The Genesis of Live Cell Imaging. SPIE Press.

Matcher, S.J., 2009. A review of some recent developments in polarization-sensitive optical imaging techniques for the study of articular cartilage. Journal of Applied Physics 105, 102041.

Matthaus, C., Boydston-White, S., Miljkovic, M., Romeo, M., Diem, M., 2006. Raman and infrared microspectral imaging of mitotic cells. Applied Spectroscopy 60, 1–8.

McNay, G., Eustace, D., Smith, W.E., Faulds, K., Graham, D., 2011. Surface-enhanced Raman scattering (SERS) and surface-enhanced resonance Raman scattering (SERRS): a review of applications. Applied Spectroscopy 65, 825–837.

Mierke, C.T., Kollmannsberger, P., Zitterbart, D.P., Diez, G., Koch, T.M., Marg, S., Ziegler, W.H., Goldmann, W.H., Fabry, B., 2010. Vinculin facilitates cell invasion into three-dimensional collagen matrices. Journal of Biological Chemistry 285, 13121–13130.

Mir, M., Bhaduri, B., Zhu, R., Popescu, G., 2012. Quantitative phase imaging. In: Wolf, E. (Ed.), Progress in Optics. Elsevier.

Mir, M., Kim, T., Majumder, A., Xiang, M., Wang, R., Liu, S.C., Gillette, M.U., Stice, S., Popescu, G., 2014. Label-free characterization of emerging human neuronal networks. Scientific Reports 4, 4434.

Monici, M., 2005. Cell and tissue autofluorescence research and diagnostic applications. Biotechnology Annual Review 11, 227–256.

Moon, J.J., Saik, J.E., Poche, R.A., Leslie-Barbick, J.E., Lee, S.-H., Smith, A.A., Dickinson, M.E., West, J.L., 2010. Biomimetic hydrogels with pro-angiogenic properties. Biomaterials 31, 3840–3847.

Mosmann, T., 1983. Rapid colorimetric assay for cellular growth and survival: application to proliferation and cytotoxicity assays. Journal of Immunological Methods 65, 55–63.

Movasaghi, Z., Rehman, S., Rehman, I.U., 2007. Raman spectroscopy of biological tissues. Applied Spectroscopy Reviews 42, 493–541.

Muller, M., 2006. Introduction to confocal fluorescence microscopy. Society of Photo-Optical Instrumentation Engineers.

Nam, S.Y., Ricles, L.M., Suggs, L.J., Emelianov, S.Y., 2015. Imaging strategies for tissue engineering applications. Tissue Engineering, Part B Reviews 21, 88–102.

Nandagawali, S.T., Yerramshetty, J.S., Akkus, O., 2007. Raman imaging for quantification of the volume fraction of biodegradable polymers in histological preparations. Journal of Biomedical Materials Research Part A 82A, 611–617.

Niesner, R.A., Hauser, A.E., 2011. Recent advances in dynamic intravital multi-photon microscopy. Cytometry Part A 79A, 789–798.

Notingher, I., Bisson, I., Bishop, A.E., Randle, W.L., Polak, J.M., Hench, L.L., 2004. In situ spectral monitoring of mRNA translation in embryonic stem cells during differentiation in vitro. Analytical Chemistry 76, 3185–3193.

Nucciotti, V., Stringari, C., Sacconi, L., Vanzi, F., Fusi, L., Linari, M., Piazzesi, G., Lombardi, V., Pavone, F.S., 2010. Probing myosin structural conformation in vivo by second-harmonic generation microscopy. Proceedings of the National Academy of Sciences of the United States of America 107, 7763–7768.

Orwin, E.J., Lee, S., Raub, C., Icenogle, T., Arman, M., Cho, A., Lovec, R., Malone, A., Haskell, R.C., Hoeling, B.M., Petersen, D.C., 2004. Optical coherence microscopy for the evaluation of a tissue-engineered artificial cornea. In: Engineering in Medicine and Biology Society, 2004. IEMBS '04. 26th Annual International Conference of the IEEE, September 1–5, 2004, pp. 1218–1221.

Palikaras, K., Tavernarakis, N., 2001. Multiphoton fluorescence light microscopy. In: eLS. John Wiley & Sons, Ltd.

Pampaloni, F., Reynaud, E.G., Stelzer, E.H.K., 2007. The third dimension bridges the gap between cell culture and live tissue. Nature Reviews Molecular Cell Biology 8, 839–845.

Pan, J., Kanade, T., Chen, M., 2009. Learning to detect different types of cells under phase contrast microscopy. In: Metaxas, D.N., Yoo, T., Rittscher, J., Tasdizien, T. (Eds.), Microscopic Image Analysis with Applications in Biology. NIH Campus, Bethesda, MD.

Park, B.H., Boer, J.F., 2008. Polarization-sensitive optical coherence tomography. In: Drexler, W., Fujimoto, J.G. (Eds.), Optical Coherence Tomography: Technology and Applications. Springer Berlin Heidelberg, Berlin, Heidelberg.

Park, Y., Best, C.A., Badizadegan, K., Dasari, R.R., Feld, M.S., Kuriabova, T., Henle, M.L., Levine, A.J., Popescu, G., 2010. Measurement of red blood cell mechanics during morphological changes. Proceedings of the National Academy of Sciences 107, 6731–6736.

Perlaki, C.M., Liu, Q., Lim, M., 2014. Raman spectroscopy based techniques in tissue engineering—an overview. Applied Spectroscopy Reviews 49, 513–532.

Popescu, G., 2011. Quantitative Phase Imaging of Cells and Tissues. McGraw-Hill Education.
Popescu, G., Park, Y., Choi, W., Dasari, R.R., Feld, M.S., Badizadegan, K., 2008. Imaging red blood cell dynamics by quantitative phase microscopy. Blood Cells, Molecules & Diseases 41, 10–16.
Raub, C.B., Suresh, V., Krasieva, T., Lyubovitsky, J., Mih, J.D., Putnam, A.J., Tromberg, B.J., George, S.C., 2007. Noninvasive assessment of collagen gel microstructure and mechanics using multiphoton microscopy. Biophysical Journal 92, 2212–2222.
Rice, W.L., Firdous, S., Gupta, S., Hunter, M., Foo, C.W.P., Wang, Y., Kim, H.J., Kaplan, D.L., Georgakoudi, I., 2008. Non-invasive characterization of structure and morphology of silk fibroin biomaterials using non-linear microscopy. Biomaterials 29, 2015–2024.
Rice, W.L., Kaplan, D.L., Georgakoudi, I., 2010. Two-photon microscopy for non-invasive, quantitative monitoring of stem cell differentiation. PLoS One 5, e10075.
Rubbens, M.P., Driessen-Mol, A., Boerboom, R.A., Koppert, M.M.J., Assen, H.C., Terhaar Romeny, B.M., Baaijens, F.P.T., Bouten, C.V.C., 2009. Quantification of the temporal evolution of collagen orientation in mechanically conditioned engineered cardiovascular tissues. Annals of Biomedical Engineering 37, 1263–1272.
Sambit, S., James Goh, C.-H., Toh, S.-L., 2007. Development of hybrid polymer scaffolds for potential applications in ligament and tendon tissue engineering. Biomedical Materials 2, 169.
Santos, M.I., Tuzlakoglu, K., Fuchs, S., Gomes, M.E., Peters, K., Unger, R.E., Piskin, E., Reis, R.L., Kirkpatrick, C.J., 2008. Endothelial cell colonization and angiogenic potential of combined nano- and micro-fibrous scaffolds for bone tissue engineering. Biomaterials 29, 4306–4313.
Scarcelli, G., Besner, S., Pineda, R., Kalout, P., Yun, S., 2015a. IN vivo biomechanical mapping of normal and keratoconus corneas. JAMA Ophthalmology 133, 480–482.
Scarcelli, G., Besner, S., Pineda, R., Yun, S.H., 2014. Biomechanical characterization of keratoconus corneas ex vivo with Brillouin microscopy. Evaluation of Brillouin microscopy for keratoconus. Investigative Ophthalmology & Visual Science 55, 4490–4495.
Scarcelli, G., Kim, P., Yun, S.H., 2011. In vivo measurement of age-related stiffening in the crystalline lens by Brillouin optical microscopy. Biophysical Journal 101, 1539–1545.
Scarcelli, G., Polacheck, W.J., Nia, H.T., Patel, K., Grodzinsky, A.J., Kamm, R.D., Yun, S.H., 2015b. Noncontact three-dimensional mapping of intracellular hydromechanical properties by Brillouin microscopy. Nature Methods 12, 1132–1134.
Scarcelli, G., Yun, S.H., 2007. Confocal Brillouin microscopy for three-dimensional mechanical imaging. Nature Photonics 2, 39–43.
Schade, R., Weiss, T., Berg, A., Schnabelrauch, M., Liefeith, K., 2010. Two-photon techniques in tissue engineering. International Journal of Artificial Organs 33, 219–227.
Schenke-Layland, K., 2008. Non-invasive multiphoton imaging of extracellular matrix structures. Journal of Biophotonics 1, 451–462.
Schenke-Layland, K., Rofail, F., Heydarkhan, S., Gluck, J.M., Ingle, N.P., Angelis, E., Choi, C.-H., Maclellan, W.R., Beygui, R.E., Shemin, R.J., Heydarkhan-Hagvall, S., 2009. The use of three-dimensional nanostructures to instruct cells to produce extracellular matrix for regenerative medicine strategies. Biomaterials 30, 4665–4675.
Schenke-Layland, K., Vasilevski, O., Opitz, F., König, K., Riemann, I., Halbhuber, K.J., Wahlers, T., Stock, U.A., 2003. Impact of decellularization of xenogeneic tissue on extracellular matrix integrity for tissue engineering of heart valves. Journal of Structural Biology 143, 201–208.
Schmedlen, R.H., Masters, K.S., West, J.L., 2002. Photocrosslinkable polyvinyl alcohol hydrogels that can be modified with cell adhesion peptides for use in tissue engineering. Biomaterials 23, 4325–4332.

Schmitt, J., 1998. OCT elastography: imaging microscopic deformation and strain of tissue. Optics Express 3, 199–211.

Schmitt, J.M., 1999. Optical coherence tomography (OCT): a review. IEEE Journal of Selected Topics in Quantum Electronics 5, 1205–1215.

Scientist, B. E. D. M. I. T. B. R. M. V. & Technology, P. S. P. M. B. E. M. I., 2008. Handbook of Biomedical Nonlinear Optical Microscopy. Oxford University Press, USA.

Shin, H., Jo, S., Mikos, A.G., 2003. Biomimetic materials for tissue engineering. Biomaterials 24, 4353–4364.

Short, K.W., Carpenter, S., Freyer, J.P., Mourant, J.R., 2005. Raman spectroscopy detects biochemical changes due to proliferation in mammalian cell cultures. Biophysical Journal 88, 4274–4288.

Skala, M.C., Crow, M.J., Wax, A., Izatt, J.A., 2008. Photothermal optical coherence tomography of epidermal growth factor receptor in live cells using immunotargeted gold nanospheres. Nano Letters 8, 3461–3467.

Smith, L.E., Smallwood, R., Macneil, S., 2010. A comparison of imaging methodologies for 3D tissue engineering. Microscopy Research and Technique 73, 1123–1133.

Snyder, J.G., Virta, R.L., Segreti, J.M., 1987. Evaluation of the phase contrast microscopy method for the detection of fibrous and other elongated mineral particulates by comparison with a STEM technique. American Industrial Hygiene Association 48, 471–477.

Spoler, F., Forst, M., Marquardt, Y., Hoeller, D., Kurz, H., Merk, H., Abuzahra, F., 2006. High-resolution optical coherence tomography as a non-destructive monitoring tool for the engineering of skin equivalents. Skin Research and Technology 12, 261–267.

Sridharan, S., Mir, M., Popescu, G., 2011. Simultaneous optical measurements of cell motility and growth. Biomedical Optics Express 2, 2815–2820.

Su, H., Yin, Z., Huh, S., Kanade, T., 2013. Cell segmentation in phase contrast microscopy images via semi-supervised classification over optics-related features. Medical Image Analysis 17, 746–765.

Sun, Y., Tan, H.-Y., Lin, S.-J., Lee, H.-S., Lin, T.-Y., Jee, S.-H., Young, T.-H., Lo, W., Chen, W.-L., Dong, C.-Y., 2008. Imaging tissue engineering scaffolds using multiphoton microscopy. Microscopy Research and Technique 71, 140–145.

Swain, R.J., Jell, G., Stevens, M.M., 2008a. Non-invasive analysis of cell cycle dynamics in single living cells with Raman micro-spectroscopy. Journal of Cellular Biochemistry 104, 1427–1438.

Swain, R.J., Kemp, S.J., Goldstraw, P., Tetley, T.D., Stevens, M.M., 2008b. Spectral monitoring of surfactant clearance during alveolar epithelial type II cell differentiation. Biophysical Journal 95, 5978–5987.

Tan, W., Oldenburg, A.L., Norman, J.J., Desai, T.A., Boppart, S.A., 2006. Optical coherence tomography of cell dynamics in three-dimensional tissue models. Optics Express 14, 7159–7171.

Tan, W., Sendemir-Urkmez, A., Fahrner, L.J., Jamison, R., Leckband, D., Boppart, S.A., 2004. Structural and functional optical imaging of three-dimensional engineered tissue development. Tissue Engineering 10, 1747–1756.

Tan, W., Vinegoni, C., Norman, J.J., Desai, T.A., Boppart, S.A., 2007. Imaging cellular responses to mechanical stimuli within three-dimensional tissue constructs. Microscopy Research and Technique 70, 361–371.

Tearney, G.J., Brezinski, M.E., Bouma, B.E., Boppart, S.A., Pitris, C., Southern, J.F., Fujimoto, J.G., 1997. In vivo endoscopic optical biopsy with optical coherence tomography. Science 276, 2037–2039.

Tucker-Schwartz, J.M., Lapierre-Landry, M., Patil, C.A., Skala, M.C., 2015. Photothermal optical lock-in optical coherence tomography for in vivo imaging. Biomedical Optics Express 6, 2268–2282.

Tucker-Schwartz, J.M., Meyer, T.A., Patil, C.A., Duvall, C.L., Skala, M.C., 2012. In vivo photothermal optical coherence tomography of gold nanorod contrast agents. Biomedical Optics Express 3, 2881–2895.

Ustione, A., Piston, D.W., 2011. A simple introduction to multiphoton microscopy. Journal of Microscopy 243, 221–226.

Van Apeldoorn, A.A., Van Manen, H.-J., Bezemer, J.M., De Bruijn, J.D., Van Blitterswijk, C.A., Otto, C., 2004. Raman imaging of PLGA microsphere degradation inside macrophages. Journal of the American Chemical Society 126, 13226–13227.

Veksler, B., Kobzev, E., Bonesi, M., Meglinski, I., 2008. Application of optical coherence tomography for imaging of scaffold structure and micro-flows characterization. Laser Physics Letters 5, 236.

Ventura, M., Franssen, G.M., Oosterwijk, E., Boerman, O.C., Jansen, J.A., Walboomers, X.F., 2014. SPECT vs. PET monitoring of bone defect healing and biomaterial performance in vivo. Journal of Tissue Engineering and Regenerative Medicine n/a-n/a.

Vielreicher, M., Schurmann, S., Detsch, R., Schmidt, M.A., Buttgereit, A., Boccaccini, A., Friedrich, O., 2013. Taking a deep look: modern microscopy technologies to optimize the design and functionality of biocompatible scaffolds for tissue engineering in regenerative medicine. Journal of the Royal Society Interface 10, 20130263.

Villa, M.M., Wang, L., Huang, J., Rowe, D.W., Wei, M., 2013. Visualizing osteogenesis in vivo within a cell–scaffold construct for bone tissue engineering using two-photon microscopy. Tissue Engineering, Part C: Methods 19, 839–849.

Voytik-Harbin, S.L., Roeder, B.A., Sturgis, J.E., Kokini, K., Robinson, J.P., 2003. Simultaneous mechanical loading and confocal reflection microscopy for three-dimensional microbiomechanical analysis of biomaterials and tissue constructs. Microscopy and Microanalysis 9, 74–85.

Wang, L.V., 2008. Tutorial on photoacoustic microscopy and computed tomography. IEEE Journal of Selected Topics in Quantum Electronics 14, 171–179.

Wang, L.V., Gao, L., 2014. Photoacoustic microscopy and computed tomography: from bench to bedside. Annual Review of Biomedical Engineering 16, 155–185.

Wang, S., Larin, K.V., 2014. Optical coherence elastography for tissue characterization: a review. Journal of Biophotonics.

Wang, S., Lopez, A.L., Morikawa, Y., Tao, G., Li, J., Larina, I.V., Martin, J.F., Larin, K.V., 2014. Noncontact quantitative biomechanical characterization of cardiac muscle using shear wave imaging optical coherence tomography. Biomedical Optics Express 5, 1980–1992.

Weeks, T., Huser, T., 2010. Raman spectroscopy of living cells. In: Jue, T. (Ed.), Biomedical Applications of Biophysics. Humana Press, Totowa, NJ.

Williams, R.M., Zipfel, W.R., Webb, W.W., 2005. Interpreting second-harmonic generation images of collagen I fibrils. Biophysical Journal 88, 1377–1386.

Xu, H., Othman, S.F., Magin, R.L., 2008. Monitoring tissue engineering using magnetic resonance imaging. Journal of Bioscience and Bioengineering 106, 515–527.

Yabushita, H., Bouma, B.E., Houser, S.L., Aretz, H.T., Jang, I.-K., Schlendorf, K.H., Kauffman, C.R., Shishkov, M., Kang, D.-H., Halpern, E.F., Tearney, G.J., 2002. Characterization of human atherosclerosis by optical coherence tomography. Circulation 106, 1640–1645.

Yanez, C.O., Morales, A.R., Yue, X., Urakami, T., Komatsu, M., Järvinen, T.A.H., Belfield, K.D., 2013. Deep vascular imaging in wounds by two-photon fluorescence microscopy. PLoS One 8, e67559.

Yang, F., Murugan, R., Wang, S., Ramakrishna, S., 2005. Electrospinning of nano/micro scale poly(l-lactic acid) aligned fibers and their potential in neural tissue engineering. Biomaterials 26, 2603–2610.

Yang, V., Gordon, M., Qi, B., Pekar, J., Lo, S., Seng-Yue, E., Mok, A., Wilson, B., Vitkin, I., 2003. High speed, wide velocity dynamic range Doppler optical coherence tomography (part I): system design, signal processing, and performance. Optics Express 11, 794–809.

Yang, Y., Bagnaninchi, P.O., Hu, B., Hampson, K., Haj, A.J.E., 2008. Characterisation of scaffold architecture and tendons using optical coherence tomography and polarisation-sensitive optical coherence tomography. IET Optoelectronics 2, 188–194.

Yang, Y., Dubois, A., Qin, X.P., Li, J., El Haj, A., Wang, R.K., 2006. Investigation of optical coherence tomography as an imaging modality in tissue engineering. Physics in Medicine & Biology 51, 1649–1659.

Yao, J., Maslov, K.I., Zhang, Y., Xia, Y., Wang, L.V., 2011. Label-free oxygen-metabolic photoacoustic microscopy in vivo. Journal of Biomedical Optics 16, 076003–076003-11.

Yao, J., Wang, L.V., 2013. Photoacoustic microscopy. Laser & Photonics Reviews 7. http://dx.doi.org/10.1002/lpor.201200060.

Yeh, A.T., Kao, B., Jung, W.G., Chen, Z., Nelson, J.S., Tromberg, B.J., 2004. Imaging wound healing using optical coherence tomography and multiphoton microscopy in an in vitro skin-equivalent tissue model. Journal of Biomedical Optics 9, 248–253.

Zernike, F., 1955. How I discovered phase contrast. Science 121, 345–349.

Zhang, H.F., Maslov, K., Stoica, G., Wang, L.V., 2006. Functional photoacoustic microscopy for high-resolution and noninvasive in vivo imaging. Nature Biotechnology 24, 848–851.

Zhang, Y., Cai, X., Choi, S.W., Kim, C., Wang, L.V., Xia, Y., 2010a. Chronic label-free volumetric photoacoustic microscopy of melanoma cells in three-dimensional porous scaffolds. Biomaterials 31, 8651–8658.

Zhang, Y., Cai, X., Wang, Y., Zhang, C., Li, L., Choi, S.-W., Wang, L.V., Xia, Y., 2011. Noninvasive photoacoustic microscopy of living cells in two and three dimensions through enhancement by a metabolite dye. Angewandte Chemie (International Edition in English) 50, 7359–7363.

Zhang, Y., Hong, H., Cai, W., 2010b. Imaging with Raman spectroscopy. Current Pharmaceutical Biotechnology 11, 654–661.

Zhou, C., Tsai, T.-H., Adler, D.C., Lee, H.-C., Cohen, D.W., Mondelblatt, A., Wang, Y., Connolly, J.L., Fujimoto, J.G., 2010. Photothermal optical coherence tomography in ex vivo human breast tissues using gold nanoshells. Optics Letters 35, 700–702.

Zoubir, A., 2012. Raman Imaging: Techniques and Applications. Springer Berlin Heidelberg.

Magnetic resonance imaging monitoring of cartilage tissue engineering in vivo

9

Mrignayani Kotecha
University of Illinois at Chicago, Chicago, IL, United States

9.1 Introduction

Cartilage injury and damage are the major causes of disability in the United States [1,2]. Arthritis, sports injuries, trauma, and developmental issues frequently cause damage in the articular cartilage of joints such as knees, hips, wrists, etc. [2–4]. Cartilage is a highly specialized connective tissue covering the bones of these joints, and its main function is to provide a frictionless smooth movement of these joints. Cartilage has an inadequate self-healing capacity in adults; therefore it often requires a surgical intervention if the tissue is damaged. Some current available surgical treatment options for the repair and restoration of damaged cartilage are microfracture, osteochondral autograft implantation, osteochondral allograft transfer, and autologous chondrocyte implantation [5–7]. However, these treatments are often inadequate in restoring the full load-bearing capabilities of joints, and they have a high failure rate [7]. The regenerated tissues often do not match the biological composition and biomechanical properties of native cartilage, thus defeating the purpose of intervention [8,9]. It is believed that cartilage tissue engineering can overcome these deficits by creating a neocartilage tissue in the lab that matches the desired properties and can be implanted at the damaged site.

Cartilage tissue engineering utilizes a typical "tissue-engineering" approach by using a combination of biomaterial-based scaffolds, appropriate cells, and growth strategies to create a neocartilage tissue that expresses a high amount of cartilage extracellular matrix proteins, proteoglycans, and collagen, type II [10]. The flexibility of choosing biopolymers with suitable mechanical properties, increasingly complex tissue growth strategies involving cells and suitable growth conditions, and an ability to print a custom tissue design are all too attractive choices for targeting patient-specific cartilage therapies. This promise has led to an explosion of research in cartilage tissue engineering. However, there is still a gap in translating these techniques from bench to bedside. Promising in vitro techniques are tested and tweaked at many stages before they can reach patients. Here the animal models are an important middle step to validate promising tissue-engineering strategies from bench to bedside. A number of animal models such as mice, rats, rabbits, sheep, dogs, and horses have been used for the purpose of validating new and developing tissue-engineering technologies and moving the promising ones to the next level of hierarchy.

Monitoring and Evaluation of Biomaterials and their Performance in vivo. http://dx.doi.org/10.1016/B978-0-08-100603-0.00009-2

One important issue in cartilage tissue engineering is how engineered cartilage tissues are evaluated. At each stage of validation, engineered tissues are typically assessed using a variety of biochemical assays, histological staining, and gene expression analysis. Once authenticated, the process moves to the next level of validation using higher animal models. Increasingly, MRI is added as an additional criterion of assessment. Because of the available contrast mechanisms and because of the depth and breadth of information produced, MRI can provide a multiscale window in tissue assessment both in vitro and in vivo [11]. There has been tremendous progress in the MRI assessment of tissue-engineered cartilage in small and large animal models and in clinics. It is expected that in the near future, MRI will be widespread and acceptable in the tissue-engineering community as a sole method to provide universal tissue assessment, thus removing the need for destructive assessment techniques.

9.2 Cartilage

Cartilage is an avascular, aneural, and alymphatic tissue with a small number of chondrocytes surrounded by a rich extracellular matrix (ECM). The ECM of cartilage is made up of tissue fluid and structural macromolecules: collagens, type II, proteoglycans, other collagens (III, VI, IX, X, XI, XII, and XIV), and noncollagenous proteins and glycoproteins [12,13]. The amount of these ECM components and cells vary according to tissue location, age, and load/nonload-bearing settings, as well as on the type of species. In hyaline articular cartilage, these macromolecules and cells are arranged in a layered three-level zonal structure throughout the tissue depth, as shown in Fig. 9.1 [11,14]. This ordered macromolecular arrangement and the high water content retained using proteoglycans is important for articular cartilage as a load-bearing tissue [15].

9.3 Cartilage tissue engineering

As stated above, cartilage tissue engineering utilizes a combination of cells, biocompatible scaffold material, growth factors, and suitable growth conditions to achieve the goal of producing a neocartilage tissue with a high amount of chondrogenic matrix proteins, proteoglycans, and collagen, type II.

9.3.1 Cells

As chondrocytes are the native cartilage cells, they are the most effective cell types when producing a high amount of chondrogenic ECM. Therefore, they are the most desirable cell types for cartilage tissue engineering and regenerative medicine [16,17]. Chondrocytes can be grown as scaffold-free pellets to produce neocartilage with a high amount of chondrogenic ECM. However, the cells in pellets have the tendency to dedifferentiate into fibroblasts over the course of tissue regeneration [18]. Therefore

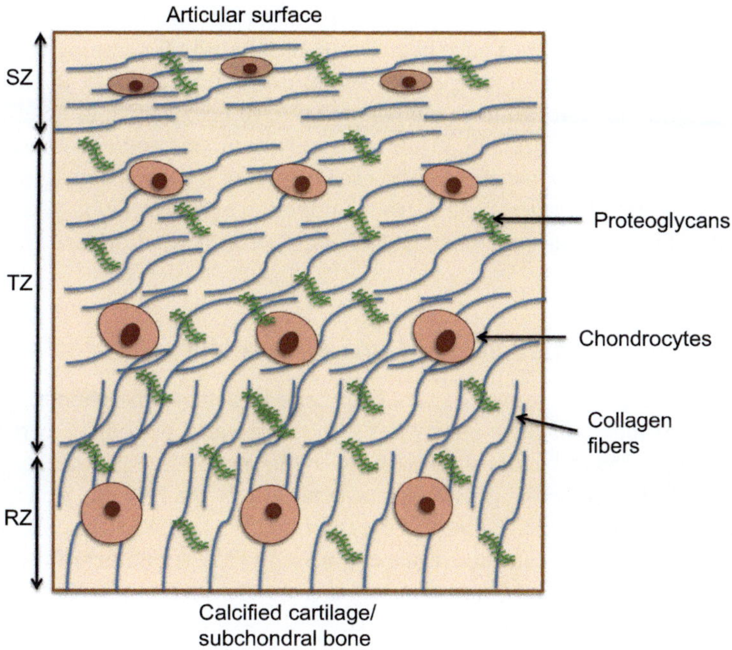

Figure 9.1 Zonal architecture of native cartilage tissue. *SZ*, superficial zone; *TZ*, transitional zone; *RZ*, radial zone.

chondrocytes are frequently embedded in porous hydrogels such as alginate, gelatin, or poly(ethylene glycol)-diacrylate (PEGDA) to maintain their phenotype and also to improve the ECM yield [19]. Even though chondrocytes are the most desirable cells for cartilage tissue engineering, harvesting enough chondrocytes for expansion and differentiation is challenging because of the small number of cells present in native tissue. Therefore stem cell-based cartilage tissue-engineering research is gaining momentum [20]. It has been shown that the bone marrow and adipose-derived stem cells are capable of chondrogenic differentiation [19–27]. The coculture of stem cells and chondrocytes have been found to be more efficient than the stem cells alone in producing a high yield of chondrogenic ECM [19,28].

9.3.2 Scaffold

Biocompatible material as scaffold is an important component in cartilage tissue engineering for developing the neocartilage with the right biochemical and mechanical properties [29,30]. Scaffold in cartilage tissue engineering is expected to provide support for tissue growth and is expected to degrade favorably when the ECM of developing tissue takes over. Scaffolds are chosen for their suitable mechanical and cell adhesion properties. Three-dimensional porous scaffold also allows upkeep of nutrient transport and waste disposal, the two important cell functions [25,31,32]. Hydrogels are considered an excellent scaffolding material because of their ability to entrap cells and bioactive molecules, as well as efficient mass transfer diffusion properties. Both natural and synthetic hydrogels have been tested successfully for cartilage tissue engineering. Among the natural hydrogels, collagen, fibrin glue, agarose, alginate, hyaluronic acid, chitosan, and cellulose are some that have been shown to be effective in cartilage tissue engineering [26,29,33]. Increasingly, synthetic and/or composite polymers are used as scaffolds because of the ease of tuning mechanical properties, pore volume, and surface characteristics. A few examples are poly(lactic-co-glycolic acid) (PLGA), PEGDA, carbon nanotubes and fibers, dacron and teflon, and PuraMatrix hydrogels [30,34].

9.3.3 Signaling molecules and growth factors

Signaling molecules and growth factors help cells to achieve the chondrogenic differentiation and maintain their phenotype. Since the early periods of cartilage tissue engineering, growth factors such as those in the insulin-like growth factor (IGF) and the TGF-β (Transforming growth factor-beta) family are found to be effective in promoting the chondrogenic differentiation of chondrocytes and stem cells and have thus become a standard in cartilage tissue engineering [35]. A number of transcription factors such as Sox9 and RunX are also found to be effective in regulating the chondrogenic differentiation of stem cells [36,37].

9.3.4 Growth conditions

Culture growth conditions affect cell differentiation in the same profound way as growth factors and signaling molecules. It has been shown that appropriate cell differentiation can be achieved using just the right mechanical properties of scaffolds without the aid of growth factors [36,38]. Several growth conditions have been tested for effectively directing the chondrogenic differentiation of cells. Native cartilage tissue is hypoxic because of its avascular nature. Using the analogy, the hypoxic condition is found to be effective in producing chondrogenic ECM of embryonic stem cells without the aid of growth factors [39–42].

9.4 Animal models in cartilage tissue engineering

Several in vivo models are successfully applied for testing new cartilage tissue-engineering and regeneration strategies [43]. Table 9.1 highlights some commonly used animal models along with their relative advantages and disadvantages. Among the small animal species, mice are the most preferable because of cost effectiveness and ease of purchasing, breeding, and housing. The athymic species offer the advantages of studying the responses of human cell lines and tissues to tissue-engineering strategies in vivo. The mice cartilage is extremely thin and not suitable for the study of partial or full cartilage defect models. Therefore murine models are the most commonly used for subcutaneous studies that provide an in vivo incubator for tissue

Table 9.1 Common animal models used in cartilage tissue engineering and regeneration studies along with their relative advantages and disadvantages

Animal models for cartilage tissue engineering	Advantages	Disadvantages	Commonly used for
Small animal models: Mice, rats, rabbits	Cost-effective, ease of handling, athymic species can be used for human cell lines, transgenic species can be used for gene therapy responses	Thin cartilage, small joint size, faster healing	Proof of concept studies
Large animal models: Goats, sheep, pigs, horses	Joint size and disease pathology closely model the human situation	Expensive, defect diameter, and cartilage size is thinner in dogs, sheep, and pigs; equine joint loading conditions are different than humans	Partial and full defect models, treatment of osteochondral defects

growth. The rats are another inexpensive species similar to mice for cartilage tissue engineering and regeneration. The bigger size of rats offers better reproducibility of results. Rabbits are the most commonly used small animal species for cartilage and osteochondral defect healing. The condyles of rabbits are large enough to create few 3–4 mm critical size defects, and they still provide the advantages of low cost and ease of maintenance, similar to mice and rats. The major disadvantage of these small animal species is that they have a high intrinsic capability to repair any defect, unlike humans, thus defeating the purpose of study. Among the large animal species, dogs have been regularly used for the study of cartilage tissue engineering. Dogs lack the intrinsic ability to heal cartilage defects, similar to humans. The canine cartilage is thin compared to humans and is most commonly used for 4 mm defect models. Goats are also preferable models because of larger joint size and limited healing capabilities. They are relatively inexpensive and easier to handle among the large animal species. Even though pigs offer large joint size and cartilage thickness close to humans, they are an aggressive species and are thus underutilized in cartilage tissue-engineering research. Finally, the most commonly used large animal species in cartilage research is the horse, because of the racing industry. With horses, it is possible to create full and partial defect models, as well as large size defect (~up to 21 mm). The major disadvantages of horses are cost, different joint loading conditions, and harder bones than humans.

9.5 Tissue assessment

The optimization loop of tissue engineering looks like Fig. 9.2. The engineered tissue is first assessed in vitro using a variety of immunohistochemical methods [44–47].

The following techniques are well established for assessing the engineered cartilage tissues:

1. DNA content measurement using Hoechst dye fluorometric assay
2. dimethylmethylene blue dye assay for Glycosaminoglycans (GAGs) measurement
3. hydroxyproline assay for collagen content measurement
4. polymerase chain reaction (PCR) for assessing mRNA extraction level

Cartilage is a load-bearing tissue, therefore mechanical characterization added to the above methods is equally important. The mechanical properties of engineered cartilage tissues are characterized by compression, tension, shear, and indentation parameters [48]. These assessment tools are the first gatekeepers of new tissue-engineering strategies. Once successful in vitro, the process moves to the next step of optimization, first using small animal models and then large animal models.

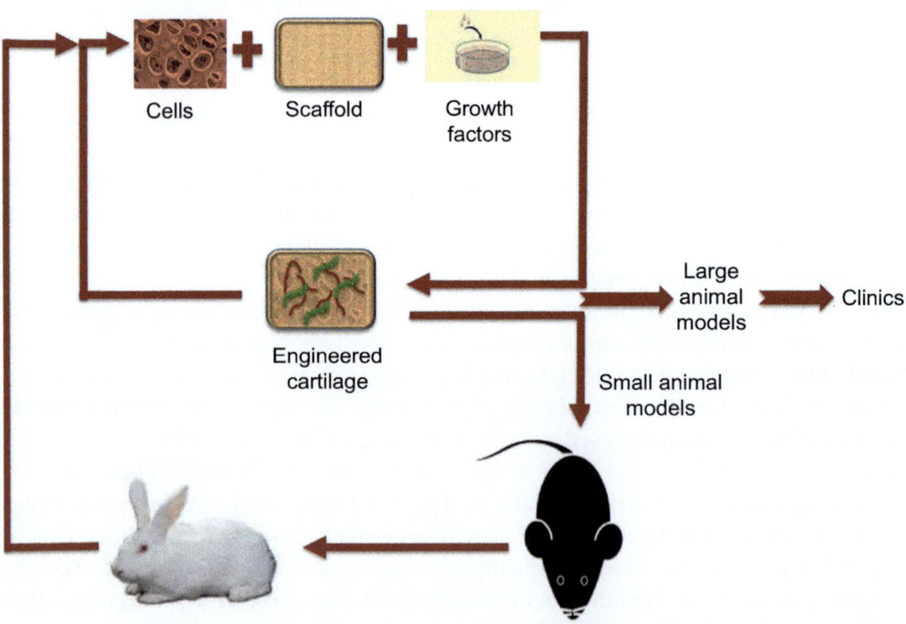

Figure 9.2 Schematic diagram showing how cartilage tissue-engineering products are optimized. The first step of optimization is in vitro by playing with a combination of cells, biomaterials, and growth factors or growth strategies. Once successful, the tissue-growth strategy is tested in small animal models, and if found successful, it is moved to large animal models before moving to clinics. At each stage, the engineered tissue is tested using many different techniques, as explained in Section 9.5. Most successful in vitro strategies do not reach clinics because of inadequate performance in vivo.

All of the aforementioned techniques to assess tissue-engineered cartilage are destructive and provide a one-time characterization. This amounts to a huge waste in terms of tissues and animals. Also, using these strategies, it is not possible to scan the samples and remove a bad sample from a batch. The ability to remove a bad sample will greatly enhance the efficiency of tissue-engineering regenerative medicine products. Therefore MRI is an excellent alternate in providing tissue assessment noninvasively. The ability to visualize native cartilage with its ordered zonal structure using parametric MRI has opened up doors for quantitative MRI monitoring of tissue-engineered cartilage [14,49,50]. MRI techniques have been shown to correlate well with proteoglycans and collagen amount in tissue-engineered cartilage in addition to providing an assessment of shear stiffness [11,51–54]. In addition, MRI techniques also have been shown to differentiate between tissue-engineered cartilage and bone right from the very early stage of development, which could be extremely helpful in animals and clinical studies [55].

9.6 Magnetic resonance imaging

MRI is a noninvasive and nonionizing imaging modality that has been extensively applied for the study of cartilage degradation and regeneration both in vitro and in vivo in animals and in clinical studies. MRI has the best soft tissue contrast among all imaging modalities. The principle of MRI is briefly discussed here (see Figure 9.3), but the readers are referred to excellent texts with detailed description elsewhere [56–58]. MRI detects nuclei that have either an odd number of protons or an odd number of neutrons. Such nuclei possess magnetic moment, $\boldsymbol{\mu}$ and angular momentum, **J**, and have a quantum mechanical property called nuclear spin (Figure 9.3 (a)). Many biologically relevant nuclei such as protons (^{1}H), sodium (^{23}Na), phosphorous (^{31}P), and carbon (^{13}C) possess nuclear spin and can therefore be observed using MRI if there is suitable hardware available. MRI involves the detailed manipulation of nuclear spins using a magnetic field, orthogonal gradient fields, and radiofrequency pulses.

The nuclear magnetic moment, $\boldsymbol{\mu}$ and angular momentum, **J**, are collinear and are related through a constant called gyromagnetic ratio γ. This is an important relationship and one that is the basis of image creation in MRI. When these nuclei are placed in a magnetic field (shown as $\mathbf{B_0}$ in Figure 9.3 (b)), they are said to be in precession around the magnetic field with the Larmor frequency ω_0 that is related to the magnetic field with ($\omega_0=\gamma \mathbf{B_0}$). Once placed in a magnetic field, nuclear state with spin I is degenerated (2I+1) fold. For example, ^{1}H with spin ½ will have two energy states (−1/2 and +1/2) and ^{23}Na with spin 3/2 will have four energy levels (−3/2, −1/2, +1/2, and +3/2), etc. In classical terms, we can say that these states are parallel and antiparallel states of nuclei with respect to the magnetic field. Using suitable radiofrequency pulses matching the Larmor frequency ω_0, resonance condition can be created, or in other words, nuclei can absorb energy and flip from antiparallel to parallel states. Since a large number of nuclei are involved, it is easy to deal with another terminology involving nuclear magnetization **M**. Those nuclei oriented toward the main magnetic field effectively

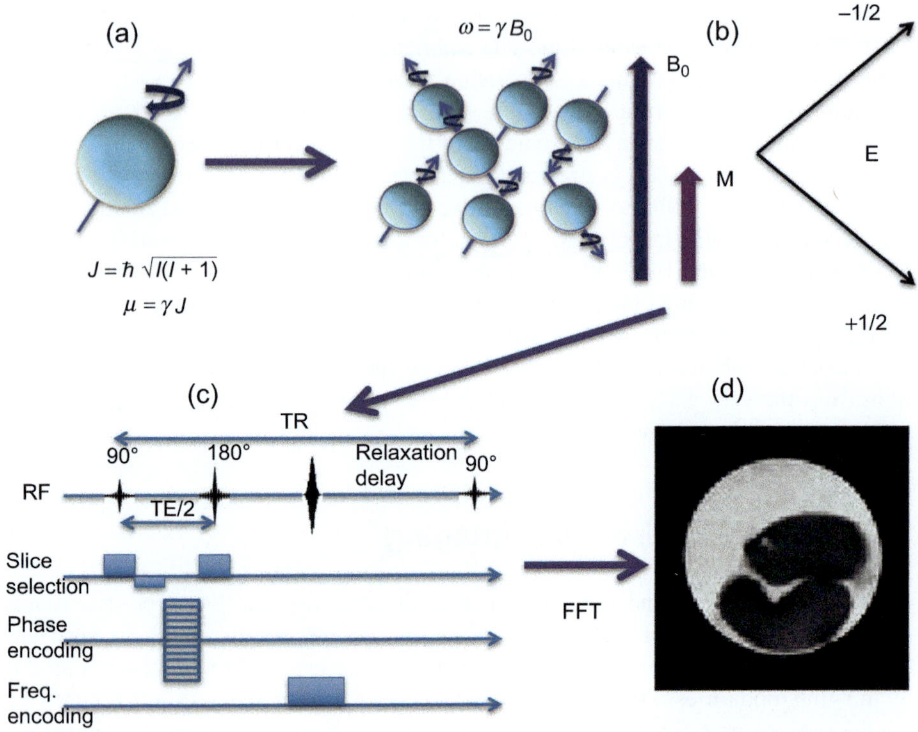

Figure 9.3 Schematic diagram depicting the basic principles of MRI acquisition. (a) a nuclear spin, (b) precessing nuclei in a magnetic field, (c) an example MRI pulse sequence for image acquisition, (d) an example MRI image of tissue engineered cartilage samples.

create what is called nuclear magnetization, denoted by **M** (Figure 9.3 (b)). The size of magnetization depends on the strength of the main magnetic field, $\mathbf{B_0}$, therefore the magnetic field strength plays a key role in MRI signal strength. The **M** can be manipulated using radiofrequency (RF) pulses.

To create an image out of this excited nuclear state, the main magnetic field $\mathbf{B_0}$ in all directions is varied with the help of gradient fields. This makes magnetization vector **M** position-dependent. Using radiofrequency pulses to manipulate the magnetization, **M**, as well as the magnetic field in all directions (as shown in Fig. 9.3(c)), one can create an image in k-space. When the fast Fourier transform is applied, the image is obtained in x–y space. Based on the pulse sequence, MRI images can have different contrasts such as water relaxation times (T_1, T_2, and T_{1rho}), apparent diffusion coefficient (ADC), magnetization transfer (MT), etc. By choosing suitable acquisition parameters, either a parameter-weighted image can be created or a parameter map can be obtained for tissue. The beauty of MRI is that the MR parameters often depend on the local environment within the tissue and are therefore representative of the tissue's physiologic state. MRI of tissue-engineered cartilage

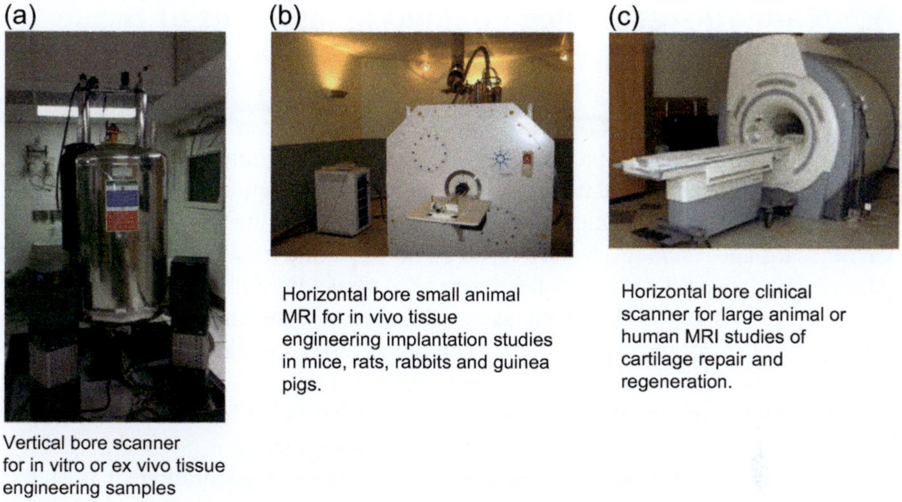

Figure 9.4 Different MRI systems are needed for the assessment of tissue-engineering cartilage in vitro and in vivo. An example of each type is given. (a) A vertical-bore NMR spectrometer suitable for in vitro MRI analysis. (b) A small animal-dedicated MRI scanner suitable for mice, rats, and rabbits. (c) A human clinical MRI scanner suitable for large animals or humans.

assessment and visualization typically uses water protons because of high water content in tissue-engineered cartilage [11]. Commonly used contrasts in MRI assessment of tissue-engineered cartilage in vitro are T_1, T_2, T_{1rho}, ADC, and MT. However, in vivo T_2 is the most favorable MR parameter for MRI assessment. Sodium MRI has also been used to assess proteoglycans in cartilage tissue engineering and regeneration [53,59].

Depending upon the choice of tissue-engineering strategy and sample size, a number of imagers can be used for the assessment of tissue-engineered cartilage, as shown in Fig. 9.4. For in vitro or ex vivo samples that are typically small in size (~few mm to few cm), wide vertical-bore NMR spectrometers (similar to one shown in Fig. 9.4(a)) can be converted to micro-MRI systems by installing additional hardware. These spectrometers can be operated at a very higher magnetic field (up to 21 Tesla) compared to clinical MRI scanners (1.5–7 Tesla). The advantages of high field micro-MRI systems are their cost effectiveness and very high resolution (~10–20 μm) due to small and dedicated RF resonators and high magnetic field. For small animal MRI, commercially available dedicated scanners similar to one shown in Fig. 9.4(b) can be used. Such scanners are typically equipped with animal monitoring systems to carry out in vivo studies and also have better resolution than clinical MRI. Finally, clinical scanners can be used for large animals and clinical studies, as shown in Fig. 9.4(c). These scanners are used with a lower resolution of the order of 2–5 mm in order to be time efficient.

9.7 Magnetic resonance imaging assessment of tissue-engineering cartilage in vivo

In the current literature, most of the in vivo MRI studies of cartilage or osteochondral defect healing after a surgical procedure do not involve any scaffolding material [60–66]. Those studies are not included in this chapter. However, there are significant numbers of animal studies where a biocompatible polymer is included in the recovery and regeneration of a cartilage lesion in vivo. As stated earlier, T_2 is the most commonly employed to observe the defect fill and assess the regenerated tissue. In addition to T_2, the gadolinium-enhanced T_1 and MT have been also used for the assessment of regenerated tissue in vivo [61,66]. A rabbit model is most commonly used for such studies because of cost effectiveness and because many biocompatible materials are still at the preclinical experimental stage of development. Goats and sheep have also been used with in vivo MRI studies of cartilage tissue engineering involving polymers.

When T_2 is used for assessing defect fill in cartilage regeneration, it is shown to decrease with fill time and converge to the natural tissue surrounding the defect fill. For example, Ramaswamy et al. observed 5 weeks of healing for full thickness chondral defect using photopolymerized PEGDA in rabbit models and found that T_2 decreases monotonically with the extent of defect bill ($r = -0.82$ between T_2 and percent of defect fill) [67]. Recently, T_2 was also used in a clinical study ($n = 15$) involving cartilage regeneration using photopolymerized PEGDA applied after standard microfracture surgery [68]. The mean T_2 was seen to decrease over the period of 6 months, suggesting better cartilage healing in biomaterial-based recovery compared to the cases where no biomaterial was involved. However, in some cases, T_2 does not seem to change with time, even though the defect fill shows normal progression. For example, Kim et al. created a 3 mm osteochondral defect in rabbits and filled it with thrombin peptide (TP-508) and PLGA microspheres [69]. Their repair tissue had significantly higher T_2 than the natural cartilage after 6 weeks and was similar to the control PLGA microspheres alone. Here we suspect that T_2 values are influenced by scaffold contribution rather than the contribution from the growing matrix [14,52]. In our publication, we have shown that once the scaffold contribution is removed, the T_2 values reflect the amount of tissue growth in vivo [70]. The advantages of using T_2 for cartilage tissue-engineering assessment in vivo are (a) easier implementation for experimental protocol, (b) short acquisition time compared to most other MR parameter acquisition, and (c) sensitivity to detect small changes in defect fill areas. In natural cartilage, T_2 is shown to be sensitive to the collagen orientation; however, in most cases, the engineered tissue is found to be less anisotropic, and therefore T_2 reveals only the extent to which the defect is filled [11,14,71].

9.8 Future directions

The future of in vivo MRI assessment of tissue-engineered cartilage looks promising. More cartilage tissue-engineering strategies are getting tested in vitro and in small animal in vivo settings, suggesting that in the future, there will be more studies in large animals and in clinical settings. As new biocompatible materials for cartilage regeneration continue to develop at a rapid pace, MRI assessment needs to keep pace. New pulse protocols and techniques to assess engineered cartilage are in continuous development. One such example is the development of magnetic resonance elastography (an MRI-based technique to measure shear stiffness) for assessment of tissue-engineered cartilage [72]. In vitro, MRI has shown promise to provide a universal assessment of engineered cartilage, such as the growth of tissue matrix, tissue anisotropy, and mechanical properties [14]. The in vivo assessment of tissue-engineered cartilage will see an extension of these techniques in animals and in clinics in coming years. Overall, the future of in vivo MRI assessment of tissue-engineered cartilage looks promising and is full of new possibilities.

References

[1] Prevalence and most common causes of disability among adults – United States. MMWR Morb Mortal Wkly Rep 2005;2009(58):421–6.
[2] CDC Report. Centers for Disease Control and Prevention, Arthritis Foundation: a national public health agenda for osteoarthritis; 2010.
[3] VanItallie TB. Gout: epitome of painful arthritis. Metabolism 2010;59:S32–6.
[4] Hunziker EB. Articular cartilage repair: basic science and clinical progress. A review of the current status and prospects. Osteoarthr Cartil 2002;10:432–63.
[5] Clair BL, Johnson AR, Howard T. Cartilage repair. Foot Ankle Spec 2009;2:179–88.
[6] Ahmed TAE, Hincke MT. Strategies for articular cartilage lesion repair and functional restoration. Tissue Eng Part B Rev 2010;16:305–29.
[7] Detterline AJ, Goldberg S, Bach Jr BR, Cole BJ. Treatment options for articular cartilage defects of the knee. Orthop Nurs 2005;24:361–6. quiz 7–8.
[8] Mithoefer K, Hambly K, Villa SD, Silvers H, Mandelbaum BR. Return to sports participation after articular cartilage repair in the knee. Am J Sports Med 2009;37:167S–76S.
[9] Duchow J, Hess T, Kohn D. Primary stability of press-fit-implanted osteochondral grafts. Am J Sports Med 2000;28:24–7.
[10] Langer R, Vacanti J. Tissue engineering. Science 1993;260:920–6.
[11] Kotecha M, Klatt D, Magin RL. Monitoring cartilage tissue engineering using magnetic resonance spectroscopy, imaging and elastography. Tissue Eng Part B Rev 2013;19:470–84.
[12] Buckwalter JA, Mankin HJ. Articular cartilage: tissue design and chondrocyte-matrix interactions. Instr Course Lect 1998;47:477–86.
[13] Eyre D. Collagen of articular cartilage. Arthritis Res 2002;4:30–5.
[14] Kotecha M, Yin Z, Magin R. Magnetic resonance in the assessment of tissue engineered cartilage. In: Xia Y, Konstantin M, editors, New developments in NMR No. 8 Biophysics and biochemistry of cartilage by NMR and MRI. Royal Society of Chemistry; 2017 (in press).
[15] Buckwalter JA, Mankin HJ, Grodzinsky AJ. Articular cartilage and osteoarthritis. Instr Course Lect 2005;54:465–80.
[16] Cheuk YC, Wong MW, Lee KM, Fu SC. Use of allogeneic scaffold-free chondrocyte pellet in repair of osteochondral defect in a rabbit model. J Orthop Res 2011;29:1343–50.
[17] Zhang Z, McCaffery JM, Spencer RG, Francomano CA. Hyaline cartilage engineered by chondrocytes in pellet culture: histological, immunohistochemical and ultrastructural analysis in comparison with cartilage explants. J Anat 2004;205:229–37.
[18] Thirion S, Berenbaum F. Culture and phenotyping of chondrocytes in primary culture. Methods Mol Med 2004;100:1–14.

[19] Georgi N, van Blitterswijk C, Karperien M. Mesenchymal stromal/stem cell-or chondrocyte-seeded microcarriers as building blocks for cartilage tissue engineering. Tissue Eng Part A 2014;20:2513–23.
[20] Johnson K, Zhu S, Tremblay MS, Payette JN, Wang J, Bouchez LC, et al. A stem cell-based approach to cartilage repair. Science 2012;336:717–21.
[21] Chao PH, Grayson W, Vunjak-Novakovic G. Engineering cartilage and bone using human mesenchymal stem cells. J Orthop Sci 2007;12:398–404.
[22] Hofmann S, Knecht S, Langer R, Kaplan DL, Vunjak-Novakovic G, Merkle HP, et al. Cartilage-like tissue engineering using silk scaffolds and mesenchymal stem cells. Tissue Eng 2006;12:2729–38.
[23] Li WJ, Tuli R, Huang X, Laquerriere P, Tuan RS. Multilineage differentiation of human mesenchymal stem cells in a three-dimensional nanofibrous scaffold. Biomaterials 2005;26:5158–66.
[24] Tuan RS, Boland G, Tuli R. Adult mesenchymal stem cells and cell-based tissue engineering. Arthritis Res Ther 2003;5:32–45.
[25] Wang Y, Kim UJ, Blasioli DJ, Kim HJ, Kaplan DL. In vitro cartilage tissue engineering with 3D porous aqueous-derived silk scaffolds and mesenchymal stem cells. Biomaterials 2005;26:7082–94.
[26] Yoneno K, Ohno S, Tanimoto K, Honda K, Tanaka N, Doi T, et al. Multidifferentiation potential of mesenchymal stem cells in three-dimensional collagen gel cultures. J Biomed Mater Res A 2005;75:733–41.
[27] Meinel L, Hofmann S, Karageorgiou V, Zichner L, Langer R, Kaplan D, et al. Engineering cartilage-like tissue using human mesenchymal stem cells and silk protein scaffolds. Biotechnol Bioeng 2004;88:379–91.
[28] Dahlin RL, Kinard LA, Lam J, Needham CJ, Lu S, Kasper FK, et al. Articular chondrocytes and mesenchymal stem cells seeded on biodegradable scaffolds for the repair of cartilage in a rat osteochondral defect model. Biomaterials 2014;35:7460–9.
[29] Cen L, Liu W, Cui L, Zhang W, Cao Y. Collagen tissue engineering: development of novel biomaterials and applications. Pediatr Res 2008;63:492–6.
[30] Moutos FT, Guilak F. Composite scaffolds for cartilage tissue engineering. Biorheology 2008;45:501–12.
[31] Li WJ, Tuli R, Okafor C, Derfoul A, Danielson KG, Hall DJ, et al. A three-dimensional nanofibrous scaffold for cartilage tissue engineering using human mesenchymal stem cells. Biomaterials 2005;26:599–609.
[32] Wise JK. Stem cell-based composite cartilage tissue engineering using nanobiomaterials. Chicago: University of Illinois at Chicago; 2008.
[33] Kirilak Y, Pavlos NJ, Willers CR, Han RZ, Feng HT, Xu JK, et al. Fibrin sealant promotes migration and proliferation of human articular chondrocytes: possible involvement of thrombin and protease-activated receptors. Int J Mol Med 2006;17:551–8.
[34] Liu SQ, Tian Q, Hedrick JL, Po Hui JH, Ee PL, Yang YY. Biomimetic hydrogels for chondrogenic differentiation of human mesenchymal stem cells to neocartilage. Biomaterials 2010;31:7298–307.
[35] Demoor M, Ollitrault D, Gomez-Leduc T, Bouyoucef M, Hervieu M, Fabre H, et al. Cartilage tissue engineering: molecular control of chondrocyte differentiation for proper cartilage matrix reconstruction. Biochim Biophys Acta 2014;1840:2414–40.
[36] Kupcsik L, Stoddart MJ, Li Z, Benneker LM, Alini M. Improving chondrogenesis: potential and limitations of SOX9 gene transfer and mechanical stimulation for cartilage tissue engineering. Tissue Eng Part A 2010;16:1845–55.
[37] Brochhausen C, Lehmann M, Halstenberg S, Meurer A, Klaus G, Kirkpatrick CJ. Signalling molecules and growth factors for tissue engineering of cartilage-what can we learn from the growth plate? J Tissue Eng Regen Med 2009;3:416–29.

[38] Stroka KM, Norman LL, Aranda-Espinoza H. Biomaterial mechanics. In: Fischer JP, Mikos AG, Bronzino JD, Peterson DR, editors. Tissue engineering: principles and practices. 1st ed. CRC Press: Taylor and Francis Group; 2012.
[39] Koay EJ, Athanasiou KA. Hypoxic chondrogenic differentiation of human embryonic stem cells enhances cartilage protein synthesis and biomechanical functionality. Osteoarthr Cartil 2008;16:1450–6.
[40] Schrobback K, Malda J, Crawford RW, Upton Z, Leavesley DI, Klein TJ. Effects of oxygen on zonal marker expression in human articular chondrocytes. Tissue Eng Part A 2012;18:920–33.
[41] Schrobback K, Klein TJ, Crawford R, Upton Z, Malda J, Leavesley DI. Effects of oxygen and culture system on in vitro propagation and redifferentiation of osteoarthritic human articular chondrocytes. Cell Tissue Res 2012;347:649–63.
[42] Saini S, Wick TM. Effect of low oxygen tension on tissue-engineered cartilage construct development in the concentric cylinder bioreactor. Tissue Eng 2004;10:825–32.
[43] Chu CR, Szczodry M, Bruno S. Animal models for cartilage regeneration and repair. Tissue Eng Part B Rev 2010;16:105–15.
[44] D'Lima DD, Kuhn K, Lotz MK. Detection of apoptosis in cartilage in situ and in isolated chondrocytes. Methods Mol Med 2004;100:275–90.
[45] Billinghurst RC, Mwale F, Hollander A, Ionescu M, Poole AR. Immunoassays for collagens in chondrocyte and cartilage explant cultures. Methods Mol Med 2004;100:251–74.
[46] McAlinden A, Haag J, Bau B, Gebhard PM, Aigner T. Quantification of mRNA expression levels in articular chondrocytes with PCR technologies. Methods Mol Med 2004;100:79–100.
[47] Hoemann CD. Molecular and biochemical assays of cartilage components. Methods Mol Med 2004;101:127–56.
[48] Chen AC, Klisch SM, Bae WC, Temple MM, McGowan KB, Gratz KR, et al. Mechanical characterization of native and tissue-engineered cartilage. Methods Mol Med 2004;101:157–90.
[49] Yin Z, Kotecha M, Schmid TM, Magin RL. High-resolution $T_{1\rho}$ and T_2 maps of articular cartilage at 11.7 T. In: The 11th International Conference on Magnetic Resonance Microscopy (ICMRM). Beijing, China. 2011.
[50] Yin Z. Magnetic resonance characterization of tissue engineered cartilage via changes in relaxation times, diffusion coefficient, and shear modulus. Crit Rev Biomed Eng 2014;42:137–91.
[51] Kotecha M, Schmid TM, Odintsov B, Magin R. Reduction of water diffusion coefficient with increased engineered cartilage matrix growth observed using MRI. In: Engineering in Medicine and Biology Society (EMBC), 2014 36th Annual International Conference of the IEEE. Chicago: IEEE; 2014. p. 3913–6.
[52] Pothirajan P, Dorcemus DL, Nukavarapu S, Kotecha M. True MRI assessment of stem cell chondrogenesis in a tissue engineered matrix. In: Ying L, editor. Engineering in Medicine and Biology Society (EMBC), 2014 36th Annual International Conference of the IEEE. Chicago: IEEE; 2014. p. 3933–6.
[53] Majumdar S, Pothirajan P, Dorcemus D, Nukavarapu S, Kotecha M. High field sodium MRI assessment of stem cell chondrogenesis in a tissue-engineered matrix. Ann Biomed Eng 2015;44(4):1120–1127.
[54] Yin Z, Schmid TM, Madsen L, Kotecha M, Magin RL. Monitoring the formation of tissue-engineered cartilage in scaffold-free pellet culture using magnetic resonance imaging. In: Proceedings of the International Society for Magnetic Resonance in Medicine (ISMRM) 20th Annual Meeting and Exhibition. Melbourne, Australia. 2012.

[55] Pothirajan P, Ravindran S, George A, Magin R, Kotecha M. Magnetic resonance spectroscopy and imaging can differentiate between engineered bone and engineered cartilage. In: Engineering in medicine and Biology Society (EMBC), 2014 36th Annual International Conference of the IEEE. Chicago: IEEE; 2014. p. 3929–32.
[56] Abragam A. Principles of nuclear magnetism. NY: Oxford University Press; 2002.
[57] Callaghan PT. Principles of magnetic resonance microscopy. Oxford: Oxford University Press; 1991.
[58] Xu HH, Othman SF, Magin RL. Monitoring tissue engineering using magnetic resonance imaging. J Biosci Bioeng 2008;106:515–27.
[59] Wheaton AJ, Borthakur A, Shapiro EM, Regatte RR, Akella SV, Kneeland JB, et al. Proteoglycan loss in human knee cartilage: quantitation with sodium MR imaging–feasibility study. Radiology 2004;231:900–5.
[60] Laurent D, O'Byrne E, Wasvary J, Pellas TC. In vivo MRI of cartilage pathogenesis in surgical models of osteoarthritis. Skelet Radiol 2006;35:555–64.
[61] Laurent D, Wasvary J, O'Byrne E, Rudin M. In vivo qualitative assessments of articular cartilage in the rabbit knee with high-resolution MRI at 3 T. Magn Reson Med 2003;50:541–9.
[62] Laurent D, Wasvary J, Rudin M, O'Byrne E, Pellas T. In vivo assessment of macromolecular content in articular cartilage of the goat knee. Magn Reson Med 2003;49:1037–46.
[63] Laurent D, Wasvary J, Yin J, Rudin M, Pellas TC, O'Byrne E. Quantitative and qualitative assessment of articular cartilage in the goat knee with magnetization transfer imaging. Magn Reson Imaging 2001;19:1279–86.
[64] O'Byrne E, Pellas T, Laurent D. Qualitative and quantitative in vivo assessment of articular cartilage using magnetic resonance imaging. Novartis Found Symp 2003;249:190–8. discussion 8-202, 34-8, 39-41.
[65] Blumenkrantz G, Majumdar S. Quantitative magnetic resonance imaging of articular cartilage in osteoarthritis. Eur Cells Mater 2007;13:76–86.
[66] Trattnig S, Winalski CS, Marlovits S, Jurvelin JS, Welsch GH, Potter HG. Magnetic resonance imaging of cartilage repair: a review. Cartilage 2011;2:5–26.
[67] Ramaswamy S, Gurkan I, Sharma B, Cascio B, Fishbein KW, Spencer RG. Assessment of tissue repair in full thickness chondral defects in the rabbit using magnetic resonance imaging transverse relaxation measurements. J Biomed Mater Res Part B Appl Biomater 2008;86:375–80.
[68] Sharma B, Fermanian S, Gibson M, Unterman S, Herzka DA, Cascio B, et al. Human cartilage repair with a photoreactive adhesive-hydrogel composite. Sci Transl Med 2013;5:167ra6.
[69] Kim M, Foo LF, Uggen C, Lyman S, Ryaby JT, Moynihan DP, et al. Evaluation of early osteochondral defect repair in a rabbit model utilizing Fourier transform-infrared imaging spectroscopy, magnetic resonance imaging, and quantitative T_2 mapping. Tissue Eng Part C Methods 2010;16:355–64.
[70] Ravindran S, Kotecha M, Huang C-C, Ye A, Pothirajan P, Yin Z, et al. Biological and MRI characterization of biomimetic ECM scaffolds for cartilage tissue regeneration. Biomaterials 2015;71:58–70.
[71] Kotecha M, Ravindran S, Schmid TM, Vaidyanathan A, George A, Magin RL. Application of sodium triple-quantum coherence NMR spectroscopy for the study of growth dynamics in cartilage tissue engineering. NMR Biomed 2013;26:709–17.
[72] Yin Z, Schmid TM, Yasar TK, Liu Y, Royston TJ, Magin RL. Mechanical characterization of tissue-engineered cartilage using microscopic magnetic resonance elastography. Tissue Eng Part C Methods 2013;20:611–9.

Noninvasive optical imaging of stem cell differentiation in biomaterials using photonic crystal surfaces

10

J.S. Choi, Y. Zhuo, B.T. Cunningham, B.A.C. Harley
University of Illinois at Urbana-Champaign, Urbana, IL, United States

10.1 Introduction

In this chapter, we describe recent advances in non-invasive optical imaging of stem cells using photonic crystal label-free biosensor surfaces. Technological progress in bioengineering approaches now enables the sophisticated control of live cells in vitro. In such applications, stem cells are often selected as the cell source as they have the capacity to expand to provide a large pool of cells with varying levels of self-renewal and differentiation potential (stem cells, progenitor cells, terminally differentiated cells) necessary to meet desired therapeutic goals. Precisely engineering stem cell fate decisions, however, has remained a challenge due to the lack of analytical tools that allow dynamic monitoring of heterogeneous stem cell populations in situ in real time at the single cell level. Currently available technologies such as fluorescence labeling or clonal expansion assays are almost always end-point analyses of ensemble populations of cells that are expensive, labor intensive, and time delayed. New optical imaging tools may increasingly permit label-free imaging of live cells for subcellular-resolution quantification of cellular activities in real time. Non-invasive optical imaging using a nanostructured photonic crystal surface in place of an ordinary glass or plastic substrate for cell growth can be easily integrated into existing bioengineering platforms such as microfluidics or microarrays and can provide a novel, alternative approach to monitor single stem cell activities in vitro. Here, we first detail the principles of photonic crystal enhanced microscopy (PCEM) then offer a detailed rationale for developing new tools that enable monitoring and screening of increasingly small populations of stem cells in vitro. Finally, we close by describing efforts to apply PCEM to characterize stem cell differentiation events via adhesion-based metrics of stem cell differentiation.

Monitoring and Evaluation of Biomaterials and their Performance in vivo. http://dx.doi.org/10.1016/B978-0-08-100603-0.00010-9

10.2 Motivation for noninvasive optical imaging of stem cells in vitro: adhesion phenotyping of stem cell differentiation

10.2.1 Material-based approaches to regulate stem cell fate decisions in vitro

Stem cell function is carefully orchestrated by an array of intrinsic and extrinsic factors [1–3]. A large number of cellular, biophysical, and chemical cues have been found to directly and indirectly impact stem cell fate decisions at different stages during development, at homeostasis, and following injuries [3]. These findings present opportunities to design and develop material-based approaches to allow better understanding of the underlying mechanisms of stem cell regulation as well as the realization of currently unmet clinical and therapeutic needs [3–5]. Combined with advances in fabrication approaches, sophisticated constructions of micro- and nanoscale features with varying material properties are now possible to selectively decouple or integrate experimental parameters that maximize the intended outcome of bioengineering applications [2,3,5].

Material-based approaches using stem cells often take advantage of the material properties to regulate stem cell function or fate decisions [4,6]. It has been reported that bulk material properties (e.g., pore size, pore alignment, stiffness, permeability) as well as surface properties (e.g., chemistry, topography, surface-bound ligand presentation, and orientation) at the cell–material interface serve as important regulators of stem cell fate: quiescence, self-renewal, differentiation, mobilization, homing, and senescence for several types of stem cells, such as mesenchymal stem cells (MSCs), embryonic stem cells (ESCs), hematopoietic stem cells (HSCs), and neuron stem cells (NSCs) [2,3].

10.2.2 Challenges associated with in vitro control of stem cell fate decisions

Advances in bioengineering approaches now allow sophisticated manipulation of live cells in vitro for a range of applications. For these applications, stem cells are often the cell source of choice as they offer several advantages [7,8]. First, stem cells can be expanded to supply a large number of cells with varying levels of self-renewal and differentiation potential. For instance, there are now well-established protocols for stem cells such as MSCs that enable precise expansion or differentiation into multiple cell lineages [9]. Second, the use of stem cells facilitates temporal control of cellular activities as they can be maintained as undifferentiated cells until appropriate extrinsic cues are presented. Third, advances in stem cell technology permit the use of patient-derived somatic cells as induced pluripotent stem cells, opening up new possibilities for patient-specific applications that may significantly enhance therapeutic outcome.

However, using stem cells is often challenging due to difficulties associated with precisely controlling stem cell fate decisions in vitro [2,3]. Despite technological advances in engineering stem cell fate decisions, underlying mechanisms of stem cell renewal and differentiation remain unclear as the critical factors required to maintain many types of stem and progenitor cells in vitro have yet to be uncovered [2]. This is particularly challenging with the use of adult stem cells as they quickly lose their stem potential in vitro [2,3]. The heterogeneity of stem and progenitor cell populations poses another challenge [2,3]. Because most stem cell populations are not homogeneous and therefore contain cells with varying functional capacity (e.g., progenitor cells, differentiating cells, terminally differentiated cells, other types of cells), stem cell populations need to be screened routinely at the single-cell level to exclude any unwanted cell populations [3]. Currently available tools (e.g., fluorescence labeling, clonal expansion assays, repopulation assays, in vivo models) rarely allow in situ screening of individual live cells for dynamic monitoring of stem cell populations because they are almost always end-point analyses of ensemble populations of cells that are expensive, labor intensive, and time delayed [2,3]. For more detailed information on stem cell engineering and currently available tools of stem cell characterization, please refer to recent reviews [2,3]. Naturally, the lack of suitable analytical approaches for quantitation of stem cell fate decisions in vitro also hampers efforts to identify factors that are essential for stem cell maintenance. These shortcomings in stem cell fate control efforts in vitro call for a new analytical approach that could spatiotemporally resolve single stem cell activities in real time.

10.2.3 Adhesion phenotyping of stem cells

Cells attach and adhere to the surrounding material surfaces to obtain material-mediated extrinsic signals that impact downstream signaling pathways [10]. As such, cell adhesion has been found to be critical in maintaining cellular activities such as growth, division, migration, and apoptosis [11,12]. Similarly, adhesion has been found to play a critical role in the regulation of stem cell activities, from proliferation and expansion to differentiation, mobilization, homing, and senescence [2,3].

As different cell populations exhibit different patterns of adhesion, a concept known as "adhesion phenotyping" has emerged [13,14]. It refers to the comprehensive and quantitative profiling of individual cells based on their adhesion characteristics to an underlying surface and it has shown promise as a new metric for cell function. For instance, adhesive profiles of individual cells have been linked to the aggressiveness of lung cancer, suggesting that adhesive properties of cell populations could be a predictive marker of pathologies [14]. Likewise, it was found that adhesive signatures of individual pluripotent stem cells could be used to isolate stem cell populations from differentiated cells [15]. These findings suggest adhesion-associated cell–material interactions contain rich information that correlates with cell function and that while still in its nascent stage, adhesion phenotyping of single cells or cell populations can provide a new functional metric for cell identification, isolation, and screening applications.

10.2.4 Noninvasive optical imaging as a potential new tool of stem cell characterization

Noninvasive optical imaging approaches may provide a novel platform that can dynamically quantify single stem cell activities in real time, in situ, by providing a means to probe individual cells in a label-free fashion [16–20]. In particular, noninvasive optical imaging allows adhesion phenotyping of live cells to dynamically quantify adhesion patterns of single cells for extended periods (up to days or weeks), which is difficult or impossible to achieve with currently available analytical techniques [16,17].

Specifically, photonic crystal enhanced microscopy (PCEM), a noninvasive optical imaging approach, enables spatially and temporally resolved quantification of single cell adhesion at the cell–surface interface by using photonic crystal (PC) surfaces as the optical transducer for biosensing, along with a modified optical microscope [16,17]. PCEM offers several advantages as a noninvasive optical imaging tool [16,17]. First, as it builds on a conventional inverted light microscope and as PC sensors are inexpensively produced via nanoreplica molding, PCEM can be set up and operated at affordable costs. Second, PCEM offers high sensitivity and high spatiotemporal resolution (submicron resolution at imaging intervals of only several seconds) that allows subcellular details of adhesion-mediated cell attachment and movement events to be imaged and quantitatively visualized. Third, PCEM can be easily integrated into many existing cell-based assay platforms including microfluidics and microarrays by simply introducing the PC element as the material interface.

These capabilities of PCEM enable the collection of adhesion footprints for a range of cell types, from adherent cells to only weakly adherent cells and even suspension culture cells traditionally regarded as nonadherent cells, to build a library of adhesion phenotypes, which may be highly useful for cell identification, isolation, and screening applications [16,17]. As evidence suggests that stem cells at different states may exhibit varying and/or distinct adhesion patterns [2,3], adhesion phenotyping of stem cells may also provide new ways to elucidate the underlying mechanisms of stem cell maintenance as well as enable dynamic screening of individual stem cells at varying stages of differentiation hierarchy to characterize stem cell fate decisions in vitro [2,3].

10.3 History: optical imaging of cells using photonic crystal enhanced microscopy (PCEM)

10.3.1 Basic principles of PCEM

The principles of PC label-free biosensor surfaces and the PCEM instrument have been described in recent publications and are briefly summarized here (Fig. 10.1) [16,17,21–24]. PCEM utilizes the sensing function of PC surfaces and is built upon a conventional benchtop inverted light microscope (e.g., Olympus BX51WI or Carl Zeiss Axio Observer Z1) by integrating it with a line-profiled and polarized light illumination source (e.g., laser or LED), a CCD camera, and a spectrometer as the detection instrument. PCEM provides a novel optical platform that enables label-free imaging of a broad range of surface-bound analytes (e.g., nanoparticles, proteins, antibodies, biomolecules). This capacity of PCEM extends to the analysis of surface-attached cells to enable sensing and imaging of whole, live cells at subcellular resolution at the cell–PC surface interface to temporally and spatially resolve adhesion-mediated cellular activities in situ in real time for life science research and engineering applications (Figs. 10.1–10.2).

The key component in PCEM is the PC biosensor, which is comprised of a periodic-modulated dielectric nanostructure as the optical transducer surface (Fig. 10.1(a) and (b))

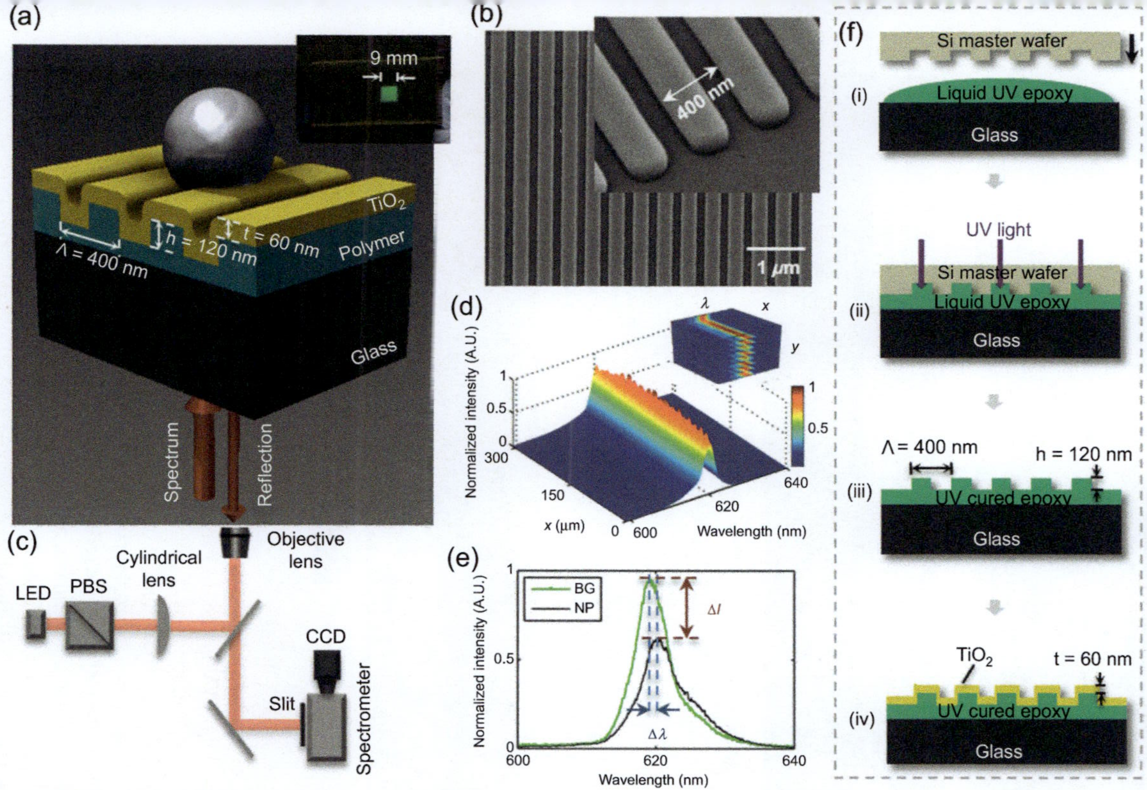

Figure 10.1 Schematic of photonic crystal enhanced microscopy. (a) A schematic of a nanoparticle attached to a photonic crystals (PC) surface. Inset: photo of a PC fabricated on a glass microscope slide. (b) SEM image of the PC surface. Inset: zoomed in to show the nanograting surface structures. (c) A schematic of the PCEM setup. (d) Normalized spectrum image (surface plot) obtained from PCEM imaging. Inset: PCEM-acquired 3-D spectrum data. (e) Example spectrum from PCEM with a peak wavelength value (PWV) shift and a peak intensity value (PIV) change with or without a nanoparticle attached on the PC surface (*BG*, background; *NP*, nanoparticle). (f) A schematic of nanoreplica molding to fabricate PCs: (i) deposition of a thin layer of liquid UV epoxy polymer between a Si wafer template and a glass substrate, (ii) hardening of the epoxy layer via exposure to UV light, (iii) removal of the Si wafer template, (iv) sputter deposition of a thin layer of TiO_2 film on top of the nanograting structure. Reprinted in part with permission from Zhuo Y, et al. Single nanoparticle detection using photonic crystal enhanced microscopy. Analyst 2014;139(5):1007–15, © 2013 RSC Publishing.

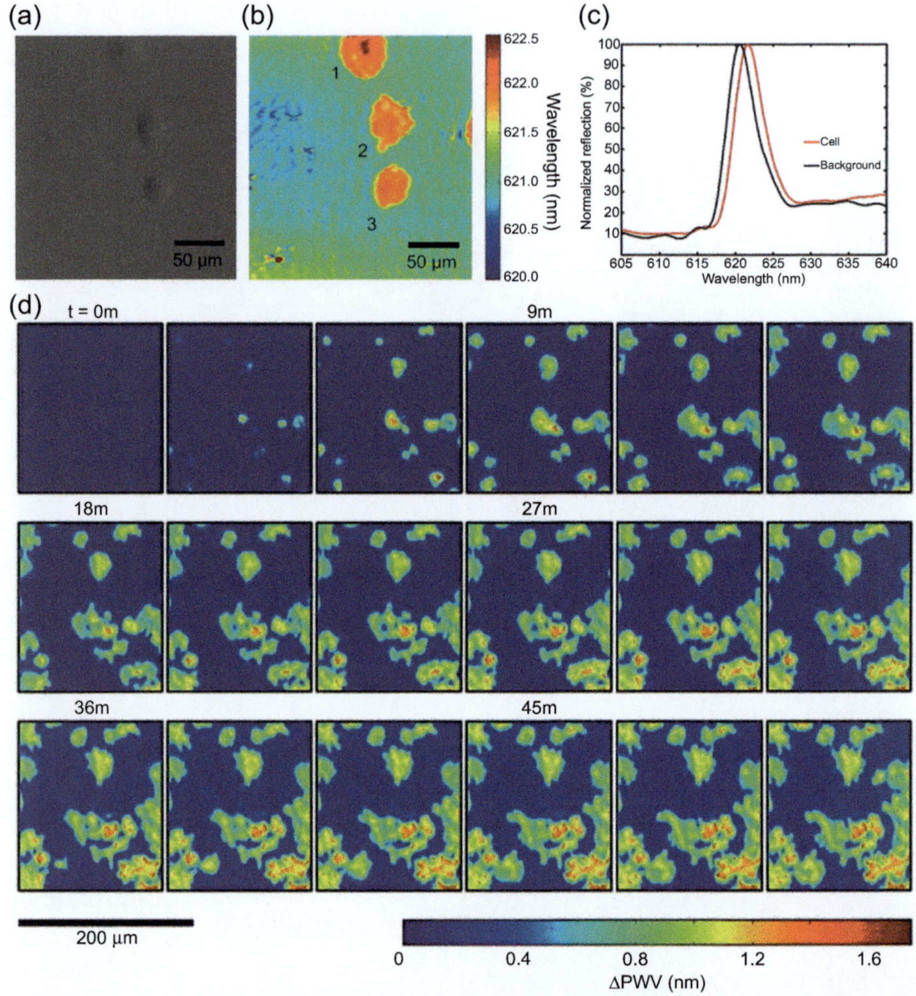

Figure 10.2 PCEM for in vitro studies of adhesion-mediated cellular behaviors. (a–b) Bright-field and the corresponding PWV images of Panc-1 cells adhered on the PC surface. PWV images clearly detail cellular protrusions at cell edges and regions of higher or lower mass distribution, noted by the differing magnitudes of the wavelength shift across the attached cell area. (c) Representative PWV spectra of the background (PC portion, nothing attached on top) versus the region where a cell is attached. (d) Time series PWS images of dental epithelial stem cells (mHAT9a) to demonstrate cellular attachment, adhesion, and movement.
Reprinted in part with permission from Chen W, et al. Photonic crystal enhanced microscopy for imaging of live cell adhesion. Analyst 2013;138(20):5886–94, © 2014 RSC Publishing.

[16,17]. The structural features of PC surfaces provide photonic band gaps, where light propagation is prohibited for specific wavelengths [25–27]. When cells attach to a PC surface, the local refractive index of the PC changes. By detecting these changes in the local refractive index of PC surfaces, it is possible to quantify the average response from the entire sensing area (biosensing) or spatially resolve localized responses that

can be differentiated from neighboring locations (bioimaging) to achieve highly sensitive label-free sensing and imaging of surface-attached analytes (Fig. 10.1(a)–(e)).

Photonic Crystal (PC) biosensors have recently been demonstrated as a highly versatile technology for a varicty of label-free assays including high-throughput screening of small molecule – protein interactions, characterization of protein–protein interactions, and measurement of cell attachment modulation by drugs [16,17,21–24]. A PC is a sub-wavelength grating structure consisting of a periodic arrangement of a low refractive index material coated with a high refractive index layer (Fig. 10.1(a)) [16]. When the PC is illuminated with a broadband light source, high order diffraction modes couple light into and out of the high index layer, destructively interfering with the zeroth-order transmitted light [17]. At a particular resonant wavelength and incident angle, complete interference occurs and no light is transmitted, resulting in 100% reflection efficiency. The resonant wavelength is modulated by the addition of biomaterial upon the PC surface, resulting in a shift to a higher wavelength. The electromagnetic standing wave that is generated at the PC surface during resonant light coupling inhibits lateral propagation, thus enabling neighboring regions on the PC surface to display a distinct resonant wavelength that is determined only by the density of biomaterial attached at that precise location. By measuring the resonant peak wavelength value (PWV) on a pixel-by-pixel basis over a PC surface, an image of cell attachment density may be recorded. PWV images of the PC may be gathered by illuminating the structure with collimated white light through the transparent substrate, while the front surface of the PC is immersed in aqueous media.

A schematic diagram of the PCEM instrument is shown in Fig. 10.1. The system is built upon the body of a standard microscope (Carl Zeiss Axio Observer Z1), but in addition to ordinary brightfield imaging, a second illumination path is provided from a fiber-coupled broadband LED (Thorlabs M617F1, $600 < \lambda < 650$ nm) [16, 28]. The fiber output is collimated and filtered by a polarizing beamsplitter cube to illuminate the PC with light that is polarized with its electric field vector oriented perpendicular to the grating lines. The polarized beam is focused by a cylindrical lens (f = 200 mm) to form a linear beam at the back focal plane of the objective lens (10x, Zeiss). After passing through the objective lens, the orientation of the line-shaped beam is rotated to illuminate the PC from below at normal incidence. The reflected light is projected, via a side port of the inverted microscope and a zoom lens, onto a narrow slit aperture at the input of an imaging spectrometer. The width of the adjustable slit can be adjusted according to the need of specific applications (e.g., 30 µm). The reflected light is collected from a linear region of the PC surface, where the width of the imaged line, 1.2 µm, is determined by the width of the entrance slit of the imaging spectrometer and the magnification power of the objective lens. The system incorporates a grating-based spectrometer (Acton Research) with a 512 x 512 pixel CCD camera (Photometrics Cascade 512). The line of reflected light, containing the resonant biosensor signal, is diffracted by the grating within the spectrometer (300 lines per mm-1) to produce a spatially resolved spectrum for each point along the line. Therefore, each pixel across the line is converted to a resonant reflection spectrum, containing a narrow bandwidth ($\Delta\lambda \approx 4$ nm) reflectance peak from the PC. The PWV of each peak is determined by fitting the spectrum to a 2nd-order polynomial function, and then mathematically determining the maximum wavelength of the function. By fitting all 512 spectra, in a process that takes 20 ms, a line comprised of 512 pixels is generated that represents one line of a PWV image of the PC surface. With an effective magnification of 26x, each pixel in the line represents a ≈0.6 μm region of the PC surface and 512 such pixels cover a total width of ≈300 μm. To generate a two-dimensional PWV image of the PC surface, a motorized stage (Applied Scientific Instruments, MS2000) translates the sensor along the axis perpendicular to the imaged line in increments of 0.6 μm per step. Using this technique, a series of lines are assembled into an image at a rate of 0.1s per line and the same area on the PC surface can be scanned repeatedly. Each image is comprised of 512 by n pixels, where n can be selected during each scan session, and each pixel represents a 0.6 x 0.6 μm region of the PC surface (Fig. 10.1(d)). A biosensor experiment involves measuring shifts in PWV. A baseline PWV image is gathered before the introduction of cells, when the PC is uniformly covered by cell media, which is aligned and mathematically subtracted from subsequent PWV images gathered during and after cell attachment (Fig. 10.1(e)).

Using nanoreplica molding, 1-D PC nanostructures can be mass produced at low cost with high reproducibility (Fig. 10.1(f)) [16,17,21–24]. The molding template is made on silicon wafers or quarts substrates via lithography. To being the process of fabricating a PC, a thin layer of ultraviolet-curable polymer (UVCP; $n_{UVCP}=1.5$) with a low refractive index (e.g., grating period of $\Lambda=400\,nm$, grating depth of $d=120\,nm$, duty cycle of $f=50\%$) is first cured on a solid support substrate (e.g., microscope slide) then a thin layer of dielectric material with a higher refractive index (e.g., TiO_2; $n_{TiO_2}=2.4$) is deposited on top (Fig. 10.1(a) and (f)). The thickness of the higher refractive index layer is selected (e.g., thickness of 60 nm) to generate a resonant reflection at a specific wavelength (e.g., resonant wavelength of $\lambda_0=620\,nm$) [21–24]. The sensitivity and the spatial resolution of the PC biosensor can be optimized by the choice of the dielectric materials and the geometry of the nanostructure features. For sensing and imaging of biological analytes, the PC surface can be further modified to immobilize application-specific biomolecules (e.g., antibodies, proteins, peptides) to enhance selectivity [17]. This nanoreplica-molding approach allows simple, rapid, and reliable fabrication of PC surfaces to offer benefits of single-use disposable detection for high-throughput screening applications. Additionally, the PC surface may be made planar by filling the nanograting structure with a polymer using a horizontal dipping process to eliminate potentially unwanted effects arising from analytes reacting to the structured surface topography [28].

10.3.2 Optical imaging of live cells using PCEM (Cunningham group publications)

PCEM provides the opportunity for noninvasive optical imaging of live cells at the cell–PC surface interface along with the potential to directly visualize and quantify adhesive contact between cells and the surface below at submicron resolution [16,17]. This is challenging for most conventional techniques such as fluorescence labeling, cytotoxic end-point analyses, or other forms of microscopy due to photobleaching [16]. PCEM is therefore particularly suitable for 2-D surface-attached cell studies aiming to characterize adhesion-mediated cellular behaviors at the cell–surface interface, including cell attachment, detachment, adhesion, chemotaxis, and migration [17].

Several configurations of PCEM instrumentation have been described for applications that include low spatial resolution imaging of biomolecular assays on a dry PC surface and high spatial resolution of cells and nanoparticles on PC surfaces covered with liquid media [21,23,28]. As a proof-of-concept, Lidstone et al. showed in 2011 that PCEM could be used to track the attachment footprint of four types of cells using collimated laser beam at $\lambda = 637$ nm from a 300-mW AlGaInP diode laser as the excitation source and 1-D PC slabs with SiO_2 (200 nm thick) and TiO_2 (~60 nm thick) layers deposited on top of a UV curable polymer layer as the sensing surface [23]. The PC surface was further coated with collagen, fibronectin, or poly-L-lysine to facilitate cell attachment. Here, PCEM imaging of cancer cells (HepG2/C3 hepatic carcinoma cells, Panc-1 pancreatic cancer cells), primary cardiomyocytes from rats, and porcine adipose-derived stem cells (ASC) showed PWS at cell attachment sites that was distinct from the spectra collected from the cell-free regions of the sensing area (Fig. 10.2(a)–(c)). Additionally, PCEM could dynamically assess when morphological changes were induced within Panc-1 pancreatic cancer cells by introducing staurosporine, an apoptosis-inducing agent. PCEM was also used to assess ASCs by replacing the cell medium with a neuronal induction medium that caused the retraction of the cell body and development of dendritic projections. These findings demonstrated the capacity of PCEM to capture transient shifts in the PC refractive index caused by cellular materials adhering and dissociating from the PC surface, which also indirectly provided a means to qualitatively assess changes in cell adhesion strength as greater PWS indicated stronger attachment to the PC surface.

In 2013, Chen et al. established an improved PCEM setup using a collimated LED light from fiber-coupled broadband LED (Thorlabs M617F1, $600 < \lambda < 650$ nm) as the light source and 1-D PC slabs with a single layer of TiO_2 (~60 nm thick) deposited on top of a UV curable polymer layer as the sensing surface [21]. This system provided improved spatial resolution that enabled optical imaging of live cells at subcellular resolution, where each pixel of the acquired image (512 × 512) corresponded to roughly 0.6 μm^2 of the PC surface. This work examined dental epithelial stem cells (mHAT9a cells) at time intervals of 3 min to monitor their attachment profiles [29]. Attached cells showed highest PWS near cell edges (Fig. 10.2(d)), consistent with the findings from other cell adhesion-based assays that show accumulation of cytoskeletal and focal adhesion-associated proteins at the cell boundary during cell adhesion events [11,30,31]. This PCEM approach also allowed label-free imaging of chemotactic migration of mHAT9a cells to agarose beads soaked in SDF1-α, a chemokine that binds CXCR4 receptors expressed on mHAT9a cells, as well as their detachment profiles in response to the administration of staurosporine, which caused apoptosis-induced detachment of cells.

More recently, Chen et al. showed the use of planar 1-D PC slabs as the sensing surface for PCEM [28]. Although the use of 1-D PC slabs with a grating surface topology allows highly sensitive noninvasive optical imaging of live cells, the structured topography introduces an additional variable that biases cell adhesion in the direction of the PC grating lines. To overcome this, Chen et al. filled TiO_2-coated PC slabs with SU-8 epoxy by a horizontal dipping process to planarize the PC surface. When 3T3 fibroblasts were imaged on fibronectin-coated planar PCs, their attachment profiles were similar to those from nonplanar counterparts, with comparable subcellular resolution.

As these publications highlight, progress in the development of PCEM imaging instrumentation and PC surfaces have enabled label-free imaging of adherent types of cells of varying size and morphology from primary and commercially available sources to spatially and temporally resolve cell–surface interactions. Such "adhesive phenotyping" of single cells using PCEM provides adhesion-associated data in real time that may be useful for basic biological research to uncover poorly understood biological mechanisms as well as for designing novel biosensing applications from identification and characterization of individual cells to high-throughput screening of cells to evaluate the efficacy of drugs.

10.4 PCEM imaging of stem cell differentiation

With PCEM established as an optical platform capable of noninvasively imaging single cell attachment and adhesion events at the cell–material interface [16,17,21–24], it is now possible to examine how such information may be used as a characterization tool. PCEM provides fast data acquisition and processing time (on the order of several seconds between images) and high spatial resolution (submicron) that enable quantitative, real-time imaging of single cells. These advances make it possible to examine dense adhesion-associated data gathered via PCEM, with the eventual goal of linking changes in cell mass distribution with adhesion strength and cell motility to dynamically trace cell attachment and adhesion kinetics [32].

Ongoing efforts are employing PCEM to establish adhesion phenotypes of single stem cells at discrete stages of differentiation and assess how they relate to their functional capacity. As a first step, we are imaging model stem cell–dental epithelial stem cells (mHAT cell line), IL-3 dependent myeloid progenitor cells (32D cell line), and porcine adipose-derived stem cells, whose differentiation protocols are well-established [20,33,34]. Here, differentiation is induced by replacing cell growth media with the defined induction media at a specified time point, providing the opportunity to use PCEM to resolve changes in cell adhesion in and around differentiation events.

PCEM allows time-lapse imaging of stem cells over the course of differentiation, which typically takes up to several weeks to complete. Preliminary findings suggest that stem cells exhibit dynamic changes in their adhesive properties during differentiation, and that PCEM can effectively image and quantify these changes to generate a large amount of adhesion-associated data. Image analysis software facilitates the processing of PCEM-generated data to extract adhesion-related parameters in spatiotemporal dimensions of interest, including cell contact/spread area, mass density/redistribution, migration speed, and migration distance. Initial analyses of adhesion and motility parameters of stem cell differentiation indicate that adhesion strength and motility of individual stem cells go through significant cell-type specific changes during the course of differentiation, suggesting that adhesion phenotyping of stem cells may provide functional metrics that would enable in situ screening of single stem cells in a high-throughput manner in vitro as well as enhance our understanding of the physiological regulation mechanisms of stem cells [32].

10.5 Conclusions and future outlook

In this chapter, we describe recent advances in noninvasive optical imaging of stem cells using photonic crystal surfaces. In particular, we detailed a type of optical imaging platform termed photonic crystal enhanced microscopy (PCEM). PCEM enables dynamic monitoring of heterogeneous stem cell populations in situ in real time at the single cell level with subcellular spatial resolution, which is difficult to achieve with currently available analytical tools and techniques (e.g., fluorescence labeling, clonal expansion assays), as they are almost always end-point ensemble analyses. PCEM employs photonic crystals as the biosensing element, whose surface properties can be easily modified to facilitate cell–surface interactions. PCEM also has the potential to be integrated into existing bioengineering platforms such as microfluidics or microarrays to provide a novel, alternative approach to monitor single stem cell activity in vitro. As PCEM noninvasively images interactions at the cell–surface interface, it is highly suitable for the characterization of cell adhesion activities as a tool for "adhesion phenotyping," a comprehensive profiling of cell attachment and adhesion-associated events. Ongoing efforts are imaging stem cells during the course of differentiation to specific lineages using several cell lines and primary cells. Here, analyses of adhesion and motility parameters suggest adhesion phenotyping during stem cell differentiation may provide important new functional metrics to enable in situ screening of single stem cells in a high-throughput manner. Such technologies would provide important new insight regarding our understanding of the physiological regulation mechanisms of stem cells.

Acknowledgments

Research reported in this publication was supported by the National Institute of Biomedical Imaging and Bioengineering of the National Institutes of Health under Award Number R21 EB018481 and the National Institute of Diabetes and Digestive and Kidney Diseases of the National Institutes of Health under Award Number R01 DK099528 , and the Beckman Institute Postdoctoral Fellowship from Arnold and Mabel Beckman Foundation. The content is solely the responsibility of the authors and does not necessarily represent the official views of the NIH.

References

[1] Zon LI. Intrinsic and extrinsic control of haematopoietic stem-cell self-renewal. Nature 2008;453(7193):306–13.
[2] Choi JS, Mahadik BP, Harley BAC. Engineering the hematopoietic stem cell niche: frontiers in biomaterial science. Biotechnol J 2015;10(10):1529–45.
[3] Choi J, Harley B. Challenges and opportunities to harnessing the (hematopoietic) stem cell niche. Curr Stem Cell Rep 2016.

[4] Vunjak-Novakovic G, Scadden DT. Biomimetic platforms for human stem cell research. Cell Stem Cell 2011;8(3):252–61.
[5] Celiz AD, et al. Materials for stem cell factories of the future. Nat Mater 2014;13(6):570–9.
[6] Dalby MJ, Gadegaard N, Oreffo ROC. Harnessing nanotopography and integrin–matrix interactions to influence stem cell fate. Nat Mater 2014;13(6):558–69.
[7] Zandstra PW, Nagy A. Stem cell bioengineering. Annu Rev Biomed Eng 2001;3(1):275–305.
[8] Yin PT, Han E, Lee K-B. Engineering stem cells for biomedical applications. Adv Healthcare Mater 2016;5(1):10–55.
[9] Caliari SR, Harley BAC. Structural and biochemical modification of a collagen scaffold to selectively enhance MSC tenogenic, chondrogenic, and osteogenic differentiation. Adv Healthcare Mater 2014;3(7):1086–96.
[10] Crowder SW, et al. Material cues as potent regulators of epigenetics and stem cell function. Cell Stem Cell 2016;18(1):39–52.
[11] Parsons JT, Horwitz AR, Schwartz MA. Cell adhesion: integrating cytoskeletal dynamics and cellular tension. Nat Rev Mol Cell Biol 2010;11(9):633–43.
[12] Ahmad Khalili A, Ahmad MR. A review of cell adhesion studies for biomedical and biological applications. Int J Mol Sci 2015;16(8):18149–84.
[13] Barney LE, et al. A cell–ECM screening method to predict breast cancer metastasis. Integr Biol Quant Biosci Nano Macro 2015;7(2):198–212.
[14] Reticker-Flynn NE, et al. A combinatorial extracellular matrix platform identifies cell-extracellular matrix interactions that correlate with metastasis. Nat Commun 2012:3.
[15] Singh A, et al. Adhesion strength-based, label-free isolation of human pluripotent stem cells. Nat Methods 2013;10(5):438–44.
[16] Zhuo Y, Cunningham B. Label-free biosensor imaging on photonic crystal surfaces. Sensors 2015;15(9):21613.
[17] Cunningham BT, et al. Recent advances in biosensing with photonic crystal surfaces: a review. IEEE Sens J 2016;16(10):3349–66.
[18] Zangle TA, Teitell MA. Live-cell mass profiling: an emerging approach in quantitative biophysics. Nat Methods 2014;11(12):1221–8.
[19] Pavlichenko I, et al. Bringing one-dimensional photonic crystals to a new light: an electrophotonic platform for chemical mass transport visualisation and cell monitoring. Mater Horiz 2015;2(3):299–308.
[20] Lifson MA, Miller BL. Photonic Crystals as Robust Label-Free Biosensors. In: Photonic Materials for Sensing, Biosensing and Display Devices. Springer International Publishing; 2016. p. 189–207.
[21] Chen W, et al. Photonic crystal enhanced microscopy for imaging of live cell adhesion. Analyst 2013;138(20):5886–94.
[22] Zhuo Y, et al. Single nanoparticle detection using photonic crystal enhanced microscopy. Analyst 2014;139(5):1007–15.
[23] Lidstone EA, et al. Label-free imaging of cell attachment with photonic crystal enhanced microscopy. Analyst 2011;136(18):3608–15.
[24] Chen W, et al. Enhanced live cell imaging via photonic crystal enhanced fluorescence microscopy. Analyst 2014;139(22):5954–63.
[25] Joannopoulos JD, Villeneuve PR, Fan S. Photonic crystals: putting a new twist on light. Nature 1997;386(6621):143–9.
[26] Joannopoulos JD, et al. Photonic crystals: molding the flow of light. Princeton university press; 2011.
[27] Liu W, Liu X, Yang B. Photonic crystals fabricated via facile methods and their applications. In: Serpe MJ, Kang Y, Zhang QM, editors. Photonic materials for sensing, biosensing and display devices; 2016. p. 101–58.

[28] Chen W, et al. Planar Photonic Crystal Biosensor for Quantitative Label-Free Cell Attachment Microscopy. Advanced Optical Materials 2015;3(11):1623–32.
[29] Otsu K, et al. Functional role of Rho-kinase in ameloblast differentiation. J Cell Physiol 2011;226(10):2527–34.
[30] Geiger B, Spatz JP, Bershadsky AD. Environmental sensing through focal adhesions. Nat Rev Mol Cell Biol 2009;10(1):21–33.
[31] Kanchanawong P, et al. Nanoscale architecture of integrin-based cell adhesions. Nature 2010;468(7323):580–4.
[32] Zhuo, Y., et al., *Quantitative and dynamic cell adhesion imaging using photonic crystal enhanced microscopy (PCEM)*. Submitted for review.
[33] Gupta D, et al. Differentiation and Characterization of Myeloid Cells. In: Current Protocols in Immunology. John Wiley & Sons, Inc; 2014.
[34] Monaco E, et al. Morphological and transcriptomic comparison of adipose and bone marrow derived porcine stem cells. The Open Tissue Engineering & Regenerative Medicine Journal 2009:20–33.

Index

'*Note*: Page numbers followed by "f" indicate figures and "t" indicate tables.'

CPI Antony Rowe
Chippenham, UK
2017-02-01 18:53